Trauma Surgery Essentials

Trauma Surgery Essentials

A Must-Know Guide to Emergency Management

ANIL K. SRIVASTAVA, MD, FACS (USA), FRCS (EDIN, UK)
Attending Surgeon: Trauma surgery/General surgery/Surgical Critical Care
Mercy Hospital, Saint Louis, MO, USA

ELSEVIER

Elsevier
1600 John F. Kennedy Blvd.
Ste 1800
Philadelphia, PA 19103-2899

TRAUMA SURGERY ESSENTIALS   ISBN: 978-0-323-87027-6

Notice

International Standard Book Number: 978-0-323-87027-6

Content Strategist: Jessica L. McCool
Content Development Specialist: Akanksha Marwah/Vaishali Singh
Publishing Services Manager: Shereen Jameel
Project Manager: Shereen Jameel
Design Direction: Ryan Cook

Printed in India

Last digit is the print number: 9 8 7 6 5 4 3 2 1

Working together
to grow libraries in
developing countries

www.elsevier.com • www.bookaid.org

Dedicated to everyone involved in the management of injured patients

FOREWORD

It is with great pleasure that I write this introduction for this book in trauma care. There is no substitute for the distilled practical thoughts of an experienced clinician such as Dr. Anil Srivastava in the management of complex trauma patients. As he points out, there are many alternatives for useful information for the care of the seriously injured – but this text is meant to be an accessible, practical guide for high-quality care across all the spectrums of places where a seriously injured patient might just show up randomly.

He has chosen a unique organizational structure to make trauma care more easily deployed with algorithms guiding the reader through must know content for trauma care. This approach simplifies and clarifies all the information needed and can be an important starting text or complement to many of the other trauma informational sources available as it gives an over arching structure to all the different topics in trauma care.

This text represents the culmination of a thoughtful, experienced clinician's observations in practice and his observations to avoid common stumbling blocks that often crop up in clinic practice. These can be avoided with forethought. By reading through the algorithm's, the reader will have a framework upon which to organize further information and refinements in trauma care to improve their trauma care methods. It is a guide, led by someone who has been there and is ready to point the way—and will help more appreciate all the work that the trauma surgery community offers.

John P. Kirby, MD, MS, FACS
Associate Professor of Acute & Critical Care Surgery
Washington University School of Medicine, St Louis, MO
January 1, 2023

I have known the author, Dr. Anil Srivastava, for a long time. He is a fellow trauma surgeon, colleague, and a good friend. So, when he approached me to write the foreword for this book, of course I could not say no. At the same time, the thought did cross my: another book; does anyone even read them anymore? Keeping my thoughts to myself, I let him explain what the book was about and show me a preliminary copy. As he started explaining, I was struck by how deeply he had thought about this and, more importantly, how he had identified a critical gap among the available resources, printed or online. This book fills a void that is often felt by a large group of practitioners all over the world who provide care to the seriously injured but are not part of a large, high-volume medical institution. Most available resources cater to practitioners who are heavily engaged in trauma care and practice at large institutions. This leaves a large swath of practitioners who provide essential trauma care, but not at a volume to keep up with the most recent advances. This book caters to them. It is a ready resource that can be utilized in a 'just in time' fashion or be used to brush up on the most recent advances in the care of the injured. After some thought, it did not surprise me that Dr. Srivastava would have the insight to be able to identify this void. He trained in multiple environments – India, a low-middle-income country with severe resource constraints; UK, a high-income country with nationalized government-provided health care; and USA, another high-income country with private insurance as the primary payor source. Additionally, complementing his diverse experience, he pursued a very broad training in the US encompassing general surgery, transplantation, burns, trauma, and surgical critical care. He trained at some of the busiest institutions in the country, providing him an insight that is in equal measure deep in subject matter, and broad in scope. After training, he has been practicing as an acute care surgeon providing care in the fields of general/trauma surgery and surgical critical care at a busy hospital in St. Louis, MO, USA.

The approach he has taken in this book of providing the absolute essential elements in a simple, easy-to-understand format, will appeal to a broad range of practitioners all over the world. The essential concepts can benefit the trainee or the practicing provider. The simple, easy-to-understand algorithms will provide a ready-to-use resource not only to the formally trained provider but also to those who have limited formal training and yet provide essential care in large parts of the world where trained providers are extremely scarce. I feel privileged that my friend asked me to write the foreword to this valuable addition to the available resources that will benefit providers and, more importantly, injured patients the world over.

Ajai K. Malhotra, MBBS (MD), MS, DNB, FRCSEd, FACS
Professor and Chief, Division of Acute Care Surgery
Department of Surgery, University of Vermont
Trauma Medical Director, Level-I Trauma Center
University of Vermont Medical Center
Chair, Vermont State Committee on Trauma

"Everything should be made as simple as possible, but not simpler."

– Albert Einstein

Trauma is one of the leading causes of death and disability worldwide. Therefore, an organized approach is essential for the management and survival of trauma patients. This requires quick evaluation, immediate lifesaving procedures, and a definitive treatment of the injuries. In the current era, there are unlimited resources on trauma-related topics: from voluminous, multi-authored textbooks, journal articles, and small pocket guidebooks to an abundance of information on the internet. With so much information, it is easy to get lost. Being a practicing trauma surgeon for many years, I strongly feel that there is a need for a book which can address this problem and simultaneously be a reliable resource. In my book, *Trauma Surgery Essentials: A Must-Know Guide to Emergency Management*, I have identified the "must-know" facts, based on information from textbooks, practice guidelines, and current peer-reviewed journals. The book has been divided into three parts: Part A covers the emergent evaluation and management of trauma patients, while Part B covers the emergency management of specific trauma problems, and Part C covers few miscellaneous topics. Each part is further subdivided into sections and chapters. All chapters contain a "Must-Know" management algorithm and descriptions of the "Must-Know Essentials" facts with relevant anatomical illustrations. This book will be a valuable resource for medical students, trainee surgical residents, trauma surgery fellows, general surgeons, trauma surgeons, ER physicians, and mid-level providers. It will also benefit non surgical physicians who are interested in the management of trauma patients. With trauma becoming an increasing global problem, the book will not only provide the much-needed resources but also aid physicians who are involved in the management of trauma patients globally.

Anil K. Srivastava, MD, FACS (USA), FRCS (Edin, UK)
Trauma surgery/General surgery/Surgical Critical Care
Mercy Hospital, Saint Louis, MO, USA

ACKNOWLEDGMENTS

I would like to thank, Bryan Troop, MD, FACS,[1] for providing suggestions, reviewing, and manuscript editing and Abbie Jensen, MD,[2] for reviews, suggestions, and editing the algorithms. I would like to thank Robert Fraser[3] for digital art illustrations. And finally, I would like to thank my wife, Priti, and my son, Rohit, for doing some of the illustrations, cover page design, and review of the manuscript.

[1] Bryan Troop, MD, FACS, Trauma Surgeon Adjunct Professor of Surgery, Department of Surgery, St. Louis University, St. Louis, Missouri, USA; Ex-Director of Trauma/General Surgery/Surgical Critical Care, Mercy Hospital, St. Louis, Missouri, USA

[2] Abbie Jensen, MD, Trauma/General Surgery/Surgical Critical Care, Mercy Hospital, Saint Louis, Missouri, USA

[3] Robert Fraser, Imperial, Missouri, USA: Digital Artist

CONTENTS

PART 1

Evaluation and Resuscitation of Trauma

Initial Evaluation
of Trauma Patients

CHAPTER 1

Death in Trauma Patients

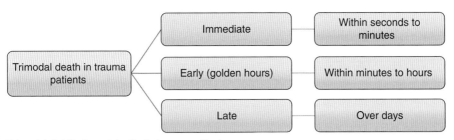

Trimodal distribution of deaths in trauma patients

Must-Know Essentials: Death in Trauma Patients

TRIMODAL DISTRIBUTION

- Immediate deaths: within seconds to minutes
- Early deaths: within minutes to hours (Golden Hours)
- Late deaths: over days

CAUSES OF IMMEDIATE DEATH

- Brain stem transection
- High spinal cord transection
- Decapitation
- Apnea due to severe brain or high spinal cord injury
- Cardiac rupture
- Rupture of aorta of large vessels
- Major tracheobronchial disruption
- Liver avulsion

CAUSES OF EARLY DEATH (GOLDEN HOURS)

- Hypoxia
  - Airway obstruction
  - Tension pneumothorax
  - Open pneumothorax
  - Massive hemothorax
  - Massive flail chest
  - Severe pulmonary contusion
  - Tracheobronchial rupture
  - Diaphragm rupture

- Major bleeding
  - External bleeding
  - Intrathoracic bleeding (hemothorax, pericardial tamponade, lung laceration)
  - Thoracic aortic rupture
  - Intraabdominal bleeding (spleen laceration, liver laceration, mesenteric laceration, major vessels injuries)
  - Bleeding from retroperitoneum
  - Pelvic fracture with massive hemorrhage
  - Postinjury coagulopathy
  - Massive facial wounds
  - Long-bone fractures
- Increased intracranial pressure
  - Diffuse brain edema
  - Cerebral hematoma (intraparenchymal or extraaxial)
  - Rapid tentorial brain herniation

CAUSES OF LATE DEATH

- Sepsis
  - Perforated hollow viscus
  - Ventilator-associated pneumonia
  - Line sepsis
  - Urinary infection
- Multiple organ failure
  - Respiratory failure
  - Cardiac failure
  - Liver failure
  - Renal failure
- Thromboembolic complications

PREVENTION OF DEATH IN TRAUMA PATIENTS

- Immediate deaths can be prevented by implementation of various trauma prevention programs.
- Early death can be prevented by prompt diagnosis and management during the "Golden Hour" of trauma.
- Late death can be prevented by thorough understanding and management of various injuries and their related complications.

CHAPTER 2

Process of Evaluation of Trauma Patients

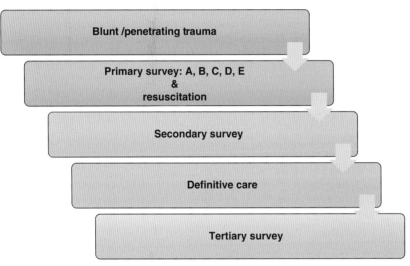

Algorithm: Evaluation of trauma patients (ATLS guidelines)

Must-Know Essentials: Process of Evaluation of Trauma Patients

PRIMARY SURVEY (A, B, C, D, E) AND RESUSCITATION

- A: Airway and cervical spine protection
- B: Breathing and ventilation
- C: Circulation and control of hemorrhage
- D: Disability: Neurological status
- E: Exposure and environmental protection

SECONDARY SURVEY

- After primary survey and management of life-threatening injuries, include:
  - AMPLE history (A: Allergy, M: Medication, P: Past medical history, L: Last meal, E: Event or environment related to injury).
  - Complete examination of the patient (head to toe).
  - Specific imaging based on clinical findings.
    - Plain x-rays
    - CT scans
    - MRI, etc.

- Lab tests including CBC, electrolytes, coagulation, drug levels, and alcohol levels.
- Identification of other injuries.

DEFINITIVE CARE

- Management of specific injury
  - Operative management
  - Nonoperative

TERTIARY SURVEY

- Essentially a repetition of the secondary survey to diagnose any missed injury
- Should be performed within 24 hours after admission
- To diagnose any missed injury
  - Missed injury is common in patients with:
    - blunt trauma.
    - altered mental status.
    - distracting injuries.
    - delayed transfer or presentation to trauma centers.

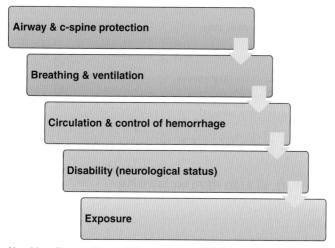

Algorithm: Primary Survey & Resuscitation (ATLS guidelines)

Must Know Essentials: Primary Survey (A, B, C, D, E) and Resuscitation

A: AIRWAY AND CERVICAL SPINE PROTECTION

- Inspect face, oropharynx, and neck.
  - Check for the patent airway by opening the airway:
    - Chin lift
    - Jaw thrust

- Check for airway obstruction.
  - Clear airway of foreign bodies.
    - Apply oropharyngeal airway if needed.
- Recognize a compromised airway.
- Recognize the need for a definitive airway.
- Apply cervical collar for c-spine protection:
  - It should be immobilized using hardboard, collar, sandbags, and tape or straps.
  - Among patients with brain injury, 5% may have an associated spine injury.
  - Inadequate immobilization can cause worsening spinal cord injury.
  - Cervical injury should be suspected in patients with blunt multisystem trauma.
  - Blunt injuries above the clavicle have a high association of cervical spine injury.

B. BREATHING AND VENTILATION

- Check the rate and depth of respiration.
- Check chest wall movements and inspect for flail chest.
- Check chest for sign of injury: open wounds, contusion, hematoma, deformity.
- Palpate chest for subcutaneous air (crepitation); palpate neck for tracheal deviation.
- Auscultate chest bilaterally.
- Administer high concentration oxygen.
- Ventilate with bag-mask device if indicated.
- Place chest tube if indicated.
- Place an occlusive dressing on an open chest wound.

C. CIRCULATION AND CONTROL OF HEMORRHAGE

- Identify source of external and internal exsanguinating bleeding.
- Check pulse and blood pressure.
- Check skin color.
- Control external bleeding.
- Establish IV access (peripheral/central/venous cut down).
- Intraosseous line if venous access is unsuccessful.
- Crystalloid infusion.
- Blood transfusion or massive transfusion protocol if indicated.
- Evaluate for persistent hypotension.
- Pelvic binder for unstable pelvic fracture.
- Introduce resuscitative endovascular balloon occlusion of the aorta (REBOA) if indicated.
- Immobilize limb for open and displaced fractures.
- Emergency thoracotomy if indicated.
- to operating room if indicated.

D. DISABILITY (NEUROLOGICAL STATUS)

- Check level of consciousness using Glasgow Coma Scale (GCS).
- Check pupils.
- Check for neurological deficit.
- Check for signs of spinal cord injury.
- Motor score of the GCS has been shown to be associated with outcome in head injury patients.

- Apart from brain injury, other causes of decreased level of consciousness in trauma patients include:
  - inadequate cerebral oxygenation.
  - impaired ventilation.
  - inadequate cerebral perfusion.
  - hypoglycemia.
  - alcohol.
  - narcotics and other drugs.
- Primary brain injury is due to structural effect of the injury to the brain.
- Secondary brain injury results due to inadequate oxygenation and perfusion to the brain.
- Goals in the management of severe brain injury based on GCS:
  - Prevent hypotension.
  - Prevent hypoxia.
    - Consider for early definitive airway.
    - Ventilate adequately.
  - Prevent hypothermia.
  - Osmotherapy to reduce intracranial pressure (ICP)
  - Prophylaxis for seizure
- Patients with spinal cord injury:
  - Consider treating neurogenic shock.
  - Consider spinal stabilization within 24 hours of the injury.

E. EXPOSURE AND ENVIRONMENTAL PROTECTION

- Expose the patient for complete examination.
- Look for any occult injuries.
- Log roll to inspect the back.
- Prevent hypothermia by:
  - warming infusion fluid.
  - increasing room temperature.
  - use of warm blanket.
- Hypothermia (core temperature less than 35°C) is a serious complication of severe trauma with hemorrhage.
  - Hypothermia is an independent predictor of survival.
    - Hypothermia may result in:
      - coagulopathy.
      - impaired oxygen delivery due to left shift of oxygen dissociation curve.
      - acidosis.
      - increased incidence of infection.
      - bradycardia.
      - cardiac arrhythmia.
      - hyperglycemia due to decrease in insulin sensitivity.

ADJUNCTS OF PRIMARY SURVEY

- Pulse oximetry
- ECG monitor
- Indwelling urinary catheter is contraindicated in the patient with:
  - blood at urethral meatus.
  - perineal ecchymosis.
  - high-riding or nonpalpable prostate.

- Nasogastric tube is contraindicated in patients with:
  - fractured cribriform plate.
  - fractured nasal bone.
- Blood gas
- Plain portable x-rays as indicated
- Focussed assessment with sonography in trauma (FAST):
  - Rapid bedside assessment of intraabdominal bleeding in patients with hypotension
  - Look for blood in the:
    - hepatorenal fossa.
    - splenorenal fossa.
    - pelvis (pouch of Douglas).
    - pericardium.
  - Is highly sensitive
  - Limitations:
    - Operator dependent
    - Distortion due to bowel gas and subcutaneous air
    - Misses diaphragm, bowel, and pancreatic injuries
- Diagnostic peritoneal lavage (DPL):
  - Rapid assessment of hypotension at bedside
  - High sensitivity
  - Disadvantages:
    - Invasive procedure
    - Misses retroperitoneal and diaphragm injury
  - Contraindications:
    - Patients with previous abdominal surgeries
    - Morbid obesity
    - Advanced cirrhosis
    - Coagulopathy
  - Criteria for positive DPL:
    - Gross blood > 10 mL
    - Gastrointestinal contents on aspiration
    - More than 100,000 RBC/mm^3
    - More than 500 WBC/mm^3
    - Gram stain positive for bacteria

CT ABDOMEN

- Indications for surgery based on CT findings
  - Pneumoperitoneum
  - Extravasation of contrast
  - Two of the following findings:
    - Free fluid in the absence of solid organ injury
    - Bowel wall thickening
    - Mesenteric fat streaking
    - Mesenteric hematoma

Resuscitation of Trauma Patients

CHAPTER 3

The Vicious Cycle of Trauma

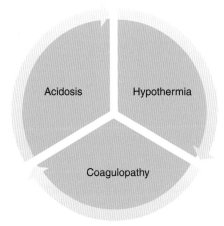

The vicious cycle of trauma and the lethal triad

Must-Know Essentials: The Vicious Cycle of Trauma and the Lethal Triad

DEFINITION

- Vicious cycle of trauma
  - Hemorrhage after trauma initiates a cycle of acidosis, hypothermia, and coagulopathy that leads to continued bleeding with eventual death.
- Lethal triad
  - A combination of hypothermia, acidosis, and coagulopathy
  - Associated with very high mortality

CAUSES OF ACIDOSIS

- Hypovolemic shock
  - Causes reduced tissue oxygen delivery and lactic acidosis
- Large volume of crystalloid infusion
  - Causes hyperchloremic acidosis
- Hypothermia
  - Causes shift of the oxygen dissociation curve to the left, resulting in tissue hypoxia and acidosis
- Coagulopathy
  - Causes ongoing bleeding, leading to tissue hypoperfusion and acidosis

CAUSES OF HYPOTHERMIA

- Environmental exposure
- Large-volume crystalloid infusion without using fluid warmer
- Loss of intrinsic thermoregulation due to tissue hypoxia in hemorrhagic shock

CAUSES OF COAGULOPATHY

- Hypothermia
  - Causes
    - Inhibition of thromboxane A2 resulting in failure of vasoconstriction, along with platelet aggregation at the injury site
    - Impairment of enzymatic process of coagulation pathways
- Hypocalcemia
  - Due to:
    - massive transfusion of stored blood.
    - massive hemorrhage leading to consumption of calcium.
  - Causes impairment of coagulation pathways
- Large-volume crystalloid infusion
  - Causes dilution of platelets and clotting factors
- Acidosis
  - Causes:
    - Fibrinolysis
    - Impairment of coagulation pathways
- Consumptive coagulopathy
  - Massive hemorrhage leading to disseminated intravascular coagulation (DIC)

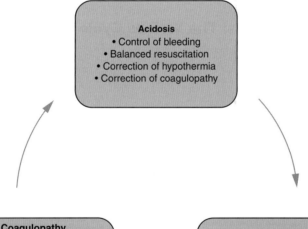

Algorithm: Prevention of the vicious cycle of trauma and the lethal triad

Must-Know Essentials: Prevention of the Vicious Cycle of Trauma and the Lethal Triad

PREVENTION OF ACIDOSIS

- Blood pH of less than 7.36 is associated with:
  - reduction of myocardial performance leading to cardiac arrhythmia, bradycardia, and cardiogenic shock.
  - coagulopathy leading to ongoing bleeding.
- Steps for the prevention of acidosis:
  - Balanced resuscitation and limited use of crystalloids
  - Management of hemorrhagic shock
  - Early control of bleeding
  - Prevention of hypothermia
  - Correction of coagulopathy

PREVENTION OF HYPOTHERMIA

- Body core temperature of <35°C (95 °F) is associated with:
  - Coagulopathy due to:
    - inhibition of thromboxane A2, resulting in reduction in local vasoconstriction and platelet aggregation at the site of injury
    - impairment of enzymatic processes of the coagulation pathways
  - Reduced tissue oxygen delivery due to the left shift of the oxygen dissociation curve; can result in reduced myocardial contractility
- Steps for the prevention of hypothermia:
  - Warming the crystalloids or plasma to 39°C (102.2 °F) before infusion, especially during large volume infusion
  - Use of external warming devices: Bair Hugger, warm blankets
  - Increase of the ambient temperature

PREVENTION OF COAGULOPATHY

- Steps for the prevention of coagulopathy:
  - Prevention of acidosis and hypothermia (as described earlier)
  - Blood transfusion:
    - Use of universally compatible RBC (blood group O Rh-negative and blood group O Rh-positive)
    - Massive blood transfusion protocol (MTP):
      - Universal RBC and plasma ratio of 1:1 and 2:1
      - RBC, plasma, and platelet ratio of 1:1:1
  - Use of viscoelastic hemostatic assay for the correction of coagulopathy
  - Correction of hypocalcemia
  - Tranexamic acid (TXA)
    - Inhibits trauma-induced hyperfibrinolysis by preventing activation of plasminogen to plasmin leading to stabilization of blood clot
    - Should be given between 1 and 3 hours after trauma
    - Limitations
      - Studies suggest that some patients develop hypercoagulable state after TXA administration.
      - Hyperfibrinolysis is not universal in trauma patients.

CHAPTER 4

Airway Assessment and Management

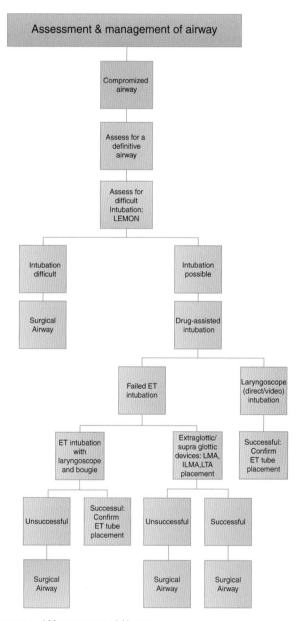

Algorithm: Assessment and Management of Airway

Must-Know Essentials: Assessment of Compromised Airway

MANIFESTATIONS OF COMPROMISED AIRWAY

- Patient unable to verbalize
- Noisy breathing
- Stridor
- Patient using or retracting accessary muscles of breathing
- Agitation
- Central nervous depression
- Tachypnea
- Cyanosis
- Low oxygen saturation

Must-Know Essentials: Definitive Airway

DEFINITION OF DEFINITIVE AIRWAY

- A tube in the trachea with a cuff inflated below the vocal cords

INDICATIONS FOR DEFINITIVE AIRWAY

- Maxillofacial trauma:
  - Midface fractures
  - Bilateral mandibular body fracture
- Inhalation injury
- Penetrating neck injury
  - Vascular trauma with significant neck hematoma
- Laryngeal injury: triad of clinical signs
  - Hoarseness
  - Subcutaneous emphysema
  - Palpable fracture
- Tracheal injury
- Risk of aspiration
  - Bleeding in the oral cavity
  - Vomiting
  - Unresponsive patients
- Need for ventilation or oxygenation
- Inadequate respiratory efforts
  - High cervical spinal cord injury
  - Severe brain injury (Glasgow Coma Scale [GCS] 8 or less)
- Apnea
  - Neuromuscular paralysis
  - Comatose patients
- Flail chest

TYPES OF DEFINITIVE AIRWAYS

- Endotracheal tubes (ETTs)

- Orotracheal
  - Rapid access to airway
  - Direct vision of the vocal cords required using a laryngoscope (direct or video laryngoscope)
  - Better suction for pulmonary toilet
  - Can perform bronchoscopy
  - Can be inserted in apneic patient
- Nasotracheal
  - Inserted blindly
  - Better tolerated in awake patients
  - May be inserted with neck in neutral position
  - Better to manage oral hygiene
  - Inability to perform bronchoscopy due to longer, thinner tube
  - Increased complications (epistaxis, maxillary sinusitis, otitis media)
  - Not indicated in apneic patients, basilar skull fracture, comminuted midface fracture
  - Must be spontaneously breathing at the time of intubation
- Surgical airways
  - Cricothyroidotomy
    - Preferred emergent surgical airway
    - Contraindicated in children <12 years of age
  - Tracheostomy
    - Indicated after failed intubation or cricothyroidotomy

Must-Know Essentials: Endotracheal Intubation

ASSESSMENT FOR A DIFFICULT INTUBATION

- LEMON Rule
  - **Look**
    - Small mouth or jaw
    - Large overbite teeth
    - Short, muscular neck
    - Obesity
  - **Evaluation** (3-3-2 rules)
    - Distance between the patient's incisor teeth should be at least 3 fingerbreadths.
    - Distance between the hyoid bone and the chin should be at least 3 fingerbreadths.
    - Distance between the thyroid notch and floor of the mouth should be at least 2 fingerbreadths.
  - **M**allampati Classification
    - Based on visualization of hypopharynx with opened mouth and protruded tongue in upright position
    - Class I: soft palate, uvula, fauces, and pillars visible
    - Class II: soft palate, uvula, and fauces visible
    - Class III: soft palate and base of uvula visible
    - Class IV: only hard palate visible
  - **O**bstruction
    - Any condition causing airway obstruction will cause difficulty in laryngoscopy and ventilation.
  - **N**eck mobility
    - Presence of C-collar
    - Neck mass
    - Cervical spondylosis

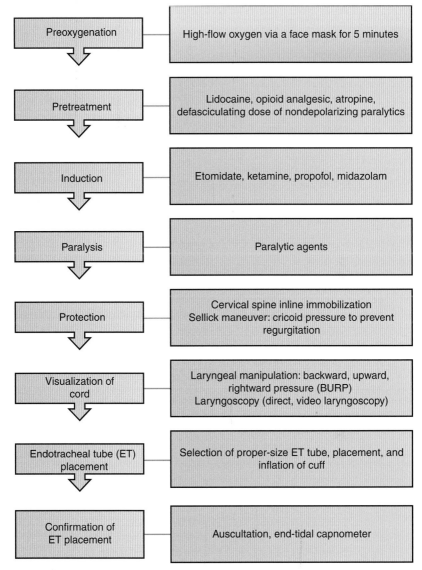

Algorithm: Steps of Drug-Assisted Intubation

STEPS OF ENDOTRACHEAL INTUBATION

- Preoxygenation
  - High-flow oxygen via a nonrebreather mask for 5 minutes
  - To maintain blood oxygenation during the apneic period of paralysis
- Pretreatment
  - Lidocaine (Xylocaine)
    - Suppresses the cough or gag reflex during laryngoscopy
    - Blunts the increase in mean arterial pressure (MAP), heart rate (HR), and intracranial pressure (ICP)

- No strong evidence but may be considered in patients with suspected intracranial hemorrhage (ICH)
- Dose: 1.5 mg/kg IV bolus
- Opioid analgesics
  - Reduces the sympathetic response of laryngoscopy and intubation
  - Fentanyl 3 mcg/kg IV bolus
  - No conclusive evidence supports the use of opioids in drug-assisted intubation.
- Atropine (Daturin)
  - May decrease the incidence of bradycardia caused by parasympathetic receptors stimulation during laryngoscopy, and succinylcholine-induced direct cardiac muscarinic receptors stimulation
  - Dose: 0.02 mg/kg IV bolus
- Defasciculation dose of nondepolarizing paralytic agents
  - May reduce the duration and intensity of muscle fasciculation caused by administration of succinylcholine (due to the stimulation of nicotinic acetylcholine receptors)
  - Recommended dose: 10% of the paralyzing dose
  - Helps to reduce increases in ICP during intubation
- Induction medications
  - Etomidate
    - Rapid onset
    - Short duration of action
    - Lack of cardiodepressant effects
    - Marked safety in patients with head injury
    - Good induction agent for patients with multiple traumas with hypotension
    - A drug of choice for virtually all cases of drug-assisted intubation due to its properties of decreasing the ICP, maintaining normal hemodynamics, and rapid onset of action
    - Lowers seizure threshold
    - Dose: 0.3 mg/kg IV bolus
    - Side effects
      - Nausea and emesis
      - Myoclonus
      - Laryngospasm
      - Transient dose-dependent suppression of adrenocortical activity
        - May last 5–15 hours
        - Clinically insignificant with single-dose bolus
  - Ketamine
    - Ideal induction agent due to rapid sedation and brief duration of action
    - Anesthesia induced in <1 minute
    - Eliminated in 2–3 hours
    - Agent of choice in patients with hypotension, as in hemorrhagic, hypovolemic, or septic shock
    - Has both analgesic and amnesic properties
    - Produces dissociative anesthetic effect
    - Agent of choice in patients with bronchospasm due to its bronchodilator effect
    - Not recommended in patients with:
      - uncontrolled hypertension.
      - elevated ICP.
      - aortic dissection.
      - aortic aneurysm.

myocardial infarction.

patients with brain injury (is a potent cerebral vasodilator, may increase ICP).

◦ Produces emergent phenomenon (delirium), characterized by:

postanesthesia visual, auditory, and proprioceptive hallucinations.

seen in 10%–30% of adults

seen rarely in children.

prevention with concomitant use of a benzodiazepine.

◦ Dose: 2 mg/kg IV bolus with clinical recovery in 10–15 minutes

- Propofol (Diprivan)
  - Causes dose-dependent sedation to coma
  - Lacks analgesic effect
  - Has amnesic properties
  - Extremely rapid (20 seconds) onset of action, with short duration (10–15 minutes) of action
  - Induction dose: 2 mg/kg/IV bolus
  - Decreases ICP.
  - Side effects
    - Decrease in systemic vascular resistance
    - Decrease in ICP
    - Respiratory depression
    - Hypotension
    - Propofol infusion syndrome
      - Associated with high dose and long term (>4 mg/kg/hr for more than 24 hrs)
      - Cardiac side effects: cardiac arrhythmia, bradycardia, asystole, and cardiac failure
      - Rhabdomyolysis
      - Metabolic acidosis
      - Renal failure
      - Hyperkalemia
      - Hyperlipidemia
      - More common in children and critically ill patients receiving catecholamines and glucocorticoids
- Midazolam (Versed)
  - Slower onset (2–3 minutes without pretreatment with opioid) and longer duration (up to several hours) of action
  - Requires titration of the dose
  - Standard dose for induction is 0.1 mg/kg, doses as high as 0.3 mg/kg may be required.
  - Mild decreases in cerebral perfusion pressure (CPP)
  - Minimal cardiovascular and respiratory effect
  - Not recommended because of its delayed induction time, as well as hypotension at induction doses and prolonged duration of action
- Paralytic agents
  - Depolarizing paralytic agent: Succinylcholine
    - An acetyl choline agonist
    - Stimulates all nicotinic and muscarinic cholinergic receptors
    - Depolarization at postsynaptic nicotinic acetylcholine receptor at the neuromuscular junction, leading to paralysis
    - Rapidly hydrolyzed in the serum by the enzyme pseudocholinesterase
    - Rapid onset (10–15 seconds) and shortest duration of action (10–15 seconds)
    - Causes transient fasciculation due to stimulation of nicotinic acetylcholine receptors

Dose
  1.5 mg/kg in adults
  2 mg/kg in children younger than 5 years
  Usual dose is 100 mg
Side effects
  Insignificant increase in ICP
  Insignificant increase in intraocular pressure
  Hyperkalemia: Patients with crush injury, major burns, electric injury, chronic renal failure, chronic paralysis, and chronic neuromuscular diseases are at risks of severe hyperkalemia.
  Bradycardia: Common in children, risk increases if a second dose of succinylcholine is administered. Because children younger than 7 years are at greatest risk; Atropine at a dose of 0.01 mg/kg in infants and 0.02 mg/kg in older children should be used to prevent this complication.
  Masseter muscle spasm: Occurs in 0.3%–1% of children.
  Certain drugs (cocaine, pyridostigmine, organophosphate) prolong paralysis when used with succinylcholine.
  Malignant hyperthermia
    Characterized by tachycardia, high fever, muscle rigidity, rhabdomyolysis, and hyperkalemia
    Contraction of the muscle fibers are due to release of stored calcium from the muscle cells
    Autosomal dominant
    Ryanodine receptor (RyR 1) genetic mutation typically located on the long arm of chromosome 19 is responsible.
    More common in men than women.
    Apart from Succinylcholine, it can be triggered by volatile anesthetic agents (Halothane, Isoflurane, and Enflurane) and rarely by physical exercise, and exposure to heat.
    A personal or family history of malignant hyperthermia is an absolute contraindication of the use of this agent.
    Susceptible individuals should be tested with muscle biopsy and caffeine-halothane contracture test or genetic testing for RYR1 mutation.
    Treatment: Dantrolene 2.5 mg/kg IV bolus, repeated as needed, followed by a maintenance dose of 1 mg/kg IV Q 4–6 hours for 36 hours. Dantrolene, a muscle relaxant, acts on RyR to prevent the release of calcium.
■ Nondepolarizing agents
  A competitive antagonist of acetylcholine; blocks the binding of acetylcholine at postsynaptic receptor and prevents depolarization leading to paralysis
  Slower onset (1–4 min)
  Longer duration of action (20–60 min). Avoid in patients where difficult intubation is anticipated.
  Rocuronium
    Fastest onset of action of all the nondepolarizing neuromuscular blockade (NMB) agents, close to that of succinylcholine
    Onset: 60–90 seconds
    Duration: 30–45 minutes
    Is an effective and safe alternative to succinylcholine
    Low incidence of histamine release
    Accumulates in hepatic dysfunction

          Some vagolytic properties

          Dose: 1–1.2 mg/kg IV bolus

        Pancuronium

          Slow onset of action (3 min) and prolonged duration (up to 60 min) of effect

          Useful in postintubation paralysis

          Cumulative effect with increasing doses

          Causes histamine release

          Accumulates in hepatic and renal dysfunction

          Vagolytic properties

          Tachycardia: most common side effect

          Dose: 0.06 to 0.1 mg/kg

        Atracurium or Cisatracurium

          Organ-independent elimination; degraded by plasma esterase hydrolysis (Hofmann elimination)

          Agent of choice in patients with renal or hepatic dysfunction

          Development of tolerance

          Histamine release with atracurium, but not with Cisatracurium

          Predisposes to seizures due to accumulation of Laudanosine (metabolites of atracurium and cisatracurium)

- Protection
  - Inline immobilization of cervical spine to protect SCI
  - Sellick maneuver
    - Pressure on cricoid to occlude esophagus and prevent regurgitation of gastric content
- Visualization of vocal cord
  - By laryngeal manipulation: backward, upward, and to the right (BURP)
  - Direct laryngoscopy
    - Macintosh blade
      - Curved, placed anterior to epiglottis, less likely to cause trauma to the teeth or epiglottis
    - Miller blade
      - Straight, placed posterior to glottis, and glottis is lifted up, gives better exposure to vocal cord opening compared to curved blade
    - No. 3 curved or straight blade is sufficient for most patients.
  - Video laryngoscopy (Glidescope)
- ETT placement
  - ETT size selection
    - Children—one of the following methods:
      - Internal diameter in mm = 16 + age/4
      - Size of the patient's little finger
      - Age (years)/2 + 12
      - Uncuffed ETT (size in mm ID [internal diameter]) = (age in years/4) + 4
      - Cuffed ETT (size in mm in ID) = (age in years/4) + 3
    - Adults
    - Largest possible, at least 7.5 F for oral and 7.0 F for nasal intubation
- Confirmation of the tube placement
  - Auscultation
  - End-tidal carbon dioxide detection
  - Calorimetric capnometer: changes color from purple to yellow with CO_2 exposure
  - Quantitative capnometer: measures CO_2 levels and can display a waveform
  - Pulse oximetry
  - Chest x-ray

Must-Know Essentials: Extraglottic Devices in Failed Intubation

SUPRAGLOTTIC

- Supraglottic devices are laryngeal masks that seal around the glottic inlet and remain superior to the larynx.
- Laryngeal mask airway (LMA)
  - A rescue device for a failed intubation
  - The inflatable cuff on the mask helps wedge the mask in the hypopharynx.
  - Does not prevent aspiration of gastric content
  - Selection of size of the tube
    - Size 3: for normal-size children ages 10–12 years, small adults weighing 30–50 kg, and most average-size women
    - Size 4: larger women, smaller men, and patients weighing 50–70 kg
    - Size 5: larger men and patients weighing over 70 kg
  - Placement technique
    - Completely deflate the cuff.
    - Apply water-soluble lubricant on the anterior and posterior surface of the cuff to facilitate insertion.
    - Open the airway and tilt the head.
    - Hold the tube with the index finger and the thumb of the dominant hand at the junction of the cuff and the shaft with the opening of the cuff toward the tongue.
    - Insert the LMA with the laryngeal surface directed caudally and by pressing the device against the hard palate.
    - Advance the device as far as the length of your index finger or long finger allows.
    - Complete the insertion by pushing the LMA farther to its final seated position.
    - Inflate the cuff with air (20 ml for size 3, 30 ml for size 4, and 40 ml for size 5). Inflate with more air if there is an air leak.
- Connect the bag valve mask (BVM) and check the chest wall movements, also verify with chest auscultation and a capnometer.

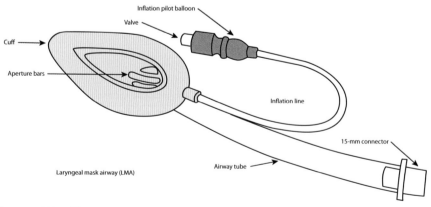

Laryngeal Mask™ Airway

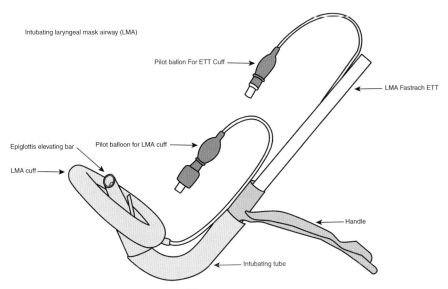

Intubating laryngeal mask airway (LMA)

Pilot ballon For ETT Cuff

LMA Fastrach ETT

Epiglottis elevating bar

Pilot balloon for LMA cuff

LMA cuff

Handle

Intubating tube

Intubating laryngeal Mask Airway (ILMA)™

- Intubating laryngeal mask airway (ILMA)
  - Placement technique
    - Insert the ILMA as described for an LMA.
    - Lubricate the ETT designed for an ILMA.
    - Insert the ETT into the ILMA, inflate the cuff, and connect to the BVM.
    - Connect the BVM, check the chest wall movements, and verify with chest auscultation and a capnometer.
    - Remove the ILMA after confirmation of the ETT placement.

RETROGLOTTIC DEVICES

- Laryngeal tubes that terminate in the upper esophagus (posterior to the glottis) and have two balloon cuffs (one pharyngeal and one esophageal), with ventilation fenestrations between the cuffs that align with the glottic opening
- These devices are used for rescue airway.
- This type of device is placed blindly in the esophagus, but a laryngoscope may be used.
- This type of device has two balloons—one seals the esophagus and the other the oropharynx, and ventilation is performed between the two balloons.
- The inflated distal esophageal balloon isolates the esophagus from laryngopharynx.
- The inflated proximal cuff isolates the laryngopharynx from the oropharynx and nasopharynx.
- Contraindicated in patients with known esophageal diseases, caustic ingestion, upper airway obstruction due to laryngeal disease, or foreign body
- Combitube
  - A dual-lumen dual-cuff tube
  - Has a proximal oropharyngeal cuff and a distal esophageal/tracheal cuff
  - The distal end of the tube has a blind end of the ventilatory part of the tube and an open end in the esophageal part of the tube.
  - Between the proximal and distal cuffs there are eight ventilating eyes for ventilation.
  - The esophageal cuff prevents aspiration.

- The Combitube comes in two sizes: 37 F for small adults and 41 F for tall adults.
- Placement technique
  - Apply a water-soluble lubricant on the tube.
  - Ask an assistant to immobilize the patient's head and neck. Do not hyperextend or hyperflex the neck.
  - Hold the tube with the dominant hand, and with the nondominant hand open the mouth and lift the chin.
  - Introduce the tip of the tube behind the base of the tongue in the midline and advance it by allowing it to follow the natural curve of the tube until the base of the connector is aligned with the patient's gum or teeth.
  - Inflate the proximal large oropharyngeal balloon with 85–100 ml air, depending on the size of the tube, and the distal balloon with 5–15 ml air.
  - Connect the blue port tube to a valve bag or vent.
  - Confirm the position of the tube by auscultation, chest wall movements, or capnometer; if the tube is not in the esophagus, ventilate through the other connecting tube.
  - Gastric decompression is possible by passing a tube through the esophageal port.
  - Secure the tube.
- Complications
  - Upper-airway hematoma
  - Pyriform sinus perforation
  - Esophageal perforation
- King Tube
  - Single lumen tube with a larger-balloon proximal oropharyngeal cuff and a smaller-balloon distal esophageal cuff
  - The proximal cuff stabilizes the tube and seals the oropharynx.
  - The distal cuff blocks the entry into the esophagus and reduces the gastric insufflation.
  - Two ventilation outlets allow ventilation, passage of bronchoscopes, and tube exchange catheters.
  - Multiple eyelets between the two cuffs supplement ventilation.
  - Both cuffs are inflated through a single small-lumen line.

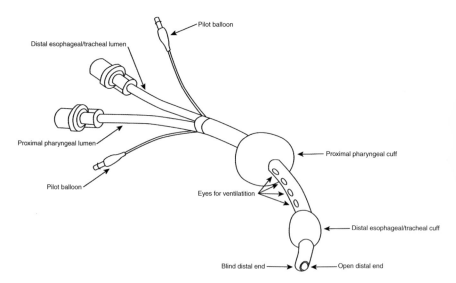

Combitube

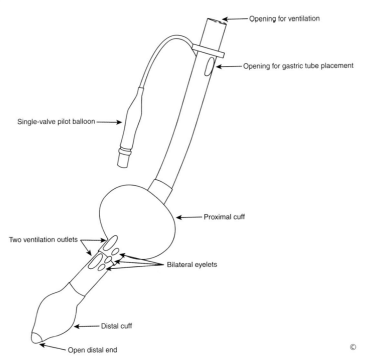

King tube

- Cuffs are inflated with volume ranging from 10 ml (size 0) to 90 ml (size 5).
- Comes in two designs: One is blind, and the other has an open distal tip that allows the passage of the gastric tube through a separate channel for gastric decompression
- Both cuffs are inflated simultaneously with a single pilot balloon.
- At the proximal end of the tube is an opening for gastric tube placement in the tubes designed with an open distal end.
- The insertion technique is similar to Combitube placement.

Must-Know Essentials: Emergency Surgical Airway

INDICATIONS

- Failed endotracheal intubation
- Contraindication of endotracheal intubation
  - Airway trauma
    - Laryngeal injury
    - Tracheal injury
    - Severe oropharyngeal hemorrhage
  - Severe glottic edema

SURGICAL ANATOMY FOR SURGICAL AIRWAY

- Anterior neck landmarks
  - Thyroid cartilage and superior thyroid notch
  - Cricoid cartilage

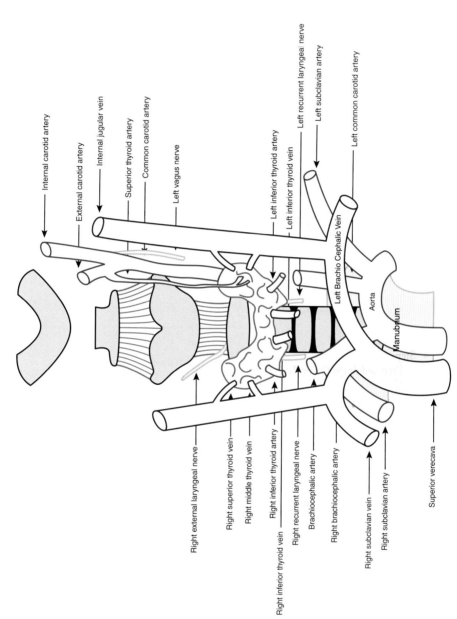

Internal carotid artery

External carotid artery

Internal jugular vein

Superior thyroid artery

Common carotid artery

Left vagus nerve

Left inferior thyroid artery

Left inferior thyroid vein

Left recurrent laryngeal nerve

Left subclavian artery

Left common carotid artery

Left Brachio Cephalic Vein

Aorta

Manubrium

Right external laryngeal nerve

Right superior thyroid vein

Right middle thyroid vein

Right inferior thyroid artery

Right inferior thyroid vein

Right recurrent laryngeal nerve

Brachiocephalic artery

Right brachiocephalic artery

Right subclavian vein

Right subclavian artery

Superior verecava

Anatomy of neck for surgical airway

- ▫ Cricothyroid membrane
- ▫ Sternal notch
- ■ Anterior neck structures
  - ▫ Thyroid gland isthmus
  - ▫ Inferior thyroid veins
- ■ Lateral neck structures
  - ▫ Common carotid arteries
  - ▫ Internal jugular veins

CRICOTHYROIDOTOMY

- ■ Fast and easier to perform
- ■ Associated with fewer complications
- ■ Contraindications
  - ▫ Patients <12 years old
  - ▫ Laryngeal fracture
  - ▫ Preexisting or acute laryngeal pathology
  - ▫ Tracheal transection with retraction of trachea into mediastinum
  - ▫ Anatomical landmarks obscured by gross hemorrhage, surgical emphysema, obesity, and so on
- ■ Types
  - ▫ Needle cricothyroidotomy
  - ▫ Percutaneous cricothyroidotomy
  - ▫ Open surgical cricothyroidotomy
- ■ Needle cricothyroidotomy
  - ▫ Steps
    - ▫ Prep and drape the neck.
    - ▫ Use local anesthetic.
    - ▫ Identify anatomic landmarks: the thyroid cartilage, the cricoid cartilage, and the cricothyroid space that contains the membrane.
    - ▫ Stabilize the larynx with the nondominant hand using the thumb and third finger and palpate the cricothyroid membrane with the index finger.
    - ▫ With the dominant hand, insert the angiographic catheter (14 G) attached to the syringe filled with normal saline into the cricothyroid membrane directing it caudally at a 45-degree angle.
    - ▫ As the needle is advanced, apply negative pressure to the syringe.
    - ▫ A distinct pop can be felt as the needle traverses the membrane and enters the trachea. In addition, air bubbles in the fluid-filled syringe confirm the entry of the needle in the trachea.
    - ▫ Advance the catheter and retract the needle.
    - ▫ Attach the jet ventilation device.
    - ▫ If a jet vent is not available, connect tubing with a side hole cut between the oxygen source and insufflate oxygen at 15 L/min with 1 second on and 4 seconds off by occluding the side hole of the tubing.
  - ▫ A needle cricothyroidotomy can usually be used for 30–45 minutes before CO_2 retention becomes significant.
  - ▫ Complications
    - ▫ Aspiration of blood
    - ▫ Esophageal injury
    - ▫ Perforation of posterior tracheal wall

- Hematoma
- Inadequate ventilation, hypoxia
- Pneumothorax
- Percutaneous cricothyroidotomy (Seldinger technique) using a kit
  - Steps
    - Prep and drape the neck.
    - Use local anesthetic.
    - Draw a small amount of water or saline into the syringe attached to the finder needle with overlying angiographic catheter.
    - Identify anatomic landmarks: thyroid cartilage, cricoid cartilage, and cricothyroid space that contains the membrane.
    - Stabilize the larynx with the nondominant hand, using the thumb and third finger, and palpate the cricothyroid membrane with the index finger.
    - Apply negative pressure while advancing the needle with catheter through the cricothyroid membrane caudally at a 45-degree angle.
    - When bubbles appear, remove the syringe and the needle, then advance the guide wire through the catheter.
    - Remove the catheter.
    - Make a small stab incision in the skin close to the guide wire.
    - Place the dilator into the airway catheter and insert the two devices together over the wire.
    - Remove both the dilator and the guide wire once the airway tube is secured in the trachea.
    - Secure the tube in place with appropriate tape.
  - Complications
    - Same as in needle cricothyroidotomy
    - Open surgical cricothyroidotomy
  - Steps
    - Prep and drape the neck.
    - Use local anesthetic.
    - Identify anatomic landmarks: thyroid cartilage, cricoid cartilage, and the cricothyroid space.
    - Stabilize the larynx with the nondominant hand using the thumb and third finger and palpate the cricothyroid membrane with the index finger.
    - With the dominant hand, make a 2–3 cm midline vertical incision using an 11-blade scalpel over the cricothyroid membrane.
    - Dissect the subcutaneous tissue with a curved hemostat.
    - Make a horizontal stab incision through the membrane. A distinct pop will be felt as the scalpel pierces the membrane and enters the trachea.
    - To avoid esophageal injury, make sure that the scalpel does not go deeper than 1 cm.
    - Avoid directing the scalpel toward the patient's head to avoid injury to the vocal cords.
    - An assistant should insert the tracheal hook at the superior end of the incision and retract the skin and membrane upward toward the patient's head. Keep the scalpel in place until the tracheal hook is inserted.
    - Dilate the incision horizontally using a Trousseau dilator or a curved hemostat with the nondominant hand.
    - With the dominant hand, insert the tracheostomy tube or an ETT.
    - Secure the tube.
    - Confirm placement through observation of chest rise, auscultation, and assessment of end-tidal CO_2.

- Complications
  - Insertion of the tube in a false passage
  - Tracheal injury
  - Vocal cord injury
  - Esophageal injury
  - Aspiration of blood
  - Bleeding
  - Laryngeal stenosis

EMERGENCY TRACHEOSTOMY

- Steps
  - Prep and drape the neck.
  - Use local anesthetic.
  - Identify anatomic landmarks: notch of the thyroid cartilage, cricoid cartilage, and sternal notch.
  - Make a 2–3 cm midline vertical incision below the cricoid cartilage.
  - Divide the platysma.
  - Split the strap muscles vertically, and retract the muscles laterally.
  - Cauterize or ligate aberrant anterior jugular veins and smaller vessels.
  - Expose the 2–4 tracheal rings by retracting the thyroid isthmus superiorly using a vein retractor, or divide the thyroid isthmus using cautery, or suture ligation using clamps.
  - Place stay sutures on each side of the trachea using 2/0 nylon sutures.
  - To facilitate the tracheal entry, place a tracheal hook on the cricoid cartilage and elevate superiorly to immobilize and elevate the tracheal wall.
  - Make a tracheotomy between the 2–3 tracheal rings using a #11 blade.
  - Spread the tracheal opening with a tracheal spreader.
  - Place the tracheostomy tube and inner cannula, and inflate the balloon.
  - Confirm the tube placement with capnography and adequate return of tidal volume.
  - Suture the tracheostomy to the skin, and also place the tracheal ties.
- Complications
  - Bleeding
  - Esophageal injury
  - Vocal cord injury
  - Pneumothorax
  - Pneumomediastinum
  - Subcutaneous emphysema
  - Tracheostomy tube blockage

CHAPTER 5

Management of Breathing and Ventilation

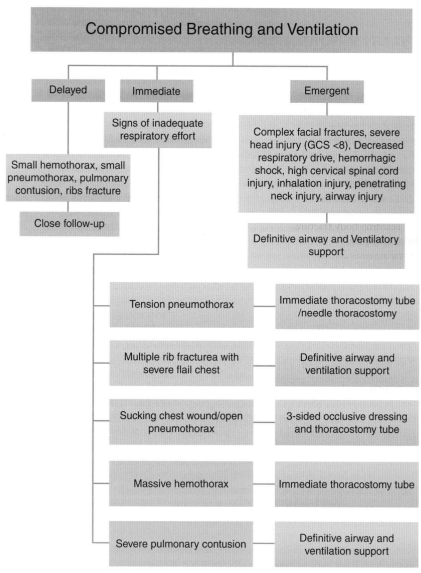

Algorithm: Compromised breathing and ventilation

Must-Know Essentials: Causes of Compromised Breathing and Ventilation

EMERGENT CONCERN OF BREATHING AND VENTILATION

- Complex maxillofacial trauma
  - Midface fractures
  - Bilateral mandibular body fracture
- Severe brain injury (GCS score <8), leading to decreased central respiratory drive
- Comatose patients
- Hemorrhagic shock
- High cervical cord injury
  - High cervical cord injury at C3/4 level may paralyze or weaken diaphragm and chest wall motion, leading to respiratory compromise.
  - High cervical injuries can cause retropharyngeal edema or hematoma with airway obstruction.
  - Common high cervical spine injuries
    - Burst fracture dislocations
    - Facet dislocations
    - Atlantooccipital injury
    - C1 ring fracture (Jefferson-type fracture)
    - C2 type III odontoid fracture
    - C2 fracture (hangman's type): fractures of bilateral pedicles with traumatic spondylolisthesis
    - Posterior arch fractures
    - Teardrop body fractures
- Inhalation injury
- Penetrating neck injury
  - Vascular trauma with significant neck hematoma
- Airway injury
  - Tracheal injury
  - Laryngeal injury

IMMEDIATE CONCERN OF BREATHING AND VENTILATION

- Massive hemothorax
- Tension pneumothorax
- Multiple rib fractures with flail chest
- Severe pulmonary contusion
- Sucking chest wound

DELAYED CONCERN OF BREATHING AND VENTILATION

- Small hemothorax
- Small pneumothorax
- Multiple rib fractures
- Pulmonary contusion

Must-Know Essentials: Clinical Findings Suggestive of Impaired Breathing and Ventilation

EXAMINATION OF THE NECK

- Distended neck veins: Tension pneumothorax
- Deviation of the trachea to the side opposite the injury is a late finding of pneumothorax.
- External signs of neck injury

EXAMINATION OF THE CHEST

- External signs of chest trauma
- Paradoxical wall motion (retraction of chest wall on inspiration): flail chest
- Chest wall deformity: multiple rib fractures
- Presence of subcutaneous air: pneumothorax
- Decreased breath sounds
  - Pneumothorax
  - Hemothorax

Must-Know Essentials: Pulse Oximetry and End-tidal CO_2

PULSE OXIMETRY

- A continuous measurement of the oxygen saturation of hemoglobin of the arterial blood
- Measures peripheral perfusion; unreliable in patients with poor peripheral perfusion such as vasoconstriction, hypotension, hypothermia
- Unreliable in severe anemia (Hb <5 g/dL)
- Not reliable in carboxyhemoglobinemia, methemoglobinemia, circulating dye (methylene blue, indocyanine green
- Does not measure partial pressure of oxygen (PaO_2)
- Pulse oxygen saturation >95% or more suggests adequate peripheral arterial oxygenation (PaO_2 > 70 mm Hg).
- Oxygen dissociation curve:
  - Relationship between partial pressure of oxygen and oxygen saturation is sigmoid in shape.
  - p50 is an oxygen tension when hemoglobin is 50% saturated.
  - When hemoglobin–oxygen affinity increases, the oxyhemoglobin dissociation curve shifts to the left and decreases p50. Factors contributing to shift to the left include:
    - decreased temperature.
    - Increased pH.
    - decreased 2,3-DPG.
    - decreased CO_2.
    - carbon monoxide.
    - methemoglobin.
  - When hemoglobin–oxygen affinity decreases, the oxyhemoglobin dissociation curve shifts to the right and increases p50. Factors contributing to the shift to the right include:
    - increased temperature.
    - decreased pH.
    - increases 2,3-DPG.
    - increased CO_2.

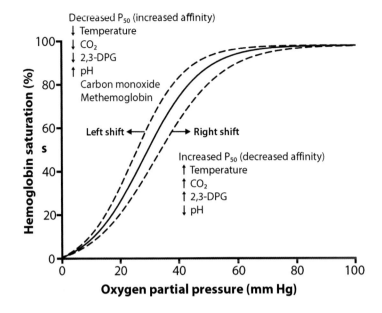

Oxygen dissociation curve

END-TIDAL CO₂ AND COMPROMISED AIRWAY

- Measurement of adequacy of ventilation
- Direct monitoring of inhaled and exhaled concentration or partial pressure of carbon dioxide
- Indirect monitor of the carbon dioxide partial pressure in the arterial blood
- Normally there is a very small difference between arterial blood and expired gas CO_2 partial pressures.
- Capnography provides information about carbon dioxide production, lung perfusion, alveolar ventilation, and elimination of carbon dioxide in patients on ventilators.

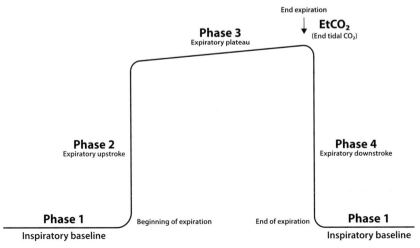

Normal capnograph

- Abnormal capnography patterns
  - Elevated $EtCO_2$
    - Decreased respiratory rate
    - Decreased tidal volume
    - Increased metabolic rate
    - Fever
  - Low $EtCO_2$
    - Increased respiratory rate
    - Increased tidal volume
    - Metabolic acidosis
  - Down-sloping phase 3
    - Severe emphysema: Destruction of alveoli causes rapid initial emptying of CO_2.
  - Prolonged phase 2/3
    - Bronchospasm
    - Chronic obstructive pulmonary disease (COPD)
    - Airway obstruction
  - Sudden drop in $EtCO_2$
    - Displaced endotracheal tube (ETT)
    - Decreased cardiac output
      - Cardiac arrhythmia
      - Pulmonary embolism
  - Dimorphic phase 2/3
    - Right mainstem intubation

Must-Know Essentials: Procedures for Compromised Breathing

THREE-SIDED OCCLUSIVE DRESSING FOR SUCKING CHEST WALL WOUND

- Normal transverse internal diameter of the trachea ranges between 1.5 and 2.5 cm in men and between 1 and 2 cm in women.
- In sucking chest wound, air is sucked into the thoracic cavity through the chest wall wound if the wound size exceeds 66% of the width of the trachea as air follows the path of least resistance.
- It can be treated with a three-sided occlusive dressing.
- A three-sided occlusive dressing prevents air from entering the pleural cavity during inhalation and allows trapped air to escape from the untapped edge during exhalation.
- Complete closure of the sucking chest wall wound can cause a tension pneumothorax.

NEEDLE THORACOSTOMY (NEEDLE DECOMPRESSION)

- Performed for life-threatening tension pneumothorax
- Technique
  - Use local anesthesia if patient is conscious and time permits.
  - Insert a 5-cm (smaller adults), 8-cm (larger adults) needle, or 14-gauge over-the-needle catheter into the 2nd intercostal space in the midclavicular line or into the 4th or 5th intercostal space in the anterior-axillary or midaxillary line.
  - Remove the needle, leave the catheter, and apply a dressing.
- Success rate is 50% to 75% in tension pneumothorax.

- Failure is due to catheter length, chest wall thickness, and kinking of the catheter.
- Complications
  - Hematoma
  - Pneumothorax
  - Lung laceration

CHEST TUBE (THORACOSTOMY TUBE)

- Anatomy of intercostal space
  - Intercostal nerve, intercostal artery, and intercostal vein runs along the lower border of the ribs.
  - Injury to the vessels can result in hemothorax.
  - Nerve injury can cause neuralgic pain.

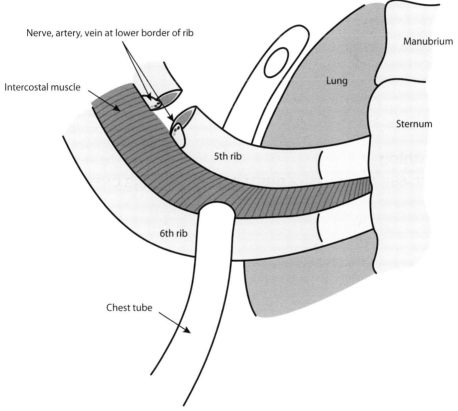

Anatomy of intercostal space

- Technique
  - Select the 5th intercostal space in men or the inframammary crease in women just anterior to the midaxillary line on the affected side.
  - Prepare and drape the chest at the insertion site.
  - Inject local anesthetic in the skin and the rib periosteum if the patient is awake.

- Make a 2–3 cm transverse (horizontal) incision at the selected site.
- A neurovascular bundle runs along the inferior border of the ribs. Dissect the subcutaneous tissue over the upper border of the rib to prevent injury of the neurovascular bundle.
- Puncture the parietal pleura with the tip of a clamp.
- Put a finger through the pleural hole and palpate for any adhesions.
- Select a chest tube: a larger tube for hemothorax, and a smaller tube for pneumothorax.
- Clamp the proximal end of the chest tube with a clamp and advance it into the pleural space through the hole in the pleura, directing the tube posteriorly and superiorly to the desired length.
- Confirm the placement by looking at the fogging in the tube and tidaling of the water column in the water seal chamber of the Pleur-evac.
- Secure the chest tube with a suture.
- Apply an occlusive dressing.
- Obtain a chest x-ray (CXR).
- Complications
  - Laceration to lungs
  - Laceration to intraabdominal organs (spleen, liver, stomach)
  - Injury to intercostal artery, vein, or nerves
  - Malposition of the tube: extrathoracic or intrathoracic
  - Chest tube kinking, clogging, or dislodgement
  - Empyema

CHAPTER 6

Assessment of Shock in Trauma Patients

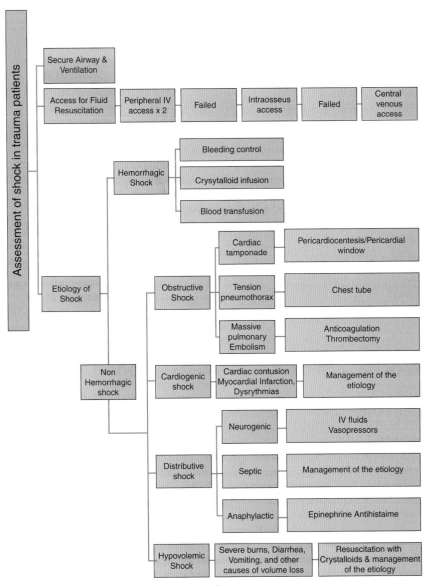

Algorithm: Assessment of shock in trauma patients

Must-Know Essentials: Shock in Trauma Patients

CLASSIFICATION OF SHOCK IN TRAUMA PATIENTS

- Hemorrhagic shock: most common in trauma patients
  - Bleeding from lacerations
  - Bleeding in the soft tissue of the extremity injuries
  - Fractures: due to bleeding at fracture sites
    - Pelvic fractures: 2000–3000 mL
    - Femur shaft fracture: 1000–1500 mL
    - Tibia fracture: 500–1000 mL
    - Humerus: up to 750 mL
    - Radius/ulna: 250–500 mL
  - Retroperitoneal bleeding
  - Intraperitoneal bleeding
  - Intrathoracic bleeding in severe chest injuries
- Nonhemorrhagic shock
  - Hypovolemia: due to volume loss
    - Severe burns
    - Other causes of volume loss
  - Obstructive shock: due to physical obstruction in the heart or great vessels
    - Cardiac tamponade
    - Tension pneumothorax
    - Massive pulmonary embolism
  - Cardiogenic shock: due to failure of the cardiac pump.
    - Cardiac contusion
    - Myocardial infarction
    - Dysrhythmias
    - Blunt cardiac injury
  - Distributive shock: impaired utilization of oxygen and failure of energy production by cells
    - Neurogenic shock
    - Distributive shock:
      - Neurogenic
      - Septic shock

CAUSES OF PERSISTENT SHOCK IN TRAUMA PATIENTS

- Exsanguinating hemorrhage
  - Major thoracic injuries
  - Major abdominal injuries
  - Retroperitoneal vascular injuries
  - Pelvic injuries
- Tension pneumothorax
- Cardiac tamponade
- Cardiogenic shock
  - Cardiac contusion
  - Myocardial infarction
- Neurogenic shock
  - Cervical or upper thoracic spinal cord injury

CLASSIFICATION OF HEMORRHAGIC SHOCK

- American College of Surgeons (ACS) classification: based on the quantity of blood loss
  - Class I: <15% blood loss

- Class II: 15%–30% blood loss
- Class III: 30%–40% blood loss
- Class IV: >40 % blood loss
- Based on response to initial crystalloid infusion:
  - Rapid responder
    - Patients with <20 % blood loss
    - Patent becomes hemodynamically stable after receiving the initial crystalloid bolus.
    - May require surgical intervention
  - Transient responder
    - Responds briefly to crystalloid bolus
    - Ongoing bleeding, 20%–40% blood loss
    - Blood and blood product transfusions are indicated.
    - Surgical intervention is indicated.
  - Minimal or nonresponder
    - Failure to respond to crystalloid or blood infusions
    - Emergent surgical intervention is required.
    - Shock may be due to nonhemorrhagic causes.
      - Cardiogenic shock: blunt cardiac injury, myocardial infarction
      - Cardiac tamponade
      - Tension pneumothorax
      - Neurogenic shock: cervical or upper thoracic spinal cord injury

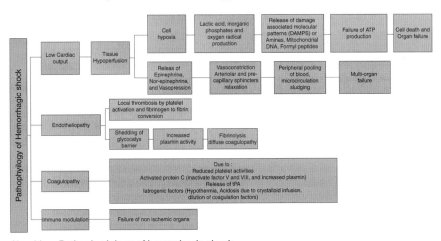

Algorithm: Pathophysiology of hemorrhagic shock.

Must-Know Essentials: Pathophysiology of Hemorrhagic Shock

DECREASED FILLING PRESSURE IN THE HEART DUE TO VOLUME LOSS

- Low ventricular filling pressure
- Decreased cardiac output, leading to hypotension
- Increased systemic vascular resistance (SVR)

INCREASED SYMPATHETIC AND DECREASED PARASYMPATHETIC OUTFLOW

- Tachycardia, except in patients on beta blockers, and athletes
- Increased cardiac contractility

- Vasoconstriction due to catecholamine release:
  - Skin pallor
  - Reduced capillary refilling

HYPOPERFUSION TO ORGANS

- Cellular hypoxia leading to cellular death and organ failure
  - Skin and muscles
    - Anaerobic metabolism causing lactic acidosis
  - Kidney
    - Initially reduced cortical function followed by renal failure
  - Bowel
    - Cellular damage
    - Failure to transport nutrients from bowel mucosa
    - Bacterial translocation from gut to portal circulation
    - Bowel may remain ischemic after flow is reestablished in the macro circulation, because of the occlusion of capillary networks caused by edema.
  - Liver
    - Hypoglycemia
    - Coagulopathy
    - Cellular necrosis
    - The liver may remain ischemic after flow is reestablished in the macro circulation, because of the occlusion of capillary networks caused by edema.
  - Lungs
    - Impaired functions to filter for toxic metabolites, inflammatory mediators released by ischemic cells, and translocated gut bacteria
    - Acute lung injury
    - Increased pulmonary resistance leading to right heart failure
  - Heart
    - Myocardial ischemia leading to hypotension and heart failure
    - Low pulse pressure

COAGULOPATHY

- Reduced platelet activities
- Activated protein C:
  - Inactivate factors V and VIII
  - Increases plasmin activities
- Release of tPA
  - Hypothermia
  - Large-volume crystalloid infusion
    - Dilution of coagulation factors
    - Acidosis

ENDOTHELIOPATHY

- Local thrombosis by platelet activation
- Fibrinogen to fibrin conversion

- Shedding of glycocalyx barrier of the endothelial cells
- Increased plasmin activity resulting in fibrinolysis

IMMUNE MODULATION

- Reperfusion following hemorrhagic shock causes release of toxic mediators into the circulation, causing immune modulation and resulting in failure of nonischemic organs (liver, lung, heart, brain, endocrine, and bone).

METABOLIC ACIDOSIS

- Lactic acid production due to anaerobic metabolism in the cells
- Large-volume crystalloid infusion

HYPOTHERMIA

- Large-volume infusion of crystalloids without warming
- Environmental exposure to cold
- Vasodilatation due to loss of energy reserve in the vascular endothelium

Must-Know Essentials: Manifestation of Hemorrhagic Shock

SKIN

- Cool, pale, diaphoretic due to vasoconstriction of skin
- Diminishes to absent capillary refilling

NEUROLOGICAL

- Mental status changes from normal, agitated, lethargic to comatose due to hypoperfusion to brain.

CARDIOVASCULAR

- Tachycardia
- Decreased systolic blood pressure
  - Young patients may lose 40% of their blood volume before systolic blood pressure (SBP) drops below 100 mm Hg.
  - Elderly patients may become hypotensive with a volume loss as little as 10%.
  - Patients with coronary artery disease may become hypotensive because of myocardial insufficiency after blood losses of less than 1500 mL.
  - Patients on beta blockers may be unable to produce an appropriate sympathetic response and become hypotensive after modest blood loss.
- Decreased pulse pressure

PULMONARY

- Tachypnea due to hypoxia and acidosis
- Acute respiratory failure

RENAL

- Oliguria, anuria, and acute kidney injury

GENERAL WEAKNESS

- Caused by hypoxia and acidosis

THIRST

- Caused by hypovolemia

NONFUNCTIONING PULSE OXIMETER

- Due to vasoconstriction

PROGRESSIVE HYPOTHERMIA

- Large-volume infusion of crystalloids without warming
- Environmental exposure to cold
- Vasodilatation due to loss of energy reserve in the vascular endothelium

PROGRESSIVE METABOLIC ACIDOSIS

- Lactic acid production due to anaerobic metabolism in the cells
- Large-volume crystalloid infusion
- Elevated base deficit

COAGULOPATHY

- Reduced platelet activities
- Activated protein C (inactivate factors V and VIII and increased plasmin)
- Release of tPA
- Hypothermia
- Large-volume crystalloid infusion
  - Acidosis
  - Dilutional coagulopathy

DECREASED MIXED VENOUS OXYGEN SATURATION (SmvO$_2$)

- Measured via pulmonary artery catheter
- Central venous oxygen saturation (ScvO$_2$) correlates well with mixed venous oxygen saturation

MANIFESTATION OF HEMORRHAGIC SHOCK BASED ON ACS GRADING

American College of Surgeons (ACS) Classification of Hemorrhagic Shock

	Class I	Class II (Mild)	Class III (Moderate)	Class IV (Severe)
Approximate blood loss	<15%	15%–30%	30%–40%	>40 %
Heart rate	Normal	Normal/High	High	High
Blood pressure	Normal	Normal	Normal/Low	Low
Pulse pressure	Normal	Low	Low	Low
Respiratory rate	Normal	Normal	Normal/Increased	Increased
Urine output (mL/hr)	Normal	Normal	Low	Very Low
Glasgow Coma Scale (Score)	Normal	Normal	Low	Low
Base deficit	0 to −2 mEq/L	−2 to −6 mEq/L	−6 to −10 mEq/L	−10 mEq/L or less
Need for blood products	Monitor	Possible	Yes	Massive transfusion

Must-Know Essentials: Differential Diagnosis of Shock in Trauma Patient

Differential Diagnosis of Shock in Trauma Patients

	Hypovolemic Shock	Cardiogenic Shock	Obstructive Shock	Distributive Shock
Heart rate	Elevated	Elevated	Elevated	Elevated
Cardiac output	Low	Low	Low	High, may be Low
Ventricular filling pressure	Low	High	High	Low
Systemic vascular resistance (SVR)	Elevated	Elevated	Elevated	Low
Pulse pressure	Low	Low	Low	High
SvO$_2$/ScvO$_2$	Low	Low	Low	Normal or High
Signs of low organ perfusion (lactic acidosis, low urine output, mental status changes)	Yes	Yes	Yes	Yes

OBSTRUCTIVE SHOCK

- Cardiac tamponade
  - Manifestations
    - Beck's triad
      - Hypotension
      - Muffled heart sounds
      - Distended neck veins
    - Pulsus paradoxus: a drop of >10 mm Hg in SBP during inspiration in cardiac tamponade
    - Tachycardia
    - Low cardiac output
    - Elevated ventricular filling pressure
    - Elevated SVR

- Low pulse pressure
- $SvO_2/ScvO_2$ ratio: low
- Echocardiography is the diagnostic test of choice. Findings include:
- Large inferior vena cava (IVC), with minimal changes during breathing
  - Right atrium collapse during systole
  - Enlarged pericardium
  - Collapsed ventricles
  - During inspiration
    - Increased pressure in the right ventricle
    - Bulge of interventricular septum toward the left ventricle, leading to decreased filling of the left ventricle
    - Marked decrease to complete collapse of the right ventricle volume
- Tension pneumothorax
  - Manifestations
    - Acute respiratory distress
    - Subcutaneous emphysema
    - Absent breath sounds
    - Hyperresonance to percussion
    - Tracheal shift
    - Findings of obstructive shock
      - Tachycardia
      - Low cardiac output
      - Elevated ventricular filling pressure
      - Elevated SVR
      - Low pulse pressure
      - $SvO_2/ScvO_2$ ratio: low
- Pulmonary embolism
  - Manifestations
    - Acute respiratory distress
    - Acute chest pain
    - Hemoptysis
    - Evidence of deep vein thrombosis (DVT)
    - Tachypnea
    - Cyanosis in more severe cases
  - Other manifestations as in obstructive shock

CARDIOGENIC SHOCK

- Myocardial infarction
  - Chest pain
  - Specific echocardiography findings
  - Elevated cardiac enzymes (creatinine phosphokincase [CK], troponin)
- Cardiac contusion
  - Tachycardia
  - Dysrhythmias
  - Echocardiography findings
- Cardiac dysrhythmias
  - Hypotension with abnormal cardiac rhythm
- Other manifestations in cardiogenic shock
  - Low cardiac output
  - High filling pressure

- Decreased pulse pressure
- High SVR
- Jugular vein distention (JVD)
- Pulmonary edema
- S3 gallop
- Decreased SmvO$_2$

DISTRIBUTIVE SHOCK

- Manifestations
  - Tachycardia
  - Cardiac output may be high or low
  - High pulse pressure
  - Low SVR
  - Normal or high mixed venous oxygen saturation (SvO$_2$)/ScvO$_2$
  - Neurogenic shock: in cervical and upper thoracic spinal cord injuries
    - Loss of sympathetic tone:
      Hypotension
      Bradycardia
    - Neurological deficit based on the level of injury
  - Septic shock
    - Early septic shock
      Modest hypotension
      Warm skin
      Wide pulse pressure
    - Late sepsis
      Cutaneous vasoconstriction
      Decreased systolic pressure
      Narrow pulse pressure

Must-Know Essentials: Systemic Inflammatory Response Syndrome (SIRS), Sepsis and Septic Shock

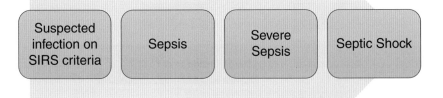

Sequence in infection

SYSTEMIC INFLAMMATORY RESPONSE SYNDROME (SIRS), SEPSIS AND SEPTIC SHOCK (AMERICAN COLLEGE OF CHEST PHYSICIANS [ACCP] / SOCIETY OF CRITICAL MARE MEDICINE [SCCM] IN 1992)

- Systemic inflammatory response syndrome (SIRS)
  - Presence of two or more of the following criteria
    - Temperature: <36°C (96.8°F) or >38°C (100.4°F)
    - Heart rate: >90/min
    - Respiratory rate: >20/min or $PaCO_2$ <32 mm Hg (4.3 kPa)
    - WBC: >12,000/mm³ or <4,000 mm³ or 10% bands
- Etiology of SIRS
  - Trauma
  - Burns
  - Ischemia
  - Hemorrhage
  - Pulmonary embolism
  - Acute pancreatitis
  - Cardiac tamponade
- Sepsis
  - SIRS with infection
- Severe sepsis
  - SIRS with evidence of sepsis-induced tissue hypoperfusion or organ dysfunction
- Septic shock
  - Caused by overwhelming systemic infection
  - Sepsis-induced hypotension (SBP <90 mm Hg or a reduction of 40 mm Hg from baseline) despite adequate fluid resuscitation
  - Perfusion abnormalities
    - Lactic acidosis
    - Oliguria
    - Alteration in mental status

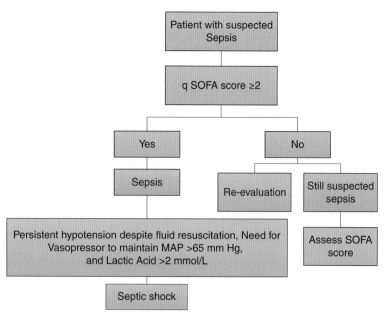

Algorithm: Assessment of septic shock (Sepsis-3, 2016 Consensus)

New Definition of Sepsis and Septic Shock (Third International Consensus Definitions for Sepsis and Septic Shock [Sepsis-3, 2016]

- Sepsis
  - Life-threatening organ dysfunction caused by a dysregulated host response to infection
  - Quick Sequential (Sepsis Related) Organ Failure Assessment (q SOFA) score ≥2
  - q SOFA score calculation criteria: 1 point for each of the following:
    - Alteration in mental status
    - Systolic blood pressure ≤100 mm Hg
    - Respiratory rate ≥22/min
  - The baseline SOFA score can be assumed to be 0 in patients not known to have preexisting organ dysfunction.
  - A SOFA score ≥2 reflects an overall mortality risk of approximately 10% in a general hospital population with suspected infection.
- Septic shock
  - Septic shock is a subset of sepsis in which underlying circulatory and cellular/metabolic abnormalities are profound enough to substantially increase mortality.
  - Sepsis with persisting hypotension despite adequate volume resuscitation with:
    - vasopressors requirement to maintain MAP ≥65 mm Hg and
    - serum lactate level >2 mmol/L (18 mg/dL)

Sequential (Sepsis Related) Organ Failure Assessment (SOFA) score calculation

Systems	0	1	2	3	4
Respiratory (PaO$_2$/FIO$_2$ mm Hg)	>400	<400	<300	<200 with respiratory support	<100 with respiratory support
Coagulation (platelets)	>150	<150	<100	<50	<20
Liver (bilirubin mg/dL)	<1.2	1.2–1.9	2–5.9	6–11.9	>12
Cardiovascular (mean arterial blood pressure [MAP] mm Hg)	>70	<70	Dopamine <5 or Dobutamine any dose	Dopamine 5.1–15 or Epinephrine <0.1 or Norepinephrine <0.1	Dopamine >15 or Epinephrine >0.1 or Norepinephrine >0.1
Central nervous systems (GCS)	15	13–14	10–12	6–9	<6
Renal (creatinine mg/dL)	<1.2	1.2–1.9	2.0–3.4	3.5–4.9	>5
Urine output (mL/day)				<500	<200

CHAPTER 7

Principles of Management of Hemorrhagic Shock

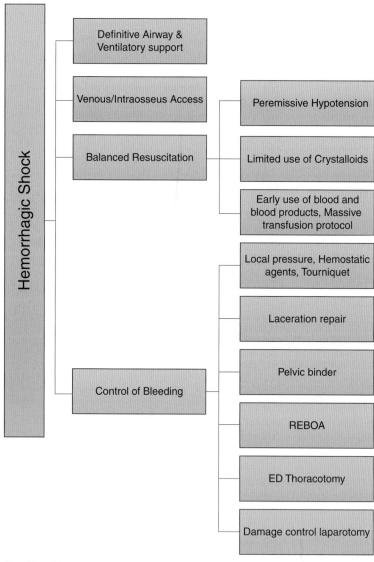

Algorithm: Management of hemorrhagic shock

Must-Know Essentials: Principles of Management of Hemorrhagic Shock

CONTROL OF AIRWAY AND VENTILATION

- Supplemental oxygen
- Definitive airway
  - Endotracheal intubation/surgical airway
- Ventilatory support

ACCESS FOR FLUID RESUSCITATION

- Peripheral line
  - Antecubital peripheral line
    - Two large-caliber (14–16 gauge) catheters
    - Short, large-caliber peripheral IV lines are preferred for rapid infusion of large volumes of fluid.
    - Rate of flow is proportional to the 4th power of the radius of the cannula and inversely related to the length (Law of Poiseuille).
- Intraosseous (IO) access
  - The bone marrow of long bones has a rich network of vessels that drain into a central venous canal, emissary veins, and, ultimately, the central circulation, providing a noncollapsible venous access.
  - Advantages
    - Rapid access in patients with failed peripheral IV line
    - Intraosseous route has roughly the same absorption rate as intravenous route.
    - Under pressure, fluid can be infused up to 200 mL/min.
    - Any medications that can be given via IV can be given per intraosseous route.
    - Needle should be removed within 3–4 hours, but it can be maintained for 24–72 hours. In practice, IO needle should be removed once an alternative vascular access is obtained.
    - The levels of drugs, chemistries, and hemoglobin, as well as acid-base status, obtained from bone marrow are reliable predictors of serum levels.
  - Contraindications
    - Fracture at the sites of insertion
  - Relative contraindications
    - Infection at the insertion site
    - Inferior vena cava injury
    - Previous attempt on the same leg bone
    - Osteogenesis imperfecta
    - Osteoporosis
  - Complications
    - Subcutaneous or subperiosteal infiltration is most common complication.
    - Pressure necrosis of skin at insertion site
    - Epiphyseal growth plate injury in children
    - Fat embolism
    - Local hematoma
    - Compartment syndrome: if the needle passes through the opposite cortex, the infused fluid enters the muscle rather than the venous system.

- Extravasation of hypertonic or caustic medications, such as sodium bicarbonate, dopamine, or calcium chloride, can result in necrosis of the muscle.
- Local infection and osteomyelitis
- Technique of IO access
  - Sites
    - Anteromedial aspect of the proximal tibia is the most common site, as it lies just under the skin and can be easily palpated and located.
    - Anterior aspect of distal femur: anterior midline 1-2 cm proximal to patella.
    - Superior iliac crest
    - Sternum
    - Proximal humerus at greater tuberosity
  - Steps of tibial IO access
    - Identify the tibial tuberosity.
    - Locate the bone 2 cm distal and slightly medial to the tibial tuberosity.
    - Support the flexed knee by placing a towel under the calf.
    - Prep and drape the patient using sterile technique.
    - If the patient is awake, inject local anesthetic (1% lidocaine) into the skin, into the subcutaneous tissue, and over the periosteum.
    - Insert the IO needle through the skin and subcutaneous tissue using automatic intraosseous device.
    - Automatic intraosseous devices
      - Quick and provides safe access
      - Deploys inject needles to a preset depth
    - Confirm the placement by aspirating bone marrow and connect the IV tubing.
- Central venous access
  - Indications
    - Failed peripheral IV
    - Failed IO line
    - Need for medications that can only be delivered centrally (certain vasopressors)
    - Consider using a short, large-bore catheter (8.5 F introducer sheath) or a double- or triple-lumen 7 F catheter.
  - Locations
    - Femoral: least sterile
    - Subclavian: avoided in patients with coagulopathy
    - Internal jugular (IJ)
  - Complications
    - Correlate directly with number of sticks
    - Arterial puncture: femoral > IJ > subclavian
    - Hematoma: femoral > IJ > subclavian
    - Pneumothorax: subclavian > IJ
    - Use of ultrasound (US) guidance: increases first-attempt success, reduces access time, reduces carotid puncture in IJ access
    - Specific complications of femoral venous access
      - Deep vein thrombosis (DVT)
      - Arterial or neurologic injury
      - Infection
      - Arteriovenous (AV) fistula
    - Specific complication of subclavian/IJ venous access
      - Pneumothorax
      - Venous thrombosis

Arterial or neurological injury
AV fistula
Chylothorax
Air embolism

BALANCED RESUSCITATION

- Limited use of crystalloids
  - Typically, normal saline (NS) or lactated Ringer's (LR) is used for initial fluid resuscitation of the trauma patients.
  - NS and LR have equivalent effects on hemodynamics and oxygen metabolism during resuscitation.
  - Resuscitation with LR has more favorable effects on fluid overload in lungs, coagulation, and acid/base balance (pH).
  - Advanced Trauma Life Support (ATLS) recommends 1 L of crystalloid as the starting point for all fluid resuscitation.
  - In penetrating trauma with hemorrhage, aggressive fluid resuscitation should be delayed until bleeding is controlled.
  - Balanced resuscitation prevents complications due to a large volume of crystalloids.
  - Infusion of large volumes of crystalloids to achieve a normal blood pressure is not recommended. Complications from large-volume crystalloid resuscitation include:
    - Prolonged ventilator dependence.
    - Increased hospital length of stay in the adult blunt trauma population.
    - Acute lung injury.
    - Acute respiratory distress syndrome (ARDS).
    - Multiorgan dysfunction.
    - Abdominal compartment syndrome.
    - Surgical Site Infections.
    - Coagulopathy due to:
      - Dilution of coagulation factors.
      - Hypothermia due to fluid stored at room temperature.
    - Large volume of normal saline causes hyperchloremic acidosis.
- Permissive hypotension:
  - Also known as hypotensive resuscitation and controlled resuscitation.
    - Goal mean arterial pressure (MAP) 40–50 mm Hg or systolic blood pressure (SBP) of 80–90 mm Hg.
    - Elevated BP causes more bleeding due to dislodgement of thrombus at the bleeding site.
  - Complications of prolonged permissive hypotension
    - Coagulation dysfunction
    - Ischemic organ dysfunction due to poor tissue perfusion
    - Mitochondrial dysfunction
    - Lactic acidosis
  - Contraindications of permissive hypotension
    - Patients with cerebrovascular disease, carotid stenosis, and compromised renal function
    - Patients with crush injury with rhabdomyolysis
    - Traumatic brain injury, and spinal cord injury. SBP >90 mm Hg is recommended in these patients.
- Early use of blood and blood products
  - Early administration of red blood cells (including uncross-matched type O) to achieve a hematocrit of 25%–30%

- Early use of plasma to maintain normal clotting factors
- Use of cryoprecipitate in coagulopathic patients
- Platelet transfusion if count <50,000
- Use of a massive transfusion protocol (MTP) using a 1:1:1 product ratio or low-titer type O whole blood.
- Use of goal-directed treatment of coagulopathy using viscoelastic assay
- Advantages of balanced resuscitation over aggressive resuscitation
  - Reduces morbidity and mortality of trauma patients with hemorrhagic shock
  - Prevents lethal triad
  - Minimizes the impact of trauma-induced coagulopathy
  - Limits blood product waste
  - Reduces the complications associated with aggressive crystalloid resuscitation

CONTROL OF BLEEDING

- Direct pressure on the bleeding wounds
- Tourniquet
- Local hemostatic agents
- Pelvic stabilization
  - Pelvic binder
  - External fixator
- Surgical hemostasis
  - External
    - Suture of bleeding laceration
    - Ligation of bleeding vessels
    - Control of bleeders with arterial clamps
  - Internal
    - Resuscitative Endovascular Balloon Occlusion of the Aorta (REBOA)
    - Angioembolization
    - Resuscitative thoracotomy
    - Damage-control celiotomy

PREVENTION OF VICIOUS CYCLE OF LETHAL TRIAD

- Lethal triad
  - Acidosis
  - Hypothermia
  - Coagulopathy

USE OF COLLOIDS FOR RESUSCITATION

- Not a fluid of choice for initial resuscitation
- More expensive than crystalloids
- Small risk of anaphylaxis
- No significant advantages over crystalloids in the early stages of resuscitation
- May be used in later part of resuscitation after a considerable capillary leak caused by the systemic inflammatory response syndrome (SIRS)
- May be associated (but no strong evidence) with less peripheral and pulmonary edema due to less capillary leak

ALBUMIN FOR RESUSCITATION IN SHOCK

- IV albumin does not have any advantage compared to crystalloid in resuscitation of hemorrhagic shock.

SODIUM BICARBONATE IN SHOCK

- No role in survival of shock
- May be indicated in pH <7.0

VASOPRESSORS IN SHOCK

- May be used to achieve a goal SBP of 80 to 90 mm Hg to maintain tissue perfusion in life-threatening hypotension
- Indicated in neurogenic shock

Must-Know Essentials: Use of Blood and Blood Products in Trauma Resuscitation

BLOOD TRANSFUSION

- Indicated to improve the oxygen-carrying capacity in patients with 30%–40% blood volume loss
- Disadvantages
  - Expensive
  - Immunosuppression
  - Short shelf life
  - Small risk of disease transmission
- Blood products are prepared after 500 mL of whole blood and 150 mL of anticoagulant are centrifuged.
  - 1 unit of packed red blood cells (PRBCs): volume 335 mL and 55% hematocrit
  - 1 unit of plasma: volume 275 mL and 80% coagulation activity
  - 1 apheresis unit of platelets: 50 mL with $3–4 \times 10^{10}$ platelets
  - 1 random donor unit of platelets constitutes 4–6 units of pooled platelets or 1 apheresis unit, both providing approximately $3–4 \times 10^{10}$ platelets
- Hemoglobin goal:
  - Normovolemic patients with good cardiopulmonary function can tolerate a hemoglobin concentration down to 7 g/dL.
  - Reduction in viscosity due to low hemoglobin may be beneficial as it helps improve cardiac output and tissue oxygenation.
  - Higher hemoglobin (8–10 g/dL):
    - Severe trauma patients
    - Patients with history of ischemic heart disease or significant respiratory disease
    - Ongoing hemorrhage
- Complications of blood transfusion
  - Coagulopathy due to:
    - hypothermia.
    - depletion of coagulation factors.
  - Thrombocytopenia
  - Thrombotic complications
  - ARDS

- Transfusion-associated circulatory overload (TACO)
  - Hydrostatic pulmonary edema
  - Incidence: 1%–8% of patients
  - One of the common causes of transfusion-related death
  - International Society of Blood Transfusion criteria for the diagnosis of TACO include:
    - Acute or worsening respiratory distress up to 12 hours after blood transfusion plus two or more of the following:
      - Acute or worsening pulmonary edema based on physical examination or chest imaging
      - Evidence of unanticipated tachycardia, hypertension, jugular venous distension, or peripheral edema
      - Evidence of fluid overload during transfusion with response to diuretic therapy
      - More than 1.5 times elevation of brain natriuretic peptide (BNP) to pretransfusion value
- Transfusion-related acute lung injury (TRALI)
  - Acute hypoxia due to noncardiogenic pulmonary edema
  - Usually within 1–2 hours, up to 6 hours after transfusion
  - Associated with all blood components in the plasma
  - Nonvolume related, even a small volume of blood can cause the symptoms
  - Associated with leukopenia/neutropenia likely due to sequestration of neutrophils in pulmonary capillaries
  - In 90% patients with TRALI, the donor blood or blood products were found to have an antibody against white blood cells (WBCs).
  - The incidence of TRALI can be mitigated by transfusion of plasma from male-only donors.
- Nonhemolytic hypersensitivity reactions to plasma proteins
  - Febrile nonhemolytic reactions due to alloimmunization from platelet or leukocyte antigens
- Serious intravascular hemolytic reactions from ABO antibodies
- Delayed extravascular hemolysis from antibody against donor Rh and non-ABO antigens
- Hypothermia
- Hyperkalemia
- Citrate complications
  - Metabolic alkalosis
  - Hypocalcemia
- Graft vs Host disease (GVHD)
  - Usually fatal.
  - Donor T-lymphocytes immune response against recipient's lymphoid tissue

MASSIVE TRANSFUSION PROTOCOL (MTP)

- Defined as use of >10 units of PRBCs in 24 hours or >4 units of PRBC in 1 hour.
- Development and implementation of MTPs have shown reduction in mortality and overall blood product use in trauma centers.
- Hemostatic resuscitation is defined as:
  - Ratio-based empiric use of packed RBCs, fresh frozen plasma (FFP), and platelets
  - Early use of platelets and FFP has shown survival benefits in trauma patients.
- American College of Surgeons (ACS) guidelines for MTP
  - Assessment of blood consumption (ABC) score: 2 or more

- ABC score is calculated using four variables: pulse >120, SBP <90, positive Focused Assessment with Sonography in Trauma (FAST), and penetrating torso injury.
- One point is given for each variable.
- Persistent hemodynamic instability
- Active bleeding requiring operation or angioembolization
- Blood transfusion in trauma bay
- Massive transfusion includes the following:
  - Use of universal blood product:
    - RBC blood group O Rh-negative
    - RBC blood group O Rh-positive
    - Universal AB plasma
  - Component transfusion: RBC, plasma, and plate ratio of 1:1:1
  - Assessment for coagulopathy, hypothermia, acidosis, and hypocalcemia
  - RBCs and plasma should be delivered by a rapid transfuser and through a blood warmer for maximum effectiveness.
  - Platelets and cryoprecipitate should not be administered through a blood warmer.
  - O Rh-negative RBCs should be used in women of childbearing age.
  - Use of cross-matched RBCs as soon as available.
  - Discontinuation of MTP:
    - If further resuscitation is futile
    - RBC transfusion: hemoglobin $\geq$10 g/dL
    - Plasma transfusion
      - Prothrombin time (PT) <18 seconds
      - Activated partial thromboplastin time (aPTT) <35 seconds
      - Platelet transfusions: platelet count >150 × 10^9/L)
      - Cryoprecipitate or fibrinogen concentrate: Fibrinogen level >180 g/L
- Use of goal-directed treatment of coagulopathy using viscoelastic assay is recommended after initial use of MTP.

Must-Know Essentials: Adjuncts to Massive Transfusion

TRANEXAMIC ACID (TXA)

- Synthetic derivative of lysine
- Is an antifibrinolytic agent
- Prevents trauma-induced hyperfibrinolysis by inhibiting activation of plasminogen to plasmin
- Effective in bleeding control after trauma (Clinical Randomisation of an Antifibrinolytic in Significant Haemorrhage [CRASH-2] trial)
- Showed 2.5% mortality reduction if given within 1 hour, and 1.3% mortality reduction if given 1–3 hours after the trauma
- Showed 1.3% increase in mortality if given more than 3 hours after the trauma
- Dose: 1 g over 10 min given within 3 hours of injury followed by an infusion of 1 g over 8 hours
- May benefit from an admission TEG to evaluate the fibrinolysis status
- Complications
  - Increased incidence of venous thromboembolism (VTE)
  - Fibrinolytic shutdown
  - Seizures

- Blurred vision
- Acute kidney injury
- Multiple system organ failure (MSOF)
- Limitations of CRASH-2 study
  - Lack of injury severity score (ISS)
  - Lack of fibrinolysis and coagulopathy status on admission
  - Some patients may develop hypercoagulable state.
  - Hyperfibrinolysis is not universal among trauma patients.

PROTHROMBIN COMPLEX

- These concentrates contain either three (II, IX, and X) or four (II, VII, IX, and X) clotting factors.
- Recommended for urgent reversal of Warfarin

RECOMBINANT FACTOR XA

- Patients on factor X inhibitors

Must-Know Essentials: Nonsurgical Methods Bleeding Control

DIRECT PRESSURE

- Direct pressure on the bleeding wounds
  - Constricts the blood vessels
  - Apply pressure using gauze pads for 5–10 minutes.
  - If bleeding stops, apply an elastic bandage over the gauze pad.
    - Wounds on the arms, shoulders, legs, groin, and neck can be effectively controlled by direct pressure.
    - If available, topical hemostatic-coated gauze may be used.

WOUND PACKING

- Indicated in areas where direct pressure may not be possible, such as cavitary wounds
- Pack the wound cavity, using gloved finger or forceps, with rolled gauze until it is tightly packed.
- If available, topical hemostatic-coated gauze may be used.

TOPICAL HEMOSTATIC AGENTS

- Commonly used topical agents
  - QuikClot (Z-Medica, Wallingford, CT, USA)
    - Nonwoven gauze coated with kaolin, which is composed of oxides of silicon, aluminum, magnesium, and sodium
      - Absorbs water when placed in a bleeding wound, thereby increasing the local concentration of clotting factors, platelets, and red blood cells
      - Promotes clotting by activating factor XII
      - Promotes exothermic reaction locally that can cause local tissue damage
      - Available as laparotomy pad and as Combat Gauze.

- HemCon (Hemorrhage Control Technologies, Portland OR, USA)
  - Composed of Chitosan, a substance derived from arthropod skeletons
  - Causes sealing of the wound and adheres to surrounding tissue
  - Available as gauze coated with HemCon, which is placed directly on the wound and secured with a pressure bandage
  - Efficacy depends entirely on the bandage adhering well to the wound; works better on flat superficial wounds
  - Difficult to use in deeper wounds

TOURNIQUET

- Indicated for uncontrolled external bleeding from either blunt or penetrating limb extremities injury when direct pressure does not control the bleeding
- Should be placed as distal as possible
- Must occlude arterial inflow; occluding only venous system can increase bleeding.
- Second tourniquet above the previous one may be needed if first tourniquet does not control bleeding.
- Occlusion pressure: 100 mm Hg more than SBP.
- Use of tourniquet should not exceed 2 hours.
- Tourniquet should be released to reassess for bleeding at 2-hour intervals.
- Tourniquets properly applied in the prehospital setting should not be removed unless adequate team support is present to manage bleeding that may occur.
- Complications
  - Rhabdomyolysis
  - Tissue ischemia and limb loss
  - Nerve injury
  - Renal failure
  - Compartment syndrome
  - Amputation

SPLINTS FOR FRACTURES

- Extremity fractures with associated open hemorrhagic wounds
  - Realign the fractures.
  - Apply pressure dressing on the bleeding wounds.
  - Place a splint.
- Displaced or comminuted long bone fractures
  - May cause significant bleeding due to motion
  - Placement of a splint to reduce motion at fracture sites

PELVIC STABILIZATION

- Indicated in pelvic fractures with:
  - hemodynamic instability.
  - anterior–posterior and vertical shearing deformations in pelvic x-rays.
  - significant pubic symphysis diastasis (>2.5 cm) in open book fractures.
  - CT scans showing:
    - active arterial extravasation (CT blush).
    - compression of the urinary bladder.
    - pelvic hematoma.

- Controls the venous and/or cancellous bone bleeding by pelvic closure and reduces pelvic volume
  - Binders do not control arterial bleeding.
  - Methods of pelvic stabilization:
    - Pelvic binder
      - Fracture of the iliac wing is an absolute contraindication.
      - It should be applied over the greater trochanters.
      - Many brands of pelvic binders are commercially available.
      - Bed sheet also can be used.
    - Pelvic C-clamp
    - External fixator

Must-Know Essentials: Surgical Methods of Bleeding Control

EXTREMITIES BLEEDING

- Extremity wounds with continued bleeding despite use of nonsurgical methods can be controlled with:
  - suture of actively bleeding lacerations.
  - ligation of bleeding vessels.
  - Foley catheter balloon to tamponade for a bleeding axillary wound.

ABDOMINAL TRAUMA WITH HEMODYNAMIC INSTABILITY

- The following procedures may be indicated:
  - Zone I REBOA
  - Damage-control celiotomy
  - Resuscitative thoracotomy and cross-clamping of aorta

PELVIC FRACTURES WITH HEMODYNAMIC INSTABILITY

- The following procedures may be indicated:
  - Zone III REBOA followed by angioembolization
  - Zone III REBOA followed by surgical control of bleeding
  - Angioembolization
  - Preperitoneal pelvic packing

CHEST INJURY WITH HEMODYNAMIC INSTABILITY

- Indications for damage-control thoracotomy
  - Blunt chest trauma
    - Continued chest tube bleeding with hemodynamic instability
    - Chest tube output >1500 mL within 24 hours
  - Penetrating chest trauma
    - Injury with high-energy weapons
    - Injury with low-energy weapons and hemodynamic instability

CHAPTER 8

Viscoelastic Hemostatic Assay

Must-Know Essentials: Viscoelastic Hemostatic Assay

THROMBOELASTOGRAPHY

- Thromboelastography (TEG) is a viscoelastic hemostatic assay technique that measures clotting activity from initiation of the clotting cascade to fibrinolysis.
- It measures the interaction of platelets with the coagulation cascade (aggregation, clot strengthening, fibrin cross-linking, and fibrinolysis).
- TEG provides a graphic representation of clot formation and lysis by assessing the viscoelastic properties of the clot over time.
- Limitations of conventional coagulation measurement
  - Conventional coagulation tests include:
    - prothrombin time (PT).
    - international normalized ratio (INR).
    - activated partial thromboplastin time (aPTT).
    - thromboplastin time (TT).
    - fibrinogen concentration.
    - platelet count.
  - PT, INR, aPTT, and TT measure only one part of the coagulation cascade: conversion of fibrinogen into fibrin.
  - INR and aPTT are performed with platelet-poor plasma; they do not measure the contribution of platelets in clot formation.
  - Conventional tests are poor predictors of bleeding and thrombosis.
  - Conventional test results take longer time (30–60 min) to perform.
- Advantages of TEG
  - It is better than conventional tests for the evaluation of coagulopathy in trauma patients with acidosis, hypothermia, and hemorrhagic shock.
  - TEG-based treatment helps in focused treatment of coagulopathy associated with hypothermia and hemorrhagic shock in trauma patients.
  - TEG helps to differentiate coagulopathy due to low fibrinogen or thrombocytopenia.
  - TEG parameters correlate with blood products.
  - TEG is a good point-of-care (POC) device, as it takes only 5–10 minutes to perform.

TECHNIQUES FOR PERFORMING TEG

- TEG kaolin (standard)
  - Measures intrinsic pathway
  - Indicated for nonoperative bleeding/clotting
  - Indicated for operative bleeding/clotting in patients not on heparin or receiving massive transfusion
  - Can be used for preoperative baseline coagulation assessment
  - TEG kaolin does not correlate with INR in patients on warfarin; despite an increased INR, TEG remains normal.

- Rapid-TEG:
  - Rapid-TEG (r-TEG) uses both tissue factor and kaolin and measures both extrinsic and intrinsic pathways of coagulation.
  - Measures activated clotting time (ACT) to initial fibrin formation
  - In this assay, the R-value is replaced by the TEG-ACT value, which is measured in seconds rather than in minutes.
  - The remainder of the TEG parameters do not differ between a standard and an r-TEG.
  - It does not correlate with INR in patients on warfarin.
  - TEG-ACT represents this initial phase of clot formation.
  - Prolongation of TEG-ACT has been associated with increased requirement of massive transfusion (MT).
- TEG with platelet mapping
  - Measures the clot strength as maximal amplitude (MA)
  - Measures platelet function, including the contribution of the adenosine diphosphate (ADP) and thromboxane A2 (TxA2) receptors in clot formation
  - Can differentiate contribution of platelet and fibrinogen in clot formation
  - Determines the degree of platelet function inhibition in patients on antiplatelets

Rapid-TEG (normal values):

ACT-time: 80–140 sec
R-time: 0.2–0.9 minutes
K-time: 0.6–1.8 minutes
Alpha angle: 70.0–82.0 degrees
MA: 57.0–72.0 mm
A30 or LY30: 0–3%
G-value: 5.3–12.4 dynes/cm²
CLT: 80–140 sec

Standard TEG (normal values):

R-time: 5–10 minutes
K-time: 1–3 minutes
Alpha angle: 53–72 degrees
MA: 50–70 mm
A30 or LY30: 0–3%
G-value: 5.3–12.4 dynes/cm²
CLT: 80–140 sec

Normal thromboelastogram

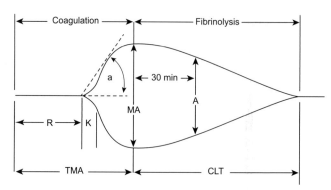

NORMAL THROMBOELASTOGRAM PARAMETERS

- R-time
  - Enzymatic reaction start time to initial fibrin clot formation
  - Measures the activity of clotting factors (intrinsic pathways)
  - Normal reaction time: 5–10 minutes
  - Normal amplitude: 2 mm
  - Prolonged R-time means coagulation factor deficiency.
  - R-time is decreased in hypercoagulable state.
- K-time
  - Kinetic time from the end of R until the clot reaches 20 mm; represents the speed of clot formation (fibrin cross-linkage)
  - Time until clot reaches a specified level of clot strength
  - Measures fibrinogen and platelet numbers
  - Normal K-time: 1–3 minutes
  - Normal amplitude: 20 mm

- Alpha angle
  - Angle from baseline to slope of tracing that represents clot formation
  - Measures fibrinogen and platelet numbers
  - Measures the rate of clot formation
  - Measures the speed at which fibrin buildup and cross-linking take place, hence assesses the rate of clot formation
  - Normal value: 53–72 degrees
- Maximum amplitude value (MA)
  - Measurement of direct function of the fibrin, platelet number, and platelet function
  - Measures maximal clot strength
  - Represents the ultimate strength of the fibrin clot (i.e., overall stability of the clot)
  - Normal value: 50–70 mm
- A30 or LY30
  - Measures clot lysis at 30 minutes after maximum clot strength (MA)
  - Measure fibrinolysis/clot stability
  - Can be an early indicator of massive hemorrhage
  - Normal range: 0%–3%.
  - Hyperfibrinolysis: A 30 greater than 3% is considered as pathological clot breakdown; seen in trauma patients with coagulopathy, and is associated higher mortality.
- TMA
  - Time to maximum amplitude
  - Lysis of the clot starts after TMA.
- G measurement
  - Measures clot strength or clot firmness
  - Is the single most important value of the entire assay, as it represents the overall function or effectiveness of the clot
  - Normal value: 5.3–12.4 dynes/cm^2
  - G value >10 dynes/cm^2 indicates increased risk of thrombosis.
  - Treatment for high G value: platelet inhibitors such as clopidogrel (Plavix) or aspirin
  - A G value <5 dynes/cm^2 indicates increased risk of hemorrhage.
- Clot lysis time (CLT)
  - Normal value: 80–140 sec

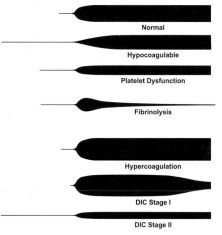

Thromboelastogram in coagulation disorders

THROMBOELASTOGRAM PATTERNS IN VARIOUS COAGULATION DISORDERS

- Hypocoagulable state: anticoagulants, hemophilia, and coagulation factor deficiency
  - Prolonged R- and K-values
  - Decreased MA
  - Decreased alpha angle
- Platelet dysfunction (thrombocytopenia, thrombocytopathy, antiplatelets)
  - Normal R-value
  - Prolonged K-value
  - Decreased MA
- Fibrinolysis (t-PA, urokinase, streptokinase)
  - Normal R-value
  - Continuous decrease of MA
  - LY30 >7.5%
- Hypercoagulation
  - Decreased R- and K-values
  - Prolonged MA
  - Prolonged alpha angle
- Disseminated intravascular coagulation (DIC)
  - Stage I: hypercoagulable state with secondary fibrinolysis
  - Stage II: hypocoagulable state

TEG-BASED TREATMENT RECOMMENDATIONS

- ACT >140 sec
  - Fresh frozen plasma (FFP)
- Increased R-time >10 minutes
  - FFP
  - FFP contains all the coagulation factors, including the labile factors V and VIII.
  - Longer R-time requires more FFP infusion.
- K-time >3 minutes
  - Cryoprecipitate
  - Cryoprecipitate contains fibrinogen, Von Willebrand factor, factor VIII, factor XIII, and fibronectin.
- Decreased MA <50 mm
  - Suggests platelets deficiency or dysfunction
  - Desmopressin (DDAVP)/cryoprecipitate/fibrinogen
  - Platelet transfusion: active bleeding
  - Slightly decreased MA value suggests depressed platelet function. Desmopressin should be given at a dose of 0.3 μg/kg intravenously. Desmopressin promotes platelet adhesion, and it functions by releasing factor VIII/von Willebrand complexes from the tissue endothelium.
- Alpha angle
  - Measures the speed of clot strengthening and estimates the fibrinogen level
  - Decrease in alpha angle <53 degrees reveals a deficiency in fibrinogen that results in a longer time to obtain maximal clot strength.
  - Treated with cryoprecipitate, which contains fibrinogen and is transfused until the alpha angle is >53 degrees

- LY30 >3%
  - Antifibrinolytic agents
    - Tranexamic acid (TXA)
    - Aminocaproic acid
  - G measurement
  - >10 dynes/cm^2: Platelet inhibitors such as clopidogrel (Plavix) or aspirin
  - <5 dynes/cm^2: Platelets

CHAPTER 9

Resuscitative Endovascular Balloon Occlusion of the Aorta

Must-Know Essentials: Resuscitative Endovascular Balloon Occlusion of the Aorta in Abdominal Trauma (Blunt/Penetrating)

BACKGROUND

- For resuscitative endovascular balloon occlusion of the aorta (REBOA), an endovascular balloon is placed in the aorta to control hemorrhage, as well as to maintain myocardial and cerebral perfusion in traumatic arrest and hemorrhagic shock by augmenting afterload.

ZONES OF AORTA FOR REBOA PLACEMENT

- Average diameter of the aorta
  - Thoracic aorta: 20 mm
  - Distal abdominal aorta: 15 mm
  - On average, the aorta is 2 mm narrower in women than in men.
- Aortic length
  - Varies among individuals
  - Abdominal aorta from the level of celiac artery to its bifurcation is approximately 13 cm long.
- Externally, the abdominal aorta can be measured from the xiphoid process to just above the umbilicus.
- Zones of REBOA
  - Aorta is divided into three separate zones for the purpose of REBOA balloon deployment.
  - Zone I
    - Extends from the origin of the left subclavian artery to the celiac artery
    - Approximately 20 cm long in adults
    - Estimated externally to extend from the medial head of the clavicle or sternal notch to the xiphisternum, or T4 vertebra to L1 vertebra, or T4 vertebra to 12th rib.
  - Zone II
    - Extends from the celiac artery to the most caudal renal artery
    - Approximately 3 cm long.
    - REBOA balloon is not recommended in this zone.
  - Zone III
    - Extends distally from the most caudal renal artery to the aortic bifurcation
    - Approximately 10 cm long
    - Estimated externally to extend from L2 vertebra to L4 vertebra, or from the xiphisternum to the umbilicus

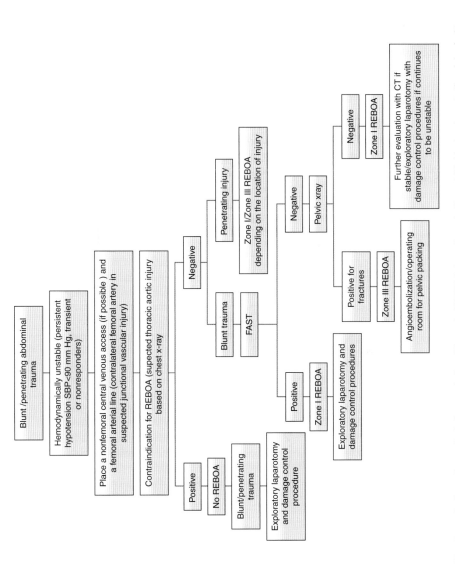

Algorithm: Resuscitative endovascular balloon occlusion of the aorta (REBOA) in hemodynamically unstable blunt and penetrating abdominal trauma

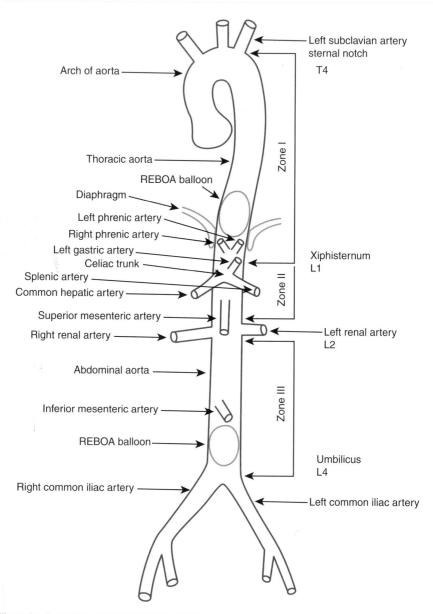

Illustration: Zones of the aorta for REBOA placement

INDICATIONS FOR REBOA BALLOON

- Blunt/penetrating life-threatening hemorrhage below the diaphragm with:
  - persistent hypotension: systolic blood pressure (SBP) <90 mm Hg.
  - hypotension unresponsive to resuscitation.
  - hypotension with transient response to resuscitation.
- In presumed life-threatening hemorrhage below the diaphragm with cardiac arrest:

- REBOA may be considered as an alternative to resuscitative thoracotomy.
- REBOA is less invasive than resuscitative thoracotomy and can be performed rapidly as compared with resuscitative thoracotomy.

CONTRAINDICATIONS FOR REBOA

- High clinical/radiological suspicion of thoracic aortic injury.
- Chest x-ray (CXR) findings suspicious for thoracic aortic injury
  - Widened mediastinum (mediastinum-to-chest-width ratio > 0.25)
  - Irregular aortic arch
  - Blurred aortic contour
  - Loss of aortopulmonary window
    - Depression of left main bronchus
    - Left pleural cap
    - left large hemothorax

LOCATIONS FOR REBOA CATHETER

- Blunt abdominal trauma
  - Zone I REBOA
    - Focused Assessment with Sonography in Trauma (FAST) suggestive for intraabdominal hemorrhage
    - Negative FAST and pelvic x-ray negative for fractures
  - Zone III REBOA
    - Negative FAST and pelvic x-ray positive for fractures
- Penetrating abdominal trauma
  - Zone I
    - Hemodynamically unstable penetrating central or upper abdominal injuries
  - Zone III REBOA
    - Pelvic or groin injury with uncontrolled hemorrhage
    - Junctional vascular injury (iliac or common femoral vessels)
    - Proximal lower-extremity hemorrhage
- Presumed life-threatening hemorrhage below the diaphragm with cardiac arrest
  - Zone I REBOA

TYPES OF REBOA CATHETERS

- Coda Balloon Catheter (Cook Medical, Bloomington, IN, USA)
  - Requires a 12 F sheath for balloon placement
  - Catheter placed using the guidewire
  - Needs repair of the arterial access site after removal of the catheter.
- ER-REBOA Catheter (Prytime Medical, Boerne, TX, USA)
  - Less invasive
  - Needs 7 F arterial line sheath for placement
  - Catheter placement does not require a guidewire.
  - Does not need repair of the arterial access site

TECHNIQUE OF ER-REBOA PLACEMENT

- Essential supplies for femoral arterial access
  - Femoral Micropuncture introducer set (Cook, Bloomington, IN, USA): 21 G/7 cm needle, .018 inch/40 cm Nitinol wire guide, and 5 F/10-cm-long cannula

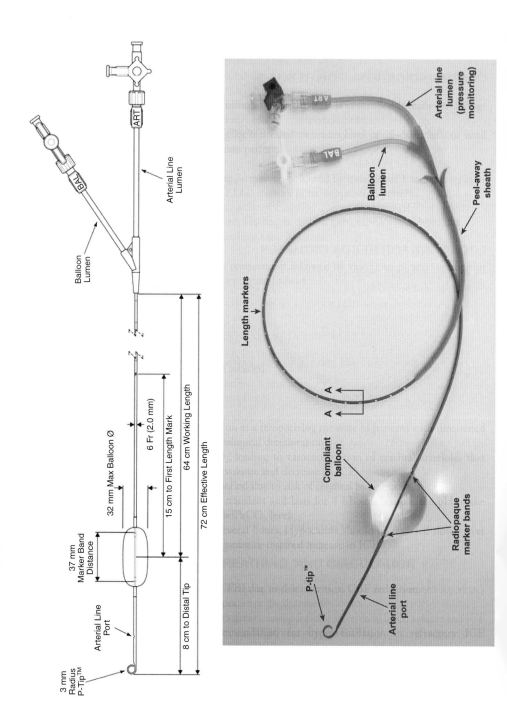

Balloon Lumen

Arterial Line Lumen

3 mm Radius P-Tip™

Arterial Line Port

37 mm Marker Band Distance

32 mm Max Balloon Ø

6 Fr (2.0 mm)

15 cm to First Length Mark

8 cm to Distal Tip

64 cm Working Length

72 cm Effective Length

Arterial line lumen (pressure monitoring)

Balloon lumen

Peel-away sheath

Length markers

Compliant balloon

P-tip™

Arterial line port

Radiopaque marker bands

A A

ART

BAL

The ER-REBOA™ Catheter Quick Reference Guide
6 REBOA Steps: ME-FIIS (Pronounced 'Me-Fiz')

Get Early CFA Access	1. Measure	2. Empty	

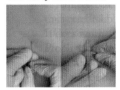 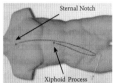 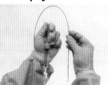 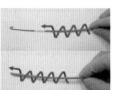

Obtain access using standard techniques

Placement depth[1,2,3,4,5,6]
• Zone 1 : ~ 46 cm
• Zone 3 : ~ 28 cm

Deflate balloon
• Ensure balloon is fully deflated
• Hold vacuum for **5 seconds and close stopcock**

Advance & twist peel-away to cover P-tip®
• Corkscrew twist to wrap balloon tightly
• Ensure the balloon and P-tip® are captured

3. Flush   4. Insert

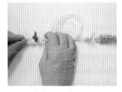 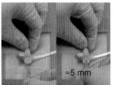 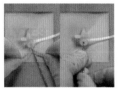 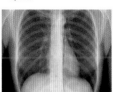

≈5 mm

Attach & flush arterial line
• Use standard techniques
• Ensure all air is purged

Insert peel-away into valve
• Approximately 5 mm

Advance catheter to desired depth
• Hold orange peel-away
• Advance blue Catheter
• Pull peel-away back after balloon passes valve

Position catheter
If available, use x-ray or fluoroscopy to confirm position using radiopaque markers

5. Inflate[1,2,3,4,5,6]   6. Secure   Provide Definitive Treatment

Inflation Volume	
Zone 1	Start with 8 cc
Zone 3	Start with 2 cc

"Start 2, Start 8, Don't Overinflate."
Start small, then check

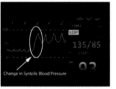 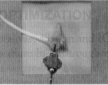 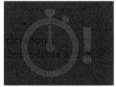

Monitor arterial waveform feedback
• Look for increase in blood pressure above balloon
• Feel for loss of contralateral pulse
• **Mark time of inflation**

Secure Catheter close to the introducer sheath

Provide definitive hemorrhage control
• The clock is ticking!
• Move quickly to definitive control

Deflate	Remove	Caution	

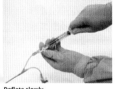 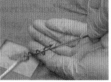 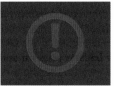 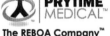

Deflate slowly
• Prepare team for potential rebound hypotension

Fully deflate balloon
• Hold vacuum for **5 seconds and close stopcock**
• Corkscrew twist the catheter to facilitate removal
• If necessary, remove catheter and introducer sheath as a unit

Check for full and equal pulse in each leg using your standard technique

PRYTIME MEDICAL™
The REBOA Company™
www.prytimemedical.com

This instruction is not a replacement for the instruction for use (IFU). The ER-REBOA™ Catheter IFU should be read in its entirety before using the device

1. Joint Trauma System Clinical Practice Guideline (JTS CPG) REBOA for Hemorrhagic Shock (CPG ID: 38)
2. Pezy P, Flaris AN, Prat NJ, Cotton F, Lundberg PW, Caillot JL, David JS, Voiglio EJ. Fixed Distance Model for Balloon Placement During Fluoroscopy-Free Resuscitative Endovascular Balloon Occlusion of the Aorta in a Civilian Population. JAMA Surg. 2016 Dec 14.
3. Linnebur M, Inaba K, Haltmeier T, Rasmussen TE, Smith J, Mendelsberg R, Grabo D, Demetriades D. Emergent non-image guided resuscitative endovascular balloon occlusion of the aorta (REBOA) catheter placement: A cadaver-based study. J Trauma Acute Care Surg. 2016 Sep;81(3):453-7.
4. MacTaggart JN, Poulson WE, Akhter M, Seas A, Thorson K, Phillips NY, Desyatova AS, Kamenskiy AV. Morphometric roadmaps to improve accurate device delivery for fluoroscopy-free resuscitative endovascular balloon occlusion of the aorta. J Trauma Acute Care Surg. 2016 Jun;80(6):941-6.
5. Morrison JJ, Stannard A, Midwinter MJ, Sharon DJ, Eliason JL, Rasmussen TE. Prospective evaluation of the correlation between torso height and aortic anatomy in respect of a fluoroscopy free aortic balloon occlusion system. Surgery. 2014 Jun;155(6):1044-51.
6. Stannard A, Morrison JJ, Sharon DJ, Eliason JL, Rasmussen TE. Morphometric analysis of torso arterial anatomy with implications for resuscitative aortic occlusion. J Trauma Acute Care Surg. 2013 Aug;75(2 Suppl 2):S169-72.

ADV-006 | Revision H

ER-REBOA Catheter (with permission from Prytime Medical)

- Femoral arterial line kit (Arrow, Centennial, CO, USA): 18 G, 16 cm length
- 7 F, 11 cm (Arrow, Teleflex Medical Incorporated, PA, USA): arterial line sheath.
- ER-REBOA balloon catheter (Prytime Medical, Boerne, TX, USA): 7 F/64 cm with peel-away sheath
- 30 ml syringe
- 10 ml syringe
- 3-way tap
- 0.9% saline 20 mL
- Omnipaque contrast solution 10 mL (optional)
- Sterile drape
- Grip-lock dressing
- Two large Tegaderm dressings
- ER-REBOA introducer sheath kit:
  - Needle 18 G/7 cm
  - Introducer sheath 7 F with .035-inch short guidewire
  - 30 cc syringe
  - 10 cc syringe, prefilled with saline
  - 5 F clamp
  - Scalpel with #11 blade
  - Nylon suture
- ER-REBOA catheter
  - 7 F or larger femoral sheath-compatible marked catheter with atraumatic distal (P-tip)
  - Length marks on the catheter shaft are measurements in cm from the middle of the balloon.
  - Does not need a guidewire for deployment
  - Has radiopaque marker bands
  - Catheter has two lumens that traverse the length of the catheter and connect to extension lines with stopcocks. One lumen is for blood pressure (BP) monitoring and the other is for occlusion balloon inflation/deflation.
  - Has a peel-away sheath loaded to the catheter to help the insertion of P-tip to the femoral arterial sheath valve.
  - Occlusion balloon can accommodate 5–24 cc (maximum) volume and expands to a maximum diameter of 32 mm.
    - 5 cc 15-mm balloon diameter
    - 8 cc 20-mm balloon diameter
    - 13 cc 25-mm balloon diameter
    - 20 cc 30-mm balloon diameter
    - 24 cc (maximum) 32-mm balloon diameter

STEPS FOR ER-REBOA PLACEMENT

- Prep and drape the groin.
- Place a 7 F arterial sheath guided by the following:
  - Access the femoral artery by using one of the following techniques
    - Anatomical landmark 2 cm below the midinguinal point (halfway between the anterior superior iliac spine to pubic tubercle)
    - Ultrasound guidance to identify the artery
    - Femoral cutdown if the common femoral artery (CFA) is not palpable or identified with ultrasound.
    - Use contralateral CFA if junctional vascular injury is suspected.

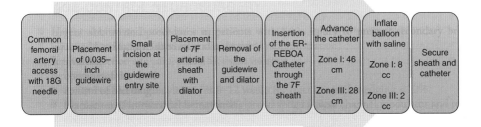

Illustration: Steps for ER-REBOA Catheter placement

- Puncture the femoral artery using a Micropuncture introducer set (21 G needle) or 18 G needle.
- If Micropuncture kit was used, place the 5 F femoral sheath to accommodate a 0.035-inch guidewire.
- Place a .035-inch guidewire either through the 5 F femoral arterial–line sheath or 18 G needle.
- Make a small incision at the guidewire site using a #11 blade.
- Place a 7 F arterial sheath with dilator over the guidewire using a Seldinger technique.
- Remove the guidewire and secure the arterial sheath with suture.
- Measure the length of the catheter.
  - Measure the ER-REBOA catheter externally for Zone 1 placement from the groin (insertion site) to the sternal notch or for Zone III placement from groin to xiphisternum.
  - Average length for Zone I is 46 cm and for Zone III is 28 cm.
- Evacuation of the catheter balloon
  - Attach a syringe with the appropriate amount of saline, then open the stopcock on the balloon lumen.
  - Purge all air from the balloon using standard techniques.
  - After complete deflation of the balloon, hold vacuum for 5 seconds and close the stopcock prior to inserting the catheter into the introducer sheath. Failure to do so may make it difficult to insert or advance the catheter.
- Flush the arterial-line lumen of the catheter.
  - Flush the arterial-line lumen with saline prior to inserting it into the introducer sheath.
  - Failure to flush the arterial line may result in an air embolism and/or poor arterial pressure monitoring.
- Insert the ER-REBOA catheter.
  - Slide the peel-away sheath toward the distal catheter tip to fully enclose and straighten the P-tip.
  - Deploy the catheter to the desired position through the 7 F arterial sheath.
  - Pull the peel-away sheath back after the balloon passes the valve.
  - If available, confirm the position with x-ray or fluoroscopy, but it is not necessary.

- Inflate the catheter balloon with saline.
  - Zone I: Start with 8 cc.
  - Zone III: Start with 2 cc.
  - Do not overinflate.
- Confirm the catheter position with inflated balloon with x-ray or fluoroscopy if possible.
- Monitor the arterial wave form.
- Secure the catheter closure to the introducer sheath using Grip-Lok catheter clamp.
- Transduce the blood pressure by connecting the BP port of the catheter.
- Document the time of REBOA balloon inflation. Maximum time with inflated balloon is up to 60 minutes.

COMPLICATIONS OF REBOA

- Complications from femoral arterial access
  - Hematoma at the access site
  - Arterial disruption
  - Arterial dissection
  - Pseudoaneurysm
  - Thromboembolism
  - Extremity ischemia
- Aortoiliac injury
  - Intimal injury
  - Thrombosis
  - Dissection
  - Arterial rupture
  - Limb loss
- Rupture of the balloon due to overinflation
- Prolonged aortic occlusion
  - Spinal cord injury due to prolonged ischemia
  - Cardiac events
  - Renal complications

REBOA MANAGEMENT GUIDELINES: AMERICAN COLLEGE OF SURGEONS COMMITTEE ON TRAUMA

- Zone I REBOA should only be performed if the anticipated time to start of an operative intervention is less than 15 minutes.
- Zone III REBOA is tolerated for longer periods of time, and may be used as an adjunct for immediate bleeding control prior to angioembolization, preperitoneal pelvic packing.
- The balloon should be deflated as soon as possible after the urgent operative or interventional hemostasis.
- Partial inflation of the balloon at either location may prolong the duration of REBOA to a maximum of 60 minutes; however, this is not well studied.
- The catheter and sheath removed as soon as possible.
- Vigilant assessment of lower-extremity perfusion must occur before, during, and after aortic occlusion, as well as after sheath removal. This monitoring must continue for at least 24 hours. If the patient leaves the OR/interventional suite with the sheath in place, demonstration by angiography of adequate extremity perfusion is recommended. Vascular surgery colleagues should participate in the assessment of distal perfusion and management and removal of the sheath.

STEPS FOR THE REMOVAL OF THE REBOA CATHETER

- Slowly but completely deflate the balloon.
- Hold the vacuum for 5 seconds and close the stopcock.
- Be prepared for possible rebound hypotension.
- Corkscrew-twist the catheter to facilitate removal through the introducer sheath.
- If necessary, remove the catheter and introducer sheath as a unit.
- Check the lower extremities for equal pulses.
- Use fluoroscopy, if possible, when manipulating (i.e., advancing, positioning, inflating, deflating, or removing) the catheter.
- If an obstruction in the vessel prevents or resists advancement of the catheter, do not force the catheter past the obstruction.
- Removal of the 7 F arterial sheath
  - After removal of the 7 F arterial sheath, apply manual compression for 30 minutes.
  - Keep the patient supine without hip or knee flexion for 6 hours after compression is completed.
  - Obtain a groin Doppler in 24–72 hours to rule out aneurysm, thrombosis, or hematoma.

CHAPTER 10

Monitoring of Resuscitation of Hemorrhagic Shock

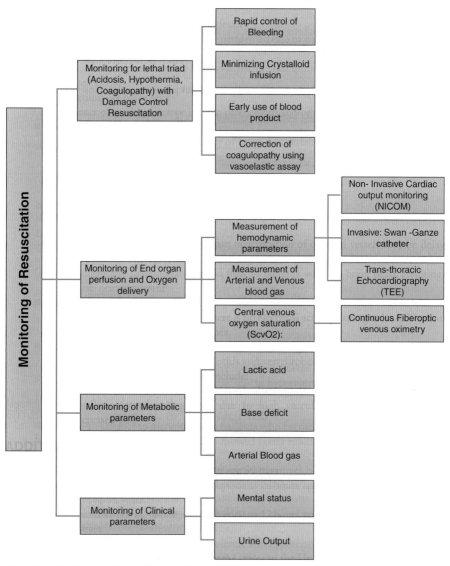

Algorithm: Monitoring of resuscitation of hemorrhagic shock

Must-Know Essentials: Monitoring of Resuscitation and Endpoint of Resuscitation

BACKGROUND

- Multiple hemodynamic, metabolic, and regional parameters are available to monitor the resuscitation of shock in trauma patients.
- No single hemodynamic or laboratory parameter can be used to define the endpoint of resuscitation.
- Traditional monitoring parameters are proven to be poor indicators of oxygen delivery secondary to compensatory mechanisms. These parameters include:
  - blood pressure (BP).
  - heart Rate (HR).
  - central venous pressure (CVP).
  - oxygen saturation (SpO_2).
- A combination of parameters should be used for the assessment of endpoint of resuscitation.

GOALS OF RESUSCITATION

- Prevention of lethal triad
  - Acidosis
  - Hypothermia
  - Coagulopathy
- Optimization of end-organ perfusion and tissue oxygen delivery
- Prevention of complications of overresuscitation.

PREVENTION OF LETHAL TRIAD

- Hypothermia, Coagulopathy, and Acidosis area associated with increased mortality in trauma patients.
- Steps for the prevention of lethal triad:
  - Monitoring, prevention, and treatment of acidosis
  - Monitoring, prevention, and treatment of hypothermia
  - Monitoring, prevention, and treatment of coagulopathy
  - Damage-control resuscitation
    - Rapid control of bleeding
    - Limited use of crystalloid infusion
    - Permissive hypotension
    - Early use of blood products

OPTIMIZATION OF END-ORGAN PERFUSION AND OXYGEN DELIVERY

- Essential to optimize the end-organ perfusion in resuscitation of shock to prevent cellular hypoxia and subsequent multiple organ dysfunction
- Basic physiology of oxygen transportation
  - Normal oxygen transportation: 640–1400 mL/min or 500–600 mL/min/m^2
  - Oxygen transport to tissue depends on:
    - arterial oxygen content (CaO_2).
    - oxygen delivery (DO_2).
    - oxygen consumption (VO_2).

- Arterial oxygen content (CaO_2)
  - Calculation: $(Hb \times 1.34 \times SaO_2/100) + (PaO_2 \times 0.003)$
    Hb (Hemoglobin): gm/100 mL of blood
    1.34: oxygen-carrying capacity in mL per gram of Hb
    SaO_2: arterial Hb oxygen saturation in decimal
    PaO_2: arterial partial pressure of oxygen in mm Hg
    0.003: Solubility coefficient of oxygen
- Venous oxygen content (CvO_2):
  - Calculation: $(Hb \times 1.34 \times S_vO_2/100) + (PvO_2 \times 0.003)$
    Hb (Hemoglobin): per gram/100 mL of blood
    1.34: oxygen-carrying capacity in mL per gram of Hb
    S_vO_2: venous Hb oxygen saturation in decimal
    PvO_2: venous partial pressure of oxygen in mm Hg
    0.003: solubility coefficient of oxygen
- Oxygen delivery (DO_2) = Cardiac index (CI) $\times$ CaO_2
- Oxygen consumption (VO_2): = Cardiac index (CI) $\times$ ($CaO_2 - CvO_2$)
- Oxygen extraction ratio (O_2 ER) = $[(CaO_2 - CvO_2)/CaO_2] = VO_2/DO_2$
- Basic Cardiac Physiology
- Cardiac Output (CO)
  - Cardiac output (CO) = Stroke volume (SV) in mL $\times$ Heart rate (HR)/minute
  - Normal cardiac output (CO): 4–8 L/min
  - Cardiac index (CI): 2.5–4 L/min/m^2
- Stroke volume (SV)
  - Blood ejected from left ventricle per heartbeat
  - Normal value: 60–70 mL
  - Stroke volume index (SVI): SV/Body surface area (BSA), 40–50 mL/beat/m^2
  - Frank-Starling curve: Stroke volume (SV) increases with increase in preload until a plateau of the Frank-Starling curve is reached.
  - Major determinants of stroke volume
    Preload
    Afterload
    Myocardial contractility
- Preload
  - Filling of heart during diastole
  - Reduction in preload decreases stroke volume and thus decreases cardiac output.
  - Causes of reduced preload
    Hemorrhagic shock
    Distributive shock: neurogenic shock, sepsis
    Obstructive shock: cardiac tamponade, tension pneumothorax
- Afterload
  - Measurement of systemic vascular resistance (SVR).
  - Normal SVR: 800–1200 dynes-sec/cm^5
  - Normal SVRI: 1970–2390 dynes-sec/cm^5/m^2
  - Increase in SVR reduces SV
  - Causes of increased SVR (increased afterload)
    Cardiogenic shock
    Hypovolemic shock
    Vasopressors

- Causes of decreased SVR (decreased afterload)
  Septic/neurogenic/anaphylactic shock
  Vasodilators
  Hyperthermia
- Cardiac contractility
  - Increased cardiac contractility improves SV
  - Decreased cardiac contractility reduces SV
  - Increased cardiac contractility
  - Inotropes
  - Decreased cardiac contractility
    Beta blockers
    Cardiomyopathy
    Cardiac ischemia
    Acidosis
    Hypoxia
    Electrolyte imbalances
- A balance between DO_2 and VO_2 to the tissue is essential for cellular homeostasis and prevention of cellular hypoxia and multiple organ dysfunction.
- Supranormal DO_2 correlates with an improved chance for survival in trauma patients.
- Overresuscitation with crystalloids to supernormal normal endpoints (CI >4.5 L/min/m^2, DO_2 >600 mL/min/m^2, and VO_2 index >170 mL/min/m^2) does not improve mortality or morbidity. *(Shoemaker WC et al: Prospective trial of supernormal value of survivors as therapeutic goals in high risk surgical patients. Chest 94:1176-1186, 1988)*
- Use of vasopressors to enhance cardiac output can cause tissue ischemia.
- Large volume of crystalloid overresuscitation is associated with:
  - coagulopathy due to dilution of platelets and clotting factors.
  - hyperchloremic acidosis.
  - acute lung injury/acute respiratory distress syndrome (ARDS).
  - multi-organ dysfunction.
  - abdominal compartment syndrome.
  - hypothermia due to fluid stored at room temperature.
- Monitoring techniques
  - CVP
    - Does not correlate with intravascular volume or right ventricular volume
    - Not reliable in patients on mechanical ventilation
    - Not reliable in patients with pulmonary hypertension
    - Right ventricular end diastolic volume index (RVEDVI) measurement may be a better indicator of adequate volume resuscitation (preload) than central venous pressure.
  - Hemodynamic monitoring
    - Invasive hemodynamic monitoring: Swan-Ganz pulmonary artery catheter
      It is used to measure pulmonary capillary wedge pressure.
      RVEDVI measurement may be a better indicator of adequate volume resuscitation (preload) than pulmonary capillary wedge pressure (PCWP).
      Use of Swan-Ganz catheter in critically ill patients does not improve survival and should not be used routinely.
    - Noninvasive cardiac output monitoring (NICOM)
      - FloTrac system (Edwards Lifesciences, Irvine, CA, USA):
        Connects to an arterial line and measures the cardiac parameters every 20 seconds
        Gives continuous measurement of SV
        Monitors and optimizes stroke volume variation (SVV) in ventilated patients

Optimizes DO_2 by continuous CO, CO/CI, SaO_2, and hemoglobin measurements.

Cheetah Starling SV (Cheetah Medical, Newton, MA, USA)

Noninvasive hemodynamic monitoring system

Four sensor pads applied on the chest wall are connected to the device for continuous hemodynamic monitoring of SVI, CI, and total peripheral resistance index (TPRI).

It optimizes SVV in ventilated patients.

Transthoracic echocardiography (TTE)

Provides dynamic measurement of intravascular volume status, and cardiac performance

Can be used for the measurement of inferior vena cava (IVC) diameter to assess the volume status

IVC diameter is measured at vena-cava atrial junction in subcostal view.

IVC diameter <2cm in patients with spontaneous breathing is considered hypovolemic despite normal BP and will respond to fluid boluses.

IVC diameter >2cm is unlikely to respond with fluid boluses.

Not reliable in the following patients:

On ventilators

Right heart failure

Increased intraabdominal pressure

Pericardial fluid

MONITORING OF METABOLIC PARAMETERS

- Lactate level
- Direct byproduct of systemic hypoperfusion
- Measurement of extent of shock
- Level of 3.4 mmol/L or greater is predictive of mortality.
- Timing of lactate clearance is more predictive of mortality than an isolated value.
  - 0%–10% mortality if cleared within 24 hours
  - 25% mortality if cleared within 24–48 hours
  - 80%–86% mortality if cleared beyond 48 hours
- Goal: achieve normal lactate level (<1.0 mmol/L) in resuscitation of shock
- Base deficit:
- Defined as the amount of base (in mmol/L) required to titrate a liter of whole arterial blood to a pH of 7.40
- Base deficit measures metabolic acidosis and tissue hypoperfusion.
- Serum bicarbonate level correlates with base deficit, but they are affected by patient's ventilatory status.
- It may be considered as a marker of elevated lactate level.
- Increasing base deficit correlates to:
  - ongoing bleeding.
  - need for blood transfusion.
  - coagulopathy.
  - Shock-related complications, including renal failure, ARDS, multiorgan failure, and acute lung injury
  - Abdominal compartment syndrome

- Mortality in patients with shock
  - Absolute base deficit can be used to measure the severity of shock, but a single value cannot be used as an endpoint.
  - Trend of base deficit over time is more useful in predicting outcomes.
- Base deficit is a superior measurement of metabolic acidosis than pH.
- Limitations: Base deficit is influenced by:
  - hyperchloremic acidosis after isotonic saline administration; it is not associated with increased mortality.
  - renal failure.
  - diabetic ketoacidosis.
  - chronic carbon dioxide (CO_2) retention.
  - ethanol intoxication.
  - administration of sodium bicarbonate.
- Severity of the base deficit
  - Mild: 2–5 mmol/L
  - Moderate: 6–14 mmol/L
  - Severe: >15 mmol/L
- Resuscitation goal
  - To achieve normal base, range from −2 to +2 mEq/L
- Arterial blood gas (ABG) and venous blood gas (VBG):
  - Persistently low pH is an early indicator of an ongoing hemorrhage or abdominal compartment syndrome.
  - Goal is to correct acidosis and achieve a normal pH range (7.35–7.45).
  - Serum pH of less than 7.36 is associated with significant morbidities.
  - Time of normalization of pH is predictive of survival.
  - Required for the measurement of:
    - CaO_2 and CvO_2.
    - DO_2.
    - VO_2.
    - O_2 ER.
  - Central venous oxygen saturation ($S_{cv}O_2$)
    - A measurement of tissue oxygen extraction and tissue hypoxia
    - Trend of $S_{cv}O_2$ correlates more with severity of shock than with an absolute value.
    - Absolute value between mixed venous oxygenation saturation (S_vO_2) using a pulmonary artery catheter and central venous oxygenation saturation ($S_{cv}O_2$) may differ, but trends between the two measurements generally correlate well.
    - Goal: to achieve >70% $S_{cv}O_2$ during resuscitation of shock
  - Continuous fiberoptic venous oximetry device
    - Monitoring device for oxygen delivery and consumption at bedside

CLINICAL PARAMETERS

- Level of consciousness; measurement of brain perfusion
- Urine output
  - Direct measurement of renal perfusion
  - Goal urine output in adults: >0.5 mL/kg
- Heart rate, respiratory rate, blood pressure, pulse pressure, and mean arterial pressure (MAP)
  - Do not quantify physiological derangements
  - Do not predict trauma outcome
  - Hypotension: predictive of a bad outcome after head injury

PART 2

Emergency Management of Regional Trauma

Head Trauma

CHAPTER 11

Evaluation of Head Injury

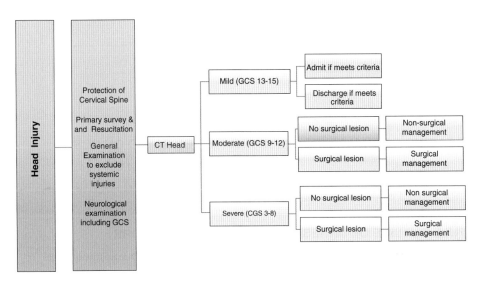

Algorithm: Evaluation of head injury

Must-Know Essentials: Evaluation of Head Injury
GLASGOW COMA SCALE (GCS)

	Score
■ Best eye-opening response	
■ Spontaneous	4
■ To speech	3
■ To pain	2
■ None	1
■ Best verbal response	
■ Oriented	5
■ Confused conversation	4
■ Inappropriate words	3
■ Incomprehensible	2
■ None	1
■ Best motor response	
■ Obeys commands	6
■ Localizes pain	5

- Flexion withdrawal to pain   4
  - Abnormal flexion (decorticate) includes: 3
  - Internal rotation of shoulder
  - Flexion of forearm and wrist with clenched fist
  - Leg extension
  - Planter flexion of foot
  - Extension (decerebrate) includes: 2
  - Adduction of arms
  - Internal rotation of shoulders
  - Pronation of forearms and extension at elbow
  - Flexion of wrist and fingers
  - Leg extension
  - Planter flexion of foot
- None (flaccid)   1

GRADING OF TRAUMATIC BRAIN INJURY (TBI) BASED ON GCS

- Mild TBI   GCS Score: 13–15
- Moderate TBI   GCS Score: 9–12
- Severe TBI: GCS Score: 3–8

FULL OUTLINE OF UNRESPONSIVENESS (FOUR) SCORE

- Useful scoring system for assessing consciousness in intubated trauma patients where components of GCS cannot be assessed
- Has a good correlation with GCS
- Assesses four responses:
  - Eyelid opening and tracking
  - Motor response
  - Brainstem reflexes
  - Respiratory drive and regularity
- Uses four domains of neurological function:
  - Eye responses
  - Motor responses
  - Brainstem reflexes
  - Breathing pattern
- Each point increase in FOUR score is associated with decrease in morbidity and mortality.
- Any decrease in these scores is associated with worsening consciousness as well as ICP.
- (E) Eye response   Score
  - Eyelids open or opened; tracking or blinking to command   4
  - Eye lids open but not tracking   3
  - Eyelids closed but open to loud voice   2
  - Eyelids closed but open to pain   1
  - Eyelids remain closed to pain   0
- (M) Motor response   Score
  - Follows commands (thumbs-ups, fist, or peace sign)   4
  - Localizes pain   3
  - Flexion response to pain   2

▪ Extension response to pain	1
▪ No response to pain or generalized myoclonus status	0
▪ (B) Brainstem reflexes	Score
▪ Pupillary and corneal reflexes present	4
▪ One pupil wide and fixed to light	3
▪ Pupillary or corneal reflexes absent	2
▪ Pupillary and corneal reflexes absent	1
▪ Pupillary, corneal, and cough reflexes absent	0
▪ (R) Respiration	Score
▪ Not intubated; regular breathing pattern	4
▪ Not intubated; Cheyne-Stokes breathing pattern	3
▪ Not intubated; irregular breathing pattern	2
▪ Intubated (endotracheal or tracheostomy tube); breathing faster than ventilator rate	1
▪ Breathing at ventilator rate or is apneic	0

TYPES OF BRAIN INJURY

- ▪ Primary brain injury
  - ▪ Injury at the time of impact
- ▪ Secondary brain injury
  - ▪ Progression of brain injury due to:
    - ▫ hypotension (systolic blood pressure [SBP] <90 mm Hg).
    - ▫ hypoxia (PaO_2 <60 mm Hg, and oxygen saturation <90%).
    - ▫ cerebral edema.
    - ▫ intracranial hypertension.
- ▪ Diffuse axonal injury
  - ▪ Associated with rotational head motion, referred to as "shearing" brain injury
  - ▪ Commonly causes coma
  - ▪ Microscopic examination of the brain reveals swollen and disconnected axons, which is a gold standard for the diagnosis.
  - ▪ Computerized tomography (CT) scan has limited value in diagnosis and may show multiple petechial foci of hemorrhage.
  - ▪ MRI is more helpful in the diagnosis.
- ▪ Brain contusion
  - ▪ Focal injury resulting in damage of capillary or other tissue components (glial cells, nerve cells, etc.)
  - ▪ CT reveals a hemorrhagic core surrounded by low-density edema.

POSTTRAUMATIC INTRACEREBRAL HEMATOMA

- ▪ Hematoma due to rupture of single or multiple vessels in the brain parenchyma

EXTRACEREBRAL HEMATOMAS

- ▪ Epidural/extradural hematoma:
  - ▪ Bleeding between the dura mater and the skull
  - ▪ Commonly due to bleeding from the middle meningeal artery
  - ▪ Frequently associated with temporal fracture

- Lucid interval
  - Temporary neurological improvement followed by deterioration after traumatic brain injury with epidural hematoma
  - Seen in 20%–50% of patients
  - Not an indication for evacuation of hematoma
- CT head: biconvex-shaped hematoma
- Subdural hematoma
  - Bleeding between dura mater and arachnoid mater
  - Usually due to rupture of bridging vein in the subdural space or bleeding from the cortical arteries
  - Common in old age with associated brain atrophy
  - CT head: crescent-shaped hematoma
- Subarachnoid hematoma
  - Usually due to rupture of cortical arteries, veins, or capillaries
  - Bleeding between the arachnoid and pia mater
  - CT head: confirms the diagnosis; may need CT angiogram if concern of nontraumatic cause of bleeding

CONCUSSION

- Transient neurologic change following a blow to the brain without neuroanatomical evidence of parenchymal injury
- Diffuse axonal injury proposed as the pathophysiologic basis of concussion
- Characteristics of cerebral concussion:
  - GCS 13–15 (mild TBI)
  - Brief period of unconsciousness or dazed consciousness
  - Posttraumatic amnesia
  - Negative neuroimaging (CT scan and MRI)
  - Most patients recover within weeks to months without sequelae or the need for specific medical intervention.
- Grading of concussion
  - Grade I
    - Transient confusion
    - No loss of consciousness
    - Symptoms resolve in <15 minutes
  - Grade II
    - Transient confusion
    - No loss of consciousness
    - Symptoms last >15 minutes
  - Grade III
    - Any loss of consciousness regardless of duration

SECOND-IMPACT SYNDROME (SIS)

- Rapid brain edema after a second concussion before symptoms from a previous concussion have subsided
- May occur within minutes, days, or weeks after an initial concussion
- Even a mildest grade of concussion can lead to SIS.
- The condition often results in severe disability or death.
- Etiology

- Exact mechanism unknown.
- May be due to metabolic changes in the brain within 15 seconds of the second concussion
- Loss of autoregulation of the cerebral vessels leads to:
  - increase in cerebral blood flow.
  - progressive cerebral edema.
  - severe intracranial hypertension leading to brain herniation.

MANAGEMENT GUIDELINES

- Indications for admission after head injury (*ATLS 10th Edition*)
  - History of prolonged loss of consciousness
  - Deteriorating level of consciousness
  - Moderate to severe headache
  - Severe alcohol or drug intoxication
  - All-penetrating head injury
  - Skull fracture
  - Cerebrospinal fluid (CSF) leak: otorrhea or rhinorrhea
  - Significant associated injury
  - No reliable companion at home
  - GCS <15
  - Persistent focal neurological deficit
  - Abnormal CT scan findings

BRAIN INJURY GUIDELINES (BIG) FOR BRAIN INJURY MANAGEMENT (*J TRAUMA ACUTE CARE SURG 2014*)

- BIG 1 (minor head injury)
  - Features include the following:
    - History of positive or negative loss of consciousness
    - Normal neurological examination
    - No intoxication
    - No anticoagulation or antiplatelets
    - No skull fractures
    - Subdural hematoma (SDH) <4 mm
    - Epidural hematoma (EDH) <4 mm
    - Intraparenchymal hematoma (IPH) <4 mm, one location
    - Subarachnoid hemorrhage (SAH): trace
    - No IVH
  - Recommendations
    - Patient may be discharged after 6 hours of observation.
    - No neurosurgery consultation
    - No repeat head CT scan
- BIG 2 (moderate injury)
  - Features include the following:
    - History of positive or negative loss of consciousness
    - Normal neurological examination
    - Positive or negative intoxication
    - No anticoagulation or antiplatelets
    - Nondisplaced skull fracture
    - SDH 5–7 mm

- EDH 5–7 mm
- IPH 3–7 mm, two locations
- SAH localized
- No IVH
  - Recommendations
    - Admit to hospital for neurological examination
    - No neurosurgery consultation
    - No repeat head CT scan
  - BIG 3 (severe head injury)
    - Features include the following:
      - Positive loss of consciousness
      - Abnormal neurological examination
      - Intoxication: yes/no
      - On anticoagulation or antiplatelets
      - Displaced skull fracture
      - SDH >8 mm
      - EDH >8 mm
      - IPH >8 mm, multiple locations
      - SAH: scattered
      - IVH: yes
    - Recommendations:
      - Admit to hospital
      - Repeat head CT scan
      - Neurosurgery consultation

INDICATIONS FOR EVACUATION OF ACUTE EPIDURAL HEMATOMA

- Regardless of GCS
  - Hematoma size >30 cm^3
  - Clot thickness >15 mm
  - Midline shift >5 mm
- Regardless of volume, thickness, or midline shift:
  - GCS <9
  - Asymmetric pupils
  - Infratentorial hematoma
  - Focal neurological deficit

INDICATIONS FOR EVACUATION IN ACUTE SUBDURAL HEMATOMA

- Regardless of GCS
  - Clot thickness >10 mm
  - Midline shift >5 mm
- Regardless of thickness or midline shift:
  - GCS <9
  - Significant mental status change with decrease in the GCS score between the time of injury and hospital admission by 2 or more points
  - Patient presents with asymmetric or fixed and dilated pupils.
  - ICP exceeds 20 mm Hg.

TRAUMATIC SUBARACHNOID HEMORRHAGE

- Evacuation of hematoma not recommended
- Incidence of posttraumatic secondary hydrocephalus approximately 0.7%–29%
- Factors contributing to the development of hydrocephalus:
  - Advanced age
  - Low GCS score at admission
  - Presence of an intraventricular hemorrhage
  - Severe traumatic SAH
- Hydrocephalus is usually of the communicating type and is managed by ventriculoperitoneal shunting.

TRAUMATIC INTRACEREBRAL HEMORRHAGE

- Surgical management of traumatic intracerebral bleeding is controversial.
- Surgical Trial In Traumatic intraCerebral Hemorrhage (STITCH-Trauma):
  - Randomized controlled trial of early surgery compared with initial conservative treatment did not show any benefit of surgical evacuation in traumatic intracerebral bleeding.

EVACUATION OF PNEUMOCEPHALUS

- If significant increase in ICP due to pneumocephalus.

CHAPTER 12

Management of Severe Brain Injury

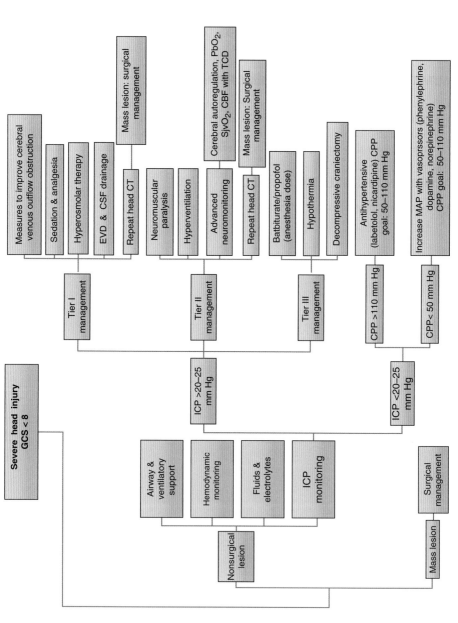

Algorithm: Management of severe head injury

Must-Know Essentials: Physiology of Cerebral Perfusion

VOLUME-PRESSURE CURVE (MONRO-KELLIE HYPOTHESIS)

- Skull is a rigid compartment and contains three components:
  - Brain
  - Blood
  - Cerebrospinal fluid (CSF)
- Average adult skull contains a total volume of 1475 mL:
  - Brain: 1300 mL
  - CSF: 65 mL
  - Arterial and venous blood: 110 mL
- An increase in the volume of one component, the volume of one or more of the another components must decrease to maintain the normal intracranial pressure (ICP). Failure of this compensatory mechanism result in an increase in ICP.
- An increase in ICP results in a decrease in cerebral perfusion leading to cerebral ischemia.

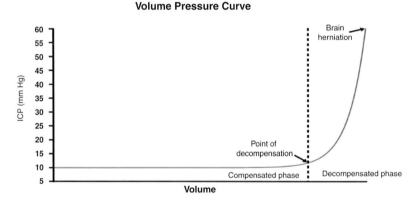

Volume pressure curve of the skull

Cerebral Perfusion Pressure

- Is the primary determinant of the cerebral blood flow (CBF)
- Cerebral perfusion pressure (CPP) = Mean arterial pressure (MAP) – Intracranial pressure (ICP)
  - MAP = Diastolic pressure + 1/3 (Systolic pressure – Diastolic pressure) or DP + 1/3 (PP)
  - Pulse pressure (PP) = Systolic pressure – Diastolic pressure
- Normal CPP: range 50–110 mm Hg
- Optimum CPP
  - >50 mm Hg to prevent ischemia
  - <110 mm Hg to prevent breakthrough hyperperfusion and cerebral edema
- Causes of reduced CPP
  - Increase in ICP
  - Decrease in blood pressure (BP)
  - Combination of above two causes

AUTOREGULATION OF CEREBRAL PERFUSION

- Pressure autoregulation
  - Intrinsic ability of brain to maintain a normal CBF with a CPP ranging from 50–110 mm Hg despite change in systolic blood pressure (SBP)
  - CPP <50 mm Hg may cause cerebral hypoperfusion, and >110 mm Hg may result in cerebral hyperperfusion leading to cerebral edema.
  - Increase in ICP increases MAP primarily through a rise in cardiac output, to maintain a steady CPP.
  - Change in MAP is regulated by reflex construction or dilation of precapillary vasculature to maintain a constant CPP, CBF, and ICP.
  - Intact autoregulation
    - Increase in MAP causes increase in CBF, CPP, and ICP. Intact autoregulation causes cerebral vasoconstriction resulting in decrease in CBF, CPP, and ICP.
    - Decrease in MAP causes decrease in CBF, CPP, and ICP. Intact autoregulation causes cerebral vasodilation leading to increase in CBF, CPP, and ICP.
  - Impaired autoregulation
    - Severe traumatic brain injury (TBI) can result in impaired autoregulation.
    - Increase in MAP causes:
      increase in CBF, CPP, and ICP.
      cerebral edema.
    - Decrease in MAP results in decrease in CPP leading to brain ischemia and infarction.
- Chemical autoregulation
  - Change in CBF in response to change in partial pressure of oxygen (PaO_2) and partial pressure of carbon dioxide ($PaCO_2$) regulates the CPP and ICP.
  - Acute hypoxia
    - It is a potent cerebral vasodilator and results in an increase in CBF.
    - CBF does not change until tissue PaO_2 falls below approximately 50 mm Hg.
    - Increases in CBF do not change cerebral metabolism but affect oxygen saturation of cerebral hemoglobin.
  - Hypercapnia
    - Causes dilation of cerebral arteries and arterioles resulting in increased blood flow
  - Hypocapnia
    - Causes constriction of cerebral arteries and arterioles resulting in decreased blood flow
  - Brain injury
    - Can cause impaired chemical autoregulation

Must-Know Essentials: Elevated Intracranial Pressure

CAUSES OF INTRACRANIAL PRESSURE

- Mass effect in head injury leading to:
  - Epidural hematoma (EDH).
  - Subdural hematoma (SDH).
  - Hemorrhagic contusion.
  - Depressed skull fractures.

- Diffuse brain edema
- Hyponatremia
- Hyperemia due to loss of autoregulation
- Disturbance of CSF circulation
  - Obstructive hydrocephalus
  - Subarachnoid hemorrhage (SAH)
- Hypoventilation
- Cerebral vasospasm
- Cerebral venous outflow obstruction
  - Increased intrathoracic pressure
  - Increased intraabdominal pressure

EFFECTS OF ELEVATED INTRACRANIAL PRESSURE

- Normal ICP: 5–15 mm Hg in lateral ventricles or lumbar subarachnoid space in supine position
- Effects of elevated ICP
  - Decrease in CPP leading to low CBF and cerebral ischemia
  - Severe increase in ICP triggers the cerebral ischemic response, also known as the Cushing reflex, which include:
    - Increase in sympathetic response leading to elevated MAP to increase CPP.
    - Reflex bradycardia.
    - Seen in late phase of intracranial hypertension (ICH), such as near brain dead/ herniation syndrome.
- Sustained ICP >40 mm Hg results in life-threatening IH.
  - May cause a shift in brain parenchyma causing cerebral herniation syndrome
  - Results in irreversible brain damage and death
- Manifestations of elevated ICP
  - Headache
  - Vomiting, with or without nausea
  - Mental status changes
    - Decrease in level of consciousness
    - Restlessness
    - Agitation
    - Confusion
  - Tachycardia
  - Dysrhythmias
  - Cushing's triad: due to pressure on medullary center
    - Increase in SBP and pulse pressure
    - Bradycardia
    - Cheyne-Stokes breathing: irregular respiration characterized by periods of slow, deep breaths followed by periods of apnea
  - Pupillary changes
    - Anisocoria (unequal pupils)
    - Sluggish reaction to light
    - No reaction to light
    - Papilledema is a reliable sign of IH but is uncommon after head injury.
    - Pupillary dilation can occur in the absence of IH.
  - Motor changes
    - Asymmetrical weakness
    - Bilateral weakness

- Posturing
- Flaccidity
- Decerebrate posturing can occur in the absence of IH.
- Brain herniation
  - Manifestation depends on the location of brain herniation.

BRAIN HERNIATION

- Displacement of brain into nearby compartments due to local ICP gradients.
- Types of brain herniation
  - Subfalcine herniation
    - Most common type of brain herniation
    - Usually due to convexity (frontal or parietal) mass lesion
    - Manifestation
      - Strangulation of the anterior cerebral artery due to movement of brain underneath the falx cerebri
      - Asymmetric (contralateral more than ipsilateral) motor posturing
      - Preserved oculocephalic reflex
  - Transtentorial herniation
    - Temporal lobe (uncal) herniation (lateral descending transtentorial hernia)
      - Usually seen due to mass lesion in the temporal lobe
      - The uncus of the temporal lobe shifts downward into the posterior fossa.
      - Manifestations
        - Ipsilateral pupillary dilation due to compression of cranial nerve III (oculomotor nerve) from herniation of the medial temporal lobe under the tentorium cerebelli causing displacement of the midbrain
        - Contralateral hemiplegia/posturing
        - Bilateral motor posturing
    - Central herniation (central descending transtentorial herniation)
      - Downward displacement of the entire brainstem through the tentorial notch due to diffuse cerebral edema
      - Manifestations:
        - Bilateral pupillary dilatation due to cranial nerve III palsy
        - Lateral gaze palsy: due to cranial nerve VI (Abducens nerve) compression leading to lateral rectus muscle palsy
        - Bilateral decorticate to decerebrate posturing
        - Decorticate posturing: stiffness of the extremities with legs held out straight, clenched fists, and bent arms on the chest
        - Decerebrate posturing: straight and rigid arms and legs, toes pointed downward, and head arched backward
        - Loss of brainstem reflexes
        - Obliteration of the suprasellar cistern in imaging
    - Ascending transtentorial herniation
      - Upward herniation of posterior fossa contents (cerebellum and brainstem) through the tentorium cerebelli.
      - Typically seen after excessive CSF ventricular drainage
      - Manifestations
        - Bilateral pupillary dilation
        - Extensor posturing

- Cerebellar/tonsillar herniation
  - Downward displacement of cerebellar tonsils through the foramen magnum due to cerebellar mass lesion resulting in compression of the medulla
  - Manifestations
    - Episodic extensor posturing
    - Cardiac dysrhythmias
    - Pupillary dilatation
    - May result in cardiopulmonary arrest
- Extracranial herniation
- Brain herniation through a traumatic or post craniotomy skull defect

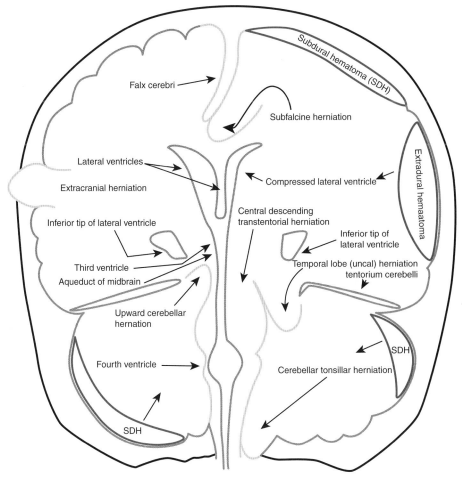

Illustration: Brain herniation

Must-Know Essentials: Monitoring of Severe Brain Injury

MRI AND CT SCAN

- Qualitative information about ICP can be obtained with CT and MRI of the brain.

- Features suggestive of increased ICP include:
  - midline shift and compression of the ventricles due to mass occupying lesion.
  - enlarged ventricles due to hydrocephalus.
  - loss of grey and white matter junction due to cerebral edema.

ELECTROENCEPHALOGRAPHY

- Triphasic wave in continuous electroencephalography (EEG) monitoring is a prognostic marker in patients with IH.
- It also is a predictor for improving cortical function in patients with elevated ICP.

INTRACRANIAL PRESSURE MONITORING

- Indications
  - Severe brain injury (Glasgow Coma Scale [GCS] <8) with initial CT evidence of:
    - structural brain damage such as hematoma or contusion.
    - increased ICP as suggested by compressed or absent basal cisterns.
  - Severe brain injury (GCS <8) with normal initial CT with two or more of the following:
    - Patient >40 years of age
    - Hypotension: SBP <90 mm Hg
    - Bilateral motor posturing
  - Brain injury with GCS >8 with computerized tomography (CT) scan evidence of structural brain damage with high risk of progression
    - Large or multiple contusions or hematoma
    - Coagulopathy
  - Brain injury with GCS >8 and extracranial injuries
    - Need for urgent surgery for extracranial injuries
    - Need for ventilation for extracranial injuries
    - Progression of pathology in CT imaging
    - Clinical deterioration
- Methods of ICP monitoring
  - External ventricular drain (EVD)
    - A catheter is placed in the lateral ventricle through a burr hole at Kocher's point (10.5 cm posterior to the nasion and 3.5 cm lateral on the midpupillary line).
    - Traditionally, the right lateral ventricle is preferred.
    - Catheter is tunneled and connected to a pressure transducer via a fluid-filled tubing at the level of the ear.
    - EVD is considered the most accurate method of ICP measurement.
    - Disadvantages
      - Catheter placement into a compressed or displaced ventricle may be difficult.
      - Risk of cerebral parenchymal bleeding during insertion of the catheter.
      - Risk of infection, such as potentially life-threatening ventriculitis
    - Advantages
      - EVD is a preferred method of ICP monitor because it is both diagnostic (measures ICP) and therapeutic (drains CSF).
      - It measures the global brain pressure.
      - It can be recalibrated after placement.
  - Nonventricular devices
    - Useful when access to the ventricle is difficult
    - Less risk of infection

- Techniques
  - Fiberoptic transducers/pressure microsensors placed outside the ventricles. Locations include:
    - Epidural
    - Intraparenchymal
    - Subarachnoid
    - Subdural
  - Subarachnoid screw
    - A catheter inserted into subarachnoid space through a hole drilled in the skull and connected to a pressure transducer
- Disadvantages
  - No therapeutic drainage
  - Reflects regional pressure rather than global brain pressure
  - Subarachnoid, subdural, and epidural ICP devices are less accurate.
  - Fiberoptic systems need external calibration to ensure constant accuracy.
- ICP waveform
  - Three components of ICP waveforms:
    - W-1:
      - Pulse pressure waveforms
    - W-2:
      - Respiratory waveforms due to respiratory cycle
    - Lundberg A, B, and C waves
      - Slow vasogenic waveforms
  - Pulse pressure (W-1) waveforms:
    - Intracranial pulse waveforms are generated by arterial pulses transmitted to brain.
    - These correlate to the arterial pressure.
    - Frequency is equal to heart rate.
    - Elevated ICP affects the characteristics of the waveform.
    - Subdivided into three waves: P1, P2, and P3
      - P1 wave
        - Also called percussion wave.
        - Due to transmitted arterial pulse through the choroid plexus into the CSF
        - High-amplitude P-wave is seen in patients with high SBP.
        - Low-amplitude P-wave is seen in low SBP.
      - P2 wave
        - Called elastance or tidal wave
        - Results from a restriction of ventricular expansion by a closed rigid skull
        - Represents cerebral compliance
        - Amplitude of P2 is increased due to decrease in brain compliance and increase in ICP.
      - P3 wave
        - Also called dicrotic wave
        - Correlates with closure of the aortic valve, equivalent of the dicrotic notch
    - Under normal circumstances: P1 > P2 > P3
    - In brain injury leading to reduced brain compliance:
      - P2 > P1
        - Sensitive predictor of poor outcome

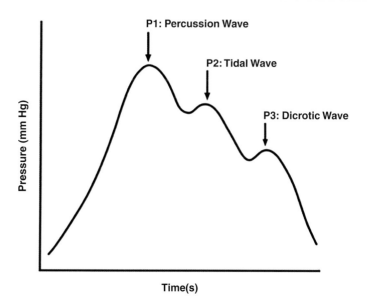

Normal ICP Waveform

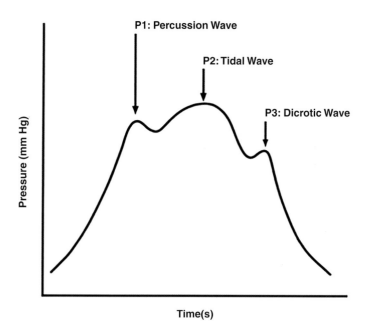

Noncompliant ICP Waveform

Illustration: ICP pulse waveforms

- Lundberg waves
  - A-wave (plateau wave)
    Sustained and severe elevation in ICP
    5–20 minutes long
    High amplitude (50–100 mm Hg)
    Suggestive of decreased intracranial compliance, compromised cerebral perfusion pressure, and global cerebral ischemia
    Considered a high risk for further (or ongoing) brain injury, with critically reduced perfusion due to a prolonged period of high ICP
    Considered pathognomonic of ICH
  - Lundberg B-wave and C-wave
    B-waves and C-waves are of less clinical significance.
  - B-wave
    Lasts for <5 minutes (usually 1–2 minutes) with 20–50 mm Hg in amplitude
    Does not represent any pathological disturbance
    Usually associated with Cheyne-Stokes respiration
    May reflect vasodilatation due to respiratory fluctuation in $PaCO_2$
    May be due to intracranial vasomotor waves causing variation of CBF
  - C-wave
    Last for 4–5 minutes
    <20 mm Hg in amplitude
    No pathological consequence
    Associated with BP-associated hemodynamic changes

ADVANCED NEUROMONITORING TECHNIQUES

- ICP monitoring alone cannot detect all potential insults; additional monitoring may be required for the management of severe TBI.
- CBF and cerebral oxygenation are important for outcomes in severe TBI.
- Low brain tissue oxygen tension (PbO_2) has been seen in patients with normal ICP and CPP.
- Techniques
  - Cerebral autoregulation measurement
    - Can be monitored by measuring cerebrovascular pressure reactivity index (PRx)
    - PRx is calculated from the MAP and ICP within a frequency range of 0.003–0.05 Hz.
    - PRx varies with the concurrent CPP in a U-shape.
    - Impaired autoregulation is characterized by PRx slope of >0.13 and lower CPP (50–60 mm Hg), and it is associated with poor outcome in TBI.
    - CPP with the lowest PRx is optimal (CPPopt) and is associated with better outcome after severe head injury with elevated ICP.
    - CPP values above CPPopt can cause hyperemia due to high CBF leading to cerebral edema and ICH.
    - CPP values below CPPopt can cause cerebral hypoperfusion and cerebral ischemia.
    - PRx can be used to guide the management of CPP and CBF in severe brain injury.
  - Brain tissue oxygen tension
    - PbO_2 can be measured using near-infrared spectroscopy (NIRS).
    - NIRS provides continuous PbO_2 and ICP monitoring.
    - Low PbO_2 (<15 mm Hg) is associated with poor outcome.
    - Management utilizing ICP and PbO_2 showed a 10% reduction in mortality and improved neurological outcome in severe TBI.

- Jugular venous oxygen saturation (SjvO2) measurement
  - SjvO$_2$ <50% associated with poor outcome in severe TBI
- Transcranial doppler ultrasonography (TCD)
  - Provides real-time monitoring of ICP and CPP
  - CBF is measured by mean blood-flow velocity (MFV), and ICP is measured by pulsatility index (PI) values of the middle cerebral artery (MCA) and the other major intracranial vessels.
  - TCD can be used to assess autoregulation with hemodynamic challenges.
  - TCD-based assessment of CBF and autoregulation has been more reliable than TCD-based ICP measurement.

Must Know Essentials: Goals in the Management of Traumatic Brain injury

RECOMMENDATIONS *(American College of Surgeons Committee on Trauma, 2015)*

- Clinical parameters
  - SBP ≥100 mm Hg
  - Temperature: 36°C–38°C (96.8°F–100.4°F)
- Monitoring parameters
  - CPP ≥60 mm Hg
  - ICP 20–25 mm Hg
  - Pulse oximetry ≥95%
  - Partial pressure of brain tissue oxygen (PbtO$_2$) ≥15 mm Hg
- Laboratory parameters
  - Glucose: 80–180 mg/dL
  - Hemoglobin: ≥7 g/dL
  - International normalized ratio (INR): <1.4
  - Sodium: 135–145 mg/dL
  - PaO$_2$: ≥100 mm Hg
  - PaCo$_2$: 35–45 mm Hg
  - pH: 7.35–7.45
  - Platelets: ≥75 × 10^3/mm^3

Must-Know Essentials: General Management of Traumatic Brain Injury

MANAGEMENT OF AIRWAY, BREATHING, AND CIRCULATION

- Important to prevent hypoxia, hypercapnia, and hypotension in order to prevent secondary brain injury
- Hypercarbia is a potent cerebral vasodilator causing increase in cerebral blood volume and ICP.
- High positive end-expiratory pressure (PEEP) can increase ICP by impeding venous return and increasing central venous pressure (CVP).
- Hypotension will result in decreased CPP

MANAGEMENT OF HYPERTENSION

- Hypertension is common in patients with head injury with ICH due to sympathetic hyperactivity.
- Systolic hypertension is greater than diastolic hypertension.

- Elevated BP may exacerbate cerebral edema.
- Correction of systolic hypertension before treating the ICH in patients with mass lesion may result in reduction of CPP.
- In patients with severe head injury with impaired autoregulation:
  - hypertension may increase CBF, CPP and ICP.
  - hypotension may decrease CBF, CPP, and ICP.
- GOAL: SBP $\geq$100 mm Hg
- Medication for hypertension
  - Sedation may resolve hypertension.
  - Vasodilating drugs such as nitroprusside, Hydralazine, and nitroglycerin should be avoided as these can increase ICP.
  - Antihypertensives of choice include:
    - Beta-blocking drugs (labetalol, esmolol), and Nicardipine
    - Central acting alpha-receptor agonists: clonidine

MANAGEMENT OF FLUIDS/ELECTROLYTES

- Hypovolemia causes reduction in CPP leading to cerebral hypoxia.
- Goal is to maintain a euvolemic state.
- Normal saline is the fluid of choice.
- Hypotonic solutions (e.g., 0.45% saline, dextrose 5% in water [D5W]) should not be used as they cause cerebral edema due to osmotic gradient in regions of the injured brain.
- Saline (2% or 3% at 1 mL/kg) can be used for resuscitation in patients at risk for increased ICP.
- Serum Na should be maintained at 135–145 mEq/L to prevent hypotonic hyponatremia.

MANAGEMENT OF HYPERTHERMIA

- Hyperthermia in head injury patients may be due to:
  - central dysregulation of body temperature due to hypothalamic injury.
  - extracranial infection or inflammatory process.
- Increases mortality due to:
  - increase in cerebral metabolic rate.
  - cerebral vasodilatation leading to increase in CBF and increase in ICP.
- Fever should be controlled with a goal temperature between 36°C and 38°C (96.8°F–100.4°F).
- Acetaminophen and cooling blankets are the first line of therapy to control temperature.
- If fever is not adequately controlled with conventional methods, advanced temperature-modulation devices—either surface or intravascular cooling catheters—should be used.

MANAGEMENT OF HYPERGLYCEMIA

- Caused by stress or brain-induced catecholamine release.
- Elevated glucose (>180 mg/dL) may aggravate ischemic insult and worsen neurologic outcome.
- Glucose control is important with a goal level of 80–180 dL.

MANAGEMENT OF ANEMIA

- Anemia has not been clearly shown to exacerbate ICP after TBI.
- Randomized trial of critically ill patients showed better outcome with a more restrictive transfusion threshold of 7 g/dL.

PROPHYLAXIS OF POSTTRAUMATIC SEIZURES IN TRAUMATIC BRAIN SEIZURES

- Classification for posttraumatic seizure (PTS)
  - Immediate: within 24 hours
  - Early: within 7 days
    - Majority: within 48 hours
    - Early seizures increase the risk of late seizures.
  - Late: after 7 days
- Incidence
  - 15%–20 % after severe brain injury
  - 35%–50% after penetrating injury
  - 50% nonconvulsive seizures in electroencephalograph (EEG) after severe TBI with elevated ICP
- Risk factors
  - Cortical contusion
  - SDH
  - Post evacuation of intracranial hematomas
  - Penetrating head injury
  - Loss of consciousness (GCS <10)
  - Amnesia lasting for >1 day
  - Prolonged coma >24 hours
  - Depressed skull fracture not elevated surgically
  - Injury with dural penetration
  - At least one nonreactive pupil
  - Age >65 years
- Effects of seizure
  - Increases cerebral metabolic rate (CMR) and CBF
  - Increases CBF leading to elevation of ICP
  - Increases release of neurotransmitters
  - Increases cerebral venous blood leading to elevation of ICP
  - Decreases brain oxygen delivery
- Severe TBI with status epilepticus is associated with high mortality rate.
- Seizure prophylaxis recommendations
  - Severe TBI (GCS <8) for 7 days
  - Used after 7 days in patients who develop late seizures
  - In severe TBI, decreases the risk of early PTS
  - Seizure medications after 7 days do not prevent late PTS.
- Medications for seizure prophylaxis
  - Both phenytoin (Dilantin) and levetiracetam (Keppra) are effective in prevention of early PTS.
  - Phenytoin
    - Not commonly used due to its multiple side effects, difficulty maintaining a therapeutic level, and numerous drug-to-drug interactions
  - Fosphenytoin (Cerebyx)
    - Prolongs recovery of activated voltage-gated Na+ channels in neuron to stabilize against repetitive neuronal firing
    - Is a water-soluble phenytoin for IV use
    - Potentially safer than IV phenytoin
    - Dosed as phenytoin equivalents (PE): 1.5 mg of fosphenytoin sodium is equivalent to 1 mg phenytoin sodium.

- Dose
  Loading dose: 10–20 mg PE/kg IV; should not exceed 150 mg PE/min
  Maintenance dose: 4–6 mg PE/kg/day IV in divided doses; should not exceed 150 mg PE/min
  Serum concentrations should be monitored for therapeutic concentration.
- Side effects
  Arrhythmias
  Hypotension (especially after rapid IV administration)
  Injection site pain, phlebitis, tissue necrosis
- Levetiracetam
  - An alternative to phenytoin
  - No clear mechanism of action, possible presynaptic calcium channel modulator and regulation of neurotransmitter release
  - Potential advantages
    - No drug–drug interactions
    - No need for serum monitoring
  - No significant advantage of seizure prevention rate compared to phenytoin in patients with severe TBI
  - Dose
    - 500–1000 mg twice daily, oral or IV, with or without a 20 mg/kg to 1 g loading dose
    - 250 mg BID in patients with renal failure on hemodialysis
  - Side effects
    - Behavioral abnormalities (agitation, irritability, depression, somnolence, asthenia, dizziness)
    - Caution is warranted in patients with psychiatric disorders.

DEEP VEIN THROMBOSIS PROPHYLAXIS IN HEAD INJURY

- Patients have risk, as high as 20%–30% even with mechanical prophylaxis of venous thromboembolism (VTE) after TBI.
- Pharmacologic deep vein thrombosis (DVT) prophylaxis should be started within the first 72 hours after TBI
- Risk of bleeding with pharmacologic prophylaxis (Modified Berne-Norwood criteria)
  - Low-risk factors
    - No moderate or high-risk factors
    - Stable head CT head after 24 hours
  - Moderate-risks factors
    - Epidural hematoma/subdural hematoma >8 mm
    - Contusion or intraventricular hemorrhage >2 cm
    - Multiple contusions per lobe
    - Subarachnoid hemorrhage with abnormal CT angiogram
    - Evidence of progression in CT head after 24 hours
  - High-risk factors
    - ICP monitor placement
    - Post craniotomy
    - Evidence of progression in CT head after 72 hours
- Pharmacologic prophylaxis using low molecular weight fractionated heparin (Enoxaparin) in TBI based on Modified Berne-Norwood criteria
  - After 24 hours in low-risk patients
  - After 72 hours in moderate-risk patients if stable CT after 72 hours
  - Not recommended in high-risk patients; inferior vena cava (IVC) filter should be considered.

NUTRITION

- Severe TBI is a hypermetabolic and hypercatabolic state.
- Early nutritional support (within 24–48 hours) has been shown to improve infection and decrease mortality.
- Nutrition should be started as soon as the patient becomes hemodynamically stable, ideally within 24–48 hours.
- Full nutritional support is recommended within 7 days after brain injury.
- Enteral feeding is preferred over parenteral feeding unless contraindicated due to GI issues.
- Postpyloric tube feeding is recommended as it is associated with a lower risk of pneumonia.

Must-Know Essentials: Three-Tier Approach for the Management of Intracranial Hypertension

COMPONENTS OF TIERED APPROACH

- Primary brain injury results in increased ICP, causing:
  - cerebral ischemia.
  - cerebral edema.
  - release of excitatory neurotransmitters, free radicals formation, and increased levels of calcium and potassium intracellularly
- Secondary brain injury: deterioration of brain functions due to hypoxia and hypotension
- Interventions in the management of TBI are aimed at decreasing ICP and improving CPP
- Stepwise approach recommended with a goal of ICP <20–25 mm Hg and CPP >50–110 mm Hg
- In tiered approach, failure to control pressure at any tier leads to next-higher-tier measures.
- Repeat CT and neurological examination is recommended to identify the surgical lesions and to guide further management.

TIER 1: SPECIFIC MANAGEMENT

- Measures to improve cerebral venous outflow obstruction to reduce ICH
- Sedation and analgesics
- Hyperosmolar therapy
- EVD placement and CSF drainage
- Repeat CT and neurological assessment
- Surgical management if indicated

TIER 2: SPECIFIC MANAGEMENT

- Hyperventilation
- Advance neuromonitoring with optimization of CPP
- Neuromuscular paralysis
- Repeat CT and neurological assessment
- Surgical management if indicated

TIER 3: SPECIFIC MANAGEMENT

- Barbiturate or propofol (Diprivan) coma
- Hypothermia
- Decompressive hemi/bilateral craniectomy

Must-Know Essentials: Specific Medical Management of Intracranial Hypertension

MEASURES TO IMPROVE CEREBRAL VENOUS OUTFLOW OBSTRUCTION TO REDUCE INTRACRANIAL HYPERTENSION

- Elevation of the head of the bed at 30 degrees
- Maintenance of head in a neutral position
- Cervical collar should be removed if it meets the criteria; otherwise keep the collar loose to prevent internal jugular vein compression.
- Reduce increased intraabdominal pressure in patients with abdominal compartment syndrome.

SEDATION AND ANALGESICS

- Beneficial effects of control of agitation in TBI include:
  - prevents elevation of ICP by reducing jugular venous pressure and systolic blood pressure.
  - protective effect due to decreases in cerebral metabolic rate of oxygen ($CMRO_2$).
- Opioids
  - Do not have any effect on $CMRO_2$ or CBF.
  - Bolus injections of opioids in patients with elevated ICP may result in transient drop in MAP and further increase in ICP due to autoregulatory cerebral vasodilation.
- Sedatives
  - Benzodiazepines cause reduction in $CMRO_2$ and CBF without any effect on ICP.
  - Midazolam (Versed) can result in tachyphylaxis.
  - There is no evidence to support the choice of sedative agents.
  - Preferred agents
    - Fentanyl for analgesia
    - Propofol for sedation
      - Ideal for periodic interruption for neurologic assessment due to its extremely short half-life
      - Can cause systemic hypotension in patients with baseline intravascular volume depletion
      - Propofol infusion syndrome can result with high dose and prolonged use.
    - Dexmedetomidine (Precedex)
      - Causes sedation and analgesia without respiratory depression
      - May cause decrease in mean ICP
      - May cause hypotension and bradycardia

HYPEROSMOLAR THERAPY

- Indicated in patients with persistent elevation of ICP despite of sedation
- Mannitol

- Commonly used for the treatment of ICH
- Mechanism of action
  - Rheological effect: Immediately after infusion, it improves regional cerebral microvascular flow and cerebral oxygenation by plasma expansion, decreasing blood viscosity, and altering red blood cells (RBCs).
  - It increases CPP due to increase in intravascular volume and cardiac output, but it does not increase ICP due to cerebral vasoconstriction in patients with intact autoregulation.
  - Osmotic diuretic effect
    - It reduces cerebral edema by creating an osmotic gradient between plasma and brain cells resulting in migration of water from the cerebral extracellular space into the vasculature space.
    - Intact blood–brain barrier is essential for this mechanism.
    - Cerebral edema may get worse with mannitol in patients with disrupted blood–brain barrier after TBI.
    - It takes 15–30 minutes until gradient is established.
- Effect on ICP is dose dependent; higher doses provide a more durable reduction in ICP.
- Peak ICP effect starts within 30–45 minutes and lasts around 1.5–6 hours.
- Relatively contraindicated in hypovolemic patients because of its diuretic effect
- Dose
  - Single rapid bolus (0.25–1.0 g/kg body weight) IV infusion over 20–30 minutes
  - When long-term reduction of ICP is needed, 0.25–0.5 g/kg can be repeated every 2–6 hours.
- Monitoring
  - Serum osmolarity should be maintained <320 mOsm/kg to prevent hypovolemia, hyperosmolarity, and renal failure.
  - Osmolar gap (OG) is more reliable to monitor mannitol therapy. An osmolar gap of 20 mOsm/kg reflects inadequate clearance of mannitol and will increase the risk of rebound rise in ICP.
  - Complications
    - Dehydration and hypotension
    - Acute renal failure
    - Hyperkalemia
    - Rebound increase in ICP due to passage of mannitol into the brain from repeated administration leading to vasogenic cerebral edema
    - Osmotic demyelination syndrome due to hypernatremia and high osmolarity.
- Hypertonic saline
  - Is an osmotic agent
  - Used as an adjunct to mannitol or in patients who become tolerant to mannitol
  - In refractory ICH, hypertonic saline showed better result in a metaanalysis.
  - Mechanism of action
    - Creates an osmotic gradient in patients with intact blood–brain barrier, resulting in passive diffusion of water from cerebral intracellular and interstitial spaces into capillaries causing reduction in ICP
    - Normalizes resting membrane potential and cell volume by restoring normal intracellular electrolyte balance in injured cells
    - Preferred over mannitol in hypovolemic and hypotensive patients
    - More beneficial in increasing MAP, CPP, and intravascular volume in patients with dehydration and in decreasing ICP

- Should be administered with caution in patients with renal insufficiency or congestive heart failure
- Effect may last for 90 minutes to 4 hours
- Dose
  - 23.4% hypertonic saline: 30 mL intermittent boluses infused over 1–2 minutes. Serum sodium above 160 mEq/dL does not provide any further benefit.
  - 3% hypertonic saline: 2.5–5 mL/kg intermittent boluses over 20–30 minutes.
  - Continuous infusion of 3% hypertonic saline for serum Na goal of 150–160 mEq/dL
  - Once serum sodium level of approximately 150 mEq/L is achieved, patient should be weaned very slowly (over several days).
  - 23.4% hypertonic saline in 30-mL boluses given as rapid IV push over 1–2 minutes is more effective in reducing high ICP than 3% sodium chloride.
  - Central line is recommended for hypertonic saline administration.
- Monitoring goals
  - ICP 20–25 mm Hg
  - CPP 50–110 mm Hg
  - Serum sodium approximately 150–160 mEq/L
  - Serum osmolality: <320 mOsm/kg
- Complications
  - Abrupt cessation of hypertonic saline can result in rebound ICH and brain herniation.
  - Renal insufficiency
  - Hyperchloremic metabolic acidosis
  - Thrombophlebitis
  - Congestive heart failure
  - Osmotic demyelination
    - Hyponatremia should be excluded before administering hypertonic saline to reduce the risk of central pontine myelinolysis.
    - Sodium level should not be increased or decreased more than 10 mEq/L over a 24-hour period to avoid the risk of central pontine myelinolysis.

DRAINAGE OF CEREBROSPINAL FLUID

- Indicated in patients with an initial GCS <6 during the first 12 hours with elevated ICP
- CSF drainage by EVD lowers ICP immediately by reducing intracranial volume.
- Drainage of even a small volume of CSF can cause significant reduction of ICP.
- Limited use in diffuse brain edema with collapsed ventricles
- In diffuse brain swelling, sudden decompression may cause collapse of the ventricles.
- Continuous drainage of CSF by an EVD may be more effective in reducing the ICP than intermittent drainage.

NEUROMUSCULAR PARALYSIS

- Nondepolarizing paralytics: cisatracurium or vecuronium
- Dose titrated by train-of-four monitoring

BARBITURATE COMA

- Used in refractory ICP elevation
- Barbiturates reduce ICP by reduction of CBF and $CMRO_2$.

- Pentobarbital or thiopentone can be used for barbiturate coma.
- Pentobarbital can cause more hypotension compared to thiopentone.
- Close hemodynamic monitoring and optimization of CPP is required during barbiturate coma.
- Dose
  - Pentobarbital
    - Bolus: 5 mg/kg every 15–30 minutes until the ICP is controlled (usually 10–20 mg/kg required)
    - Continuous infusion: 1–4 mg/kg/h titrated to serum level of 30–50 µg/mL or until EEG shows a burst-suppression pattern
  - Thiopentone
    - Loading dose of 5 mg/kg over 30 minutes followed by infusion of 1 to 5 mg/kg/hour until electroencephalogram (EEG) shows a burst-suppression pattern.
- Complications
  - Hypotension
    - Most common complication
    - Due to cardiac suppression
    - Initially treated with volume replacement followed by vasopressors, and inotropes if necessary
  - Reduced CPP
  - Respiratory depression
  - Hypokalemia
  - Hepatic dysfunction
  - Renal dysfunction
  - Ileus: Enteral feeding should be avoided.

HYPERVENTILATION

- Indicated in refractory ICP elevation as a temporizing measure in patients with threatened cerebral herniation or sudden neurological deterioration.
- Hyperventilation decreases $PaCO_2$, leading to vasoconstriction of cerebral arterioles that causes reduction in cerebral blood volume and decrease in ICP.
- It should be used for a very brief period due to risk of cerebral ischemia.
- Its effect is immediate, and often transient and lasts for 4-6 hours because the pH of the CSF rapidly equilibrates to the new $PaCO_2$ level.
- If hyperventilation was used for several hours, Hypocarbia should be reversed slowly over several days to prevent rebound hyperemia-induced increase in ICP.
- It is not recommended:
  - for ICH prophylaxis.
  - in the first 24 hours after severe TBI due to risk of critical CBF reduction.
  - for prolonged periods: >4–6 hours.
  - without PbO_2 monitoring.
- Brain trauma foundation recommendation for hyperventilation in refractory ICP elevation:
  - Brief period (15–30 min) of hyperventilation
  - Target $PaCO_2$ 30–35 mm Hg
  - Pulse oximetry ≥95%
  - PaO_2 ≥80 mm Hg

HYPOTHERMIA

- Hypothermia (33°C–35°C [91.4°F–95°F]) may be used as salvaged therapy to control ICP refractory to other medical therapy.
- It reduces ICP by lowering cerebral metabolic rate of oxygen ($CMRO_2$) requirement and thus cerebral blood volume (CBV).
- It does not have any benefit on mortality or functional outcome.
- Prophylactic hypothermia early (within 2.5 hours) or in the short term (48 hours postinjury) is not recommended to improve outcomes in patients with diffuse TBI.
- Methods of hypothermia
  - Cold saline infusion: Rapid infusion of 0.9 % normal saline at 30 mL/kg cooled to 4°C–5°C (39.2°F–41°F)
  - Various surface and endovascular cooling methods are also available.
  - Complications of hypothermia
    - Shivering
    - Cardiac arrhythmias
    - Hypokalemia
    - Coagulopathy
    - Nosocomial infection
    - Hyperglycemia
  - Rewarming
    - Can cause rebound elevation of ICP
    - Must be done slowly (0.10°C–0.3°C/h) and in a controlled fashion

CEREBRAL PERFUSION PRESSURE OPTIMIZATION

- Low CPP (<50 mm Hg) causes reflex cerebral vasodilation and ICP elevation.
- High CPP (>110 mm Hg) can sometimes cause breakthrough cerebral edema and ICP elevation.
- CPP should be maintained between 50 and 110 mm Hg.
- Vasopressors to raise BP and CPP include:
  - phenylephrine: 2–10 µg/kg/min.
  - dopamine: 5–30 µg/kg/min.
  - norepinephrine: 0.01–0.6 µg/kg/min.
- Medications to lower BP and CPP include:
  - labetalol: 5–150 mg/h.
  - nicardipine: 5–15 mg/h.
  - Nitroprusside is not recommended because it causes cerebral vasodilatation leading to elevation of ICP.

SYMPATHETIC STORMING AFTER TBI

- Incidence: 33% after severe TBI but, also seen in less severe injury
- Etiology: Hypothalamic stimulation of the sympathetic nervous system and adrenal glands resulting in increase in circulating corticoids and catecholamines, or may be due to stress response.
- Manifestations are due to exaggerated sympathetic response leading to:
  - altered level of consciousness.
  - dystonic posturing.
  - hypertension.
  - tachycardia.
  - tachypnea.

- high fever.
- diaphoresis.
- pupillary dilation.
- Management
  - Bromocriptine (Parlodel)
  - Nonselective beta blockers such as labetalol (Trandate) or propranolol (Inderal)
  - Morphine
  - May be helpful:
    - dantrolene (Dantrium)
    - clonidine (Catapres)
  - Continuous IV sedation for severe refractory cases

Must-Know Essentials: Specific Surgical Management of Intracranial Hypertension

RESECTION OF MASS LESIONS

- Is performed for a definitive therapy and to decrease the ICP in mass lesions
- Indications for evacuation in acute EDH:
  - Regardless of GCS:
    - Hematoma size: >30 cm³
    - Clot thickness >15 mm
    - Midline shift >5 mm
  - Regardless of volume, thickness, or midline shift:
    - GCS <9
    - Asymmetric pupils
    - Infratentorial hematoma
    - Focal neurological deficit
- Indications for evacuation in acute SDH:
  - Regardless of GCS:
    - Clot thickness >1 cm in greatest thickness
    - Midline shift >5 mm
  - Regardless of thickness or midline shift:
    - GCS <9
    - Significant mental status change with decrease in the GCS score between the time of injury and hospital admission by 2 or more points
    - Patient presents with asymmetric or fixed and dilated pupils.
    - ICP exceeds 25 mm Hg.

SURGERY IN TRAUMATIC SUBARACHNOID HEMORRHAGE

- Evacuation of hematoma is not recommended.
- May develop communicating-type secondary hydrocephalus requiring ventriculoperitoneal shunt.

SURGERY IN TRAUMATIC INTRACEREBRAL HEMORRHAGE OR CEREBRAL CONTUSION

- Surgical management of traumatic intracerebral bleeding is controversial.
- Surgical management may be considered in cerebral contusion or intracerebral hemorrhage with significant mass or elevation of ICP
- Surgical Trial In Traumatic intraCerebral Haemorrhage (STITCH-Trauma)
  - Randomized controlled trial of early surgery compared with initial conservative treatment did not show any benefit of surgical evacuation in traumatic intracerebral bleeding.

SURGERY IN PNEUMOCEPHALUS

- Evacuation is indicated for significant increase in ICP (tension pneumocephalus).

DAMAGE-CONTROL NEUROSURGERY

- Urgent abbreviated procedures in patients with brain injury to prevent secondary brain injury and to improve survival and outcome.
- It involves:
  - opening of the skull.
  - control of bleeding.
  - evacuation of intracranial hematomas.
  - debridement of compound wounds.
  - closure or leaving the dura open.
  - immediate replacement of skull bone flap (craniotomy) or removal of the bone flap with delayed replacement (craniectomy).
  - closure of scalp.
  - delayed definitive surgery once swelling subsides.
    - May require dural expansion with pericranium, temporalis fascia, or synthetic dura
    - May require hard-acrylic implant in a cranioplasty procedure

DECOMPRESSIVE CRANIECTOMY

- It is recommended as tier-3 management in adult patients with severe TBI with refractory ICP to other treatments.
- It prevents secondary brain injury by reducing increased ICP with subsequent improvement in brain oxygenation.
- Decompressive Craniectomy (DECRA) in Diffuse Traumatic Brain Injury trial
  - No benefit in functional outcome at 6 months after bifrontal decompressive craniectomy (DC)
  - Decreases ICP and length of stay in the ICU
- Decompressive Craniectomy for Traumatic ICH (RESCUEicp) trial
  - Significant reduction in mortality
  - Associated with a higher rate of disability
  - Higher rate of vegetative state and severe disability than medical malmanagement
- Technique of decompressive craniectomy
  - Bifrontal craniectomy:
    - Indicated in TBI with diffuse brain edema without midline shift
    - Involves the removal of a bone flap extending from the floor of the anterior cranial fossa to the coronal suture, and to the middle cranial fossa floor bilaterally with opening of the dura
  - Unilateral craniectomy:
    - Also known as hemicraniectomy, unilateral DC, or frontotemporoparietal craniectomy
    - Indicated in TBI with unilateral hemisphere swelling with midline shift
    - Involves removal of a large frontotemporoparietal bone flap
    - Size of the craniectomy is of critical importance.
      - Small craniectomies can cause brain herniation with venous infarction and increased edema at the bone margins.

　　　　Resection of a larger bone fragment is recommended for greater dural expansion
　　　and lower risk of herniation.
- DC is sometimes combined with a simultaneous lobectomy, which could reduce the ICP
  rapidly but produces a very poor result.
- Dura must be opened to achieve decompression.
- Scalp is closed over the widely opened dura mater.
- Complications of DC
  - Hemorrhagic swelling ipsilateral to the craniectomy site
  - Brain herniation through the craniectomy defect
  - Subdural hygroma
  - Seizures
  - Intracranial infection
  - CSF leak through the scalp incision

Must-Know Essentials: Brain Death

DEFINITION OF BRAIN DEATH

- Irreversible cessation of all brain functions, including cortical and brainstem functions

REQUIREMENTS FOR THE BRAIN-DEATH EXAMINATION *(The American Academy of Neurology Guideline, 2010)*

- Irreversible coma from a known cause
- Neuro imaging suggestive of irreversible loss of all brain functions
- Core body temperature >36°C (96.8 °F)
- No CNS depressants, including sedatives, illegal drugs, and alcohol, in the system
  - Subtherapeutic drug level if available
  - If drug level not available, five half-lives of the drug should be calculated (if kidney and liver functions are normal).
  - For patients with alcohol ingestion, blood alcohol level should be <0.08%.
- No residual effects of paralytics
  - Nerve stimulator for train-of-four test if paralytics were used
- SBP ≥100 mm Hg
- Absence of severe electrolyte, acid-base, or endocrine disturbances
- No spontaneous respiration

CLINICAL EXAMINATION

- Clinical examination, including cold caloric and apnea test is the most sensitive and specific tool for the diagnosis of brain death.
- Absent cortical functions
  - Irreversible coma
    - No response to noxious stimuli such as compression of the supraorbital nerves, forceful nail-bed pressure, and temporomandibular joint compression
    - Spinal reflexes may be present and compatible with brain death, including:
      　deep tendon reflexes.
      　plantar flexion reflex.
      　planter withdrawal reflex.
      　triple flexion reflex (flexion of the thigh and leg and dorsiflexion of the foot upon noxious stimulus of the foot

- Decorticate (flexor) posturing
- Decerebrate (extensor) posturing
- Absence of brainstem functions
  - Midbrain
    - Absent pupillary light reflex
    - Dilated fixed pupil (typically midposition at 5–7 mm)
  - Pons
    - Absent corneal reflex (both saline jet and tissue touch)
    - Absent oculocephalic reflex
      - Eyes immobile (doll's-eye movement), eyes move in opposite direction of the head movement.
      - Rule out cervical spine and skull base fracture before this test.
    - Absent oculovestibular reflex
      - Cold caloric test: 30–50 mL ice water each ear
      - Perform otoscopy before irrigation to exclude perforation of tympanic membrane.
      - Observe for 1 minute.
      - Wait for 5 minutes before testing the contralateral ear.
      - Normal response is tonic gaze deviation towards the side of the ear irrigated with cold water.
      - No deviation of the eyes to irrigation in each ear with 50 mL of cold water is considered a positive test.
    - Absent facial sensation and facial motor response
      - After gentle nasal and periorbital tickle
      - Corneal reflex
      - Grimacing to deep pressure on nail bed, supraorbital ridge, or temporomandibular joint
  - Medulla
    - Absent pharyngeal and tracheal reflexes
      - Absent cough reflex
      - Absent gag reflexes
      - No response to tracheal suctioning
    - No spontaneous breathing
    - Positive apnea test

APNEA TEST

- Principles of apnea test
  - No ventilatory effort after maximum CO_2 stimulation ($PaCO_2$ >60 mm Hg)
  - $PaCO_2$ >60 mm Hg stimulates ventilatory drive within 60 seconds in a functioning brainstem.
  - Without spontaneous respiration, PCO_2 rises by 2–3 mm Hg/min; in 10 minutes it should rise to 60 mm Hg. In chronic carbon dioxide retainers, an increase of 20 mm Hg from the baseline $PaCO_2$ is considered an acceptable stimulus.
- Steps
  - Preoxygenate the patient with 100% fraction of inspired oxygen (FiO_2) for 15 minutes to eliminate the stores of respiratory nitrogen.
    - Obtain a baseline arterial blood gas (ABG).
  - Prestudy $PaCO_2$ should be 40 mm Hg; if not, adjust the vent rate and recheck the ABG.
  - Disconnect the ventilator and place the patient on 100% FiO_2 through an endotracheal tube (ET) or by a nasal cannula at 6 L/minute O_2 or by a T-piece.
  - An increase in CO_2 usually occurs at a rate of 2–3 mm Hg/min.

- Obtain ABG in 10 minutes.
- Return patient to prestudy ventilatory settings after 10 minutes if PCO_2 level reaches > 60 mm Hg.
- PCO_2 >60 mm Hg after 10 minutes without any spontaneous respiration confirms a positive apnea test.
- Patient can be declared brain dead if apnea test is positive.
- Test is terminated if patient develops spontaneous respiration or hemodynamic instability.

ANCILLARY TESTS

- None of the ancillary tests should replace a clinical assessment.
- It is not a requirement for brain death.
- Indications for ancillary tests for brain death
  - Clinical examination cannot be fully performed due to patient factors.
  - Inconclusive apnea test
  - Termination of apnea test due to hemodynamic instability.
- Types of tests
  - Technetium-99 brain scan
    - Absence of uptake of isotope in brain parenchyma and/or vasculature confirms brain death.
  - Angiography
    - No intracranial blood flow at entry of carotid or vertebral artery
    - Four-vessel angiography
      - Gold standard
      - 100% accurate
      - Difficult to perform in a critically ill, unstable patient
    - CT angiography
      - May not confirm brain death
      - Uses venous injection of contrast; opacification of cerebral vessels may be delayed in patients with elevated ICP resulting in false-positive result
      - Commonly demonstrates blood flow in patients who are brain dead, resulting in false-negative result
  - Encephalography
    - Brain death can be confirmed if there is no electrical activity during at least 30 minutes of recording based on the guidelines.
  - Transcranial Doppler ultrasound
    - Should be performed for both carotids and vertebrobasilar arteries
    - Findings to confirm brain death include:
      - absence of blood flow in middle cerebral artery.
      - oscillation/reverberating flow due to high vascular resistance associated with increased ICP

ADDITIONAL REQUIREMENTS

- Newborn (gestational age ≥37 weeks) to age 30 days
  - Two examinations by two separate physicians 24 hours apart
- Age 30 days to 18 years
  - Two examinations by two separate physicians 12 hours apart
- Age ≥18 years
  - One examination
  - A second examination is needed in some states in the United States.

CHAPTER 13

Scalp Laceration, Skull Fractures, and Facial Fractures

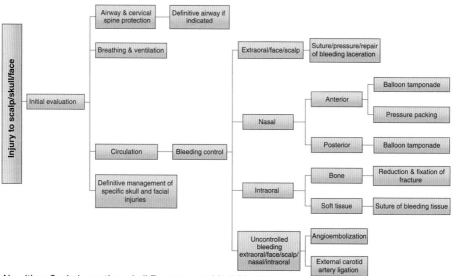

Algorithm: Scalp laceration, skull Fractures, and facial fractures

Must-Know Essentials: Evaluation of Skull and Maxillofacial Injuries

AIRWAY AND C-SPINE PROTECTION

- Complex skull and facial injuries are usually complicated by a compromised airway.
- Contributing factors
  - Head injury with diminished level of consciousness
  - Alcohol, and/or drug intoxication
  - High risk of aspiration
  - Presence of broken teeth, dentures, foreign bodies, avulsed tissues
  - Multiple mandibular fractures
  - Massive edema of glottis
  - Maxillofacial injury where there is constant risk of the displacement of tissue, bleeding, and swelling

- Consider airway protection and early definitive airway.
  - Nasotracheal intubation is not indicated in comminuted midface or skull base injury.
  - Nasotracheal intubation may be indicated in the injury of lower face, or where mouth opening is inadequate.
  - Traction movements during intubation may increase the risk of bleeding and associated damage.
  - Bag-mask ventilation may be potentially hazardous in Le Fort type II, Le Fort type III, and nasoethmoidal fractures with suspected fracture of the anterior cranial fossa due to risk of:
    - forcing infectious material into a basilar skull fracture.
    - displacing nasal debris and foreign particles into the brain.
    - tension pneumocephalus due to associated dural tear with basilar skull fracture leading to rapid deterioration of neuro status.
- C-spine protection
  - Complex maxillofacial trauma has a high risk of associated cervical spine fracture.
  - Almost 15% of skull fractures are associated with cervical spine injury.

CIRCULATION

- Sources of massive bleeding
  - Maxillofacial fractures
    - Cause oral and nasal bleeding
    - Source of bleeding may be from ethmoid artery, ophthalmic artery, vidian branch of maxillary artery
    - Most bleeding is easily controlled, but rarely, severe epistasis from the maxillary artery, may be difficult to control.
  - Skull base fractures, and laceration of pharynx causing oral bleeding
  - Scalp laceration
- Methods to control bleeding
  - Extraoral/face/scalp laceration
    - Pressure at the bleeding site(s)
    - Repair of laceration
    - Suture ligation of bleeders
  - Nasal bleeding due to maxillofacial fracture
    - Pressure packing: First choice is usually anterior and posterior packing.
    - Balloon tamponade using Foley catheter
      - Balloon tamponade should be used with caution in comminuted midface fracture because it may cause displacement of fractured fragment into orbits and brain.
    - Manual reduction of fractures
    - Selective angioembolization for continued bleeding control with packing
      - Complications
        - Cranial nerve VII palsy
        - Trismus
        - Necrosis of tongue
        - Blindness
        - Migration of emboli into internal carotid, and eventually stroke
    - Direct external carotid artery (ECA) ligation
      - May be ineffective in nasoorbital ethmoidal fracture due to collaterals from the internal carotid artery

Must-Know Essentials: Scalp Laceration

ANATOMY OF THE SCALP

- Layers of the scalp from superficial to deep
  - S: Skin
  - C: Connective tissue: dense tissue with vessels and nerves
  - A: Aponeurosis: galea (aponeurosis of occipitofrontal muscle)
  - L: Loose areolar tissue: emissary veins (dangerous zone for extracranial and intracranial infections)
  - P: Pericranium

REPAIR OF SCALP LACERATION

- Deep lacerations may result in massive bleeding from the vessels between galea and deep dermal layer, leading to hemorrhagic shock.
- Galea must be repaired to prevent:
  - facial asymmetry and asymmetrical facial expression in frontal scalp laceration.
  - subgaleal infections leading to diffuse scalp infection.
- Technique of scalp laceration repair
  - Galea is involved in:
    - single-layer repair including both galea and skin together with sutures.
    - two-layers repair: repair of galea with 3/0 or 4/0 absorbable sutures (Vicryl or Monocryl) followed by skin closure with sutures or staples.
  - Simple scalp laceration
    - Repair with staples or sutures.
  - Significant tissue loss
    - May require Z-Plasty or other plastic surgery techniques

Must-Know Essentials: Skull Fractures

CLASSIFICATION

- Based on anatomical location
  - Basilar skull fracture
  - Skull vault fracture
- Based on fracture lines/fragments
  - Linear
  - Comminuted
- Based on overlying wound
  - Open (compound)
  - Closed
- Based on degree of displacement
  - Nondisplaced
  - Displaced (depressed)

COMPLICATIONS OF SKULL FRACTURES

- Vascular injuries
  - Arterial dissection, occlusion, or rupture
  - Arterial epidural hematoma (EDH): middle meningeal artery injury in squamous temporal bone fracture

- Arteriovenous fistula (e.g., caroticocavernous fistula)
- Dural venous injury
- Venous EDH
- Dural venous sinus thrombosis
  - Common in patients with fractures extending to a dural venous sinus or the jugular foramen
- Cerebral hemorrhagic contusion
- Extension through cranial nerve foramina or canals with neural damage
- Dural tear leading to cerebrospinal fluid (CSF) leak and intracranial hypotension

SPECIFIC SKULL FRACTURES

- Linear skull fracture
  - Most common
  - Involves full thickness of the skull from the outer to the inner table
  - Complications
    - Suture diastasis
    - Venous sinus thrombosis
      - If fractures involve venous sinus groove
      - Frontal bone fracture associated with frontal sinus thrombosis
    - Epidural hematoma
      - If fracture involves vascular channels
      - Temporal bone linear fracture commonly associated with middle meningeal artery causing EDH; rare in elderly, likely due to adherence of dura to the bone
    - Cerebral contusion
    - Subarachnoid hemorrhage
- Depressed skull fracture
  - Bone fragments depressed inward into the cerebral parenchyma
  - High risk of associated injuries to the meninges, blood vessels, and brain
  - Complications
    - High incidence of compound fractures
    - Seizures
    - Neurological deficit
    - Intracranial hematoma
    - Venous sinus thrombosis
- Diastatic fracture
  - Fracture through the sutures of the skull
  - Common in infants and children under age 3 where sutures are not fused.
  - In adults
    - Usually caused by severe injuries
    - Mainly affects the lambdoidal suture because this suture fuses late
    - May cause widening of the suture and collapse of the surrounding bones
- Basilar skull fractures
  - Linear factures at the base of the skull
  - Common in severe head injury
  - Manifestations/complications of basilar skull fractures
    - Anterior cranial fossa
    - CSF rhinorrhea due to dural tear
    - Periorbital ecchymosis (raccoon eyes) due to blood leakage from the fracture site
    - Blood in the sinuses

- Middle cranial fossa
  - Retroauricular ecchymosis (Battle sign) due to bruising of the mastoid process
  - CSF otorrhea: cerebrospinal fluid leak from the ear due to tear in dura
  - Otorrhagia: bleeding from external acoustic meatus
  - Sensorineural hearing loss
  - Facial palsy due to facial (cranial nerve VII) injury
- Posterior cranial fossa
  - Occipital condyle fracture
    - Asymmetry in tongue protrusion due to cranial nerve XII injury
  - Clivus fracture
    - Most anterior portion of the basilar occipital bone
    - Problem with abduction of eye movement due to cranial nerve VI palsy.
  - Transsphenoidal basilar fracture
    - Internal carotid artery injury
    - Carotid-cavernous fistula
    - Cranial nerve injury including optic cranial nerve injury (cranial nerve II), oculomotor (cranial nerve III), trochlear (cranial nerve IV), and abducens (cranial nerve VI)
    - High incidence of dural tear with CSF leak
    - Cerebral venous thrombosis involving dural venous thrombosis, cortical vein thrombosis, and deep cerebral vein thrombosis
- Compound skull fracture
  - Associated with:
    - scalp laceration.
    - CSF otorrhea or rhinorrhea due to meningeal tear.
    - involvement of paranasal sinuses.
    - intracranial air (pneumocephalus).
  - High risk of meningitis
- Temporal bone fracture
  - Fracture of squamous part may cause epidural hematoma due to middle meningeal artery injury.
  - Features of fracture of the Petrous part
    - Retroauricular ecchymosis (Battle sign) due to bruising of the mastoid process
    - CSF otorrhea: cerebrospinal fluid leak from the ear due to tear in dura
    - Otorrhagia: bleeding from external auditory canal
    - Injury to ear ossicles leading to deafness
    - Facial palsy due to facial (cranial nerve VII injury)
    - Trigeminal nerve (cranial nerve V) injury: Fracture of the tip of the petrous temporal bone may involve the Gasserian ganglion of the trigeminal nerve.
    - Injury to otic capsule
      - Sensorineural hearing loss
      - Vestibular dysfunction including vertigo, and balance disturbance
    - Posttraumatic cholesteatoma
  - Computed tomography (CT) of the temporal bone is the imaging of choice.
- Occipital condyle fracture
  - May cause lower cranial injuries including glossopharyngeal nerve (IX), vagus nerve (X), accessory nerve (XI), and hypoglossal nerve (XII)
  - May have associated cervical spine fracture
  - May be unilateral or bilateral
  - May result in occipitocervical dissociation (atlantooccipital dislocation)

■ Occipital condyle articulates with lateral mass of C1 (atlas) vertebra, which is stabilized by:
   atlantooccipital joint capsule ligament (anterior and posterior atlantooccipital ligaments)
   lateral atlantooccipital ligaments
   alar ligaments (dens to each occipital condyle)
   apical dental ligament
■ CT scan is the best imaging for the evaluation of fracture.
■ MRI is recommended to evaluate spinal cord and ligament injuries.
■ Classification
   ■ Based on the mechanism of injury (Anderson and Montesano classification)
      Type I
         Nondisplaced comminuted
         Impaction fracture of occipital condyle
         Associated with axial compression injury
         Stable fracture
      Type II
         Basilar skull fracture extending into occipital condyle
         Associated with direct blow to lower skull
         Stable injury
      Type III
         Condylar avulsion fracture at the alar ligament attachment
         Caused by forced contralateral bending and rotation
         Potentially unstable injury
   ■ Clinical classification (Tuli classification):
      Type I: nondisplaced fracture; does not require stabilization
      Type II: displaced fracture
      IIA: no ligamentous instability; treated with external stabilization
      IIB: ligamentous instability; should be treated with surgical fixation

MANAGEMENT OF SKULL FRACTURES

■ Nonoperative management
   ■ Nondisplaced linear fractures of the vault of skull in neurologically intact patients
   ■ Linear basilar fractures in neurologically intact patients
   ■ Depressed fracture over the venous sinus in neurologically intact patient
   ■ Depressed skull fractures with depressed segment <5 mm below the inner table of adjacent bone
   ■ Temporal bone fractures
   ■ Types I and II (Anderson and Montesano classification) occipital condyle fractures; external stabilization with cervical collar
■ Operative management: indications
   ■ Depressed fractures
      ■ With cosmetic deformity, such as forehead fracture
      ■ Depression greater than the depth of the adjacent inner table
      ■ Depressed segment >5 mm below the inner table of adjacent bone
         Due to increased incidence of dural injury
         Reduces incidence of posttraumatic seizures
      ■ Significant underlying hematoma

- Open depressed skull fracture
- Fracture over the venous sinus usually treated nonoperatively due to risk of uncontrolled bleeding but should be operated in neurologically unstable patient
- Any type of open (compound) skull fracture will significant contamination
- Fractures with pneumocephalus due to dural tear
- Basilar skull fracture with persistent CSF leak after failed nonoperative management
- Temporal bone fracture
  - Immediate facial nerve injury
    - Delayed onset or incomplete facial paralysis almost always resolves with nonoperative treatment including corticosteroids.
  - Hearing loss
  - Vestibular dysfunction
  - CSF leakage
- Occipital fractures
  - Type III (Anderson and Montesano classification) or Type IIB (Tuli classification): occipitocervical fusion

Must-Know Essentials: Midface Le Fort Fractures

CLASSIFICATION

- Le Fort type I fracture
  - Transverse fracture just above the alveolar ridge of the upper teeth
  - Causes separation of hard palate from the maxilla, causing floating palate
  - Fracture lines involve:
    - pterygoid plates just above the floor of the nose.
    - inferior nasal septum.
    - lateral bony margin of the nasal opening.
    - medial and lateral walls of the maxillary sinus
- Le Fort type II fracture
  - Pyramidal fracture through the nasofrontal suture, nasal bones, medial-anterior orbital wall, orbital floor, inferior orbital rims, posterior maxilla, and pterygoid plates
  - Causes floating maxilla
- Le Fort type III fracture
  - Transverse fracture of the midface that results in craniofacial dissociation, leading to floating face
  - Separates the maxilla from the skull base
  - Fracture line passes through the nasofrontal suture, medial orbital wall, zygomaticofrontal suture, zygomatic arch, maxillofrontal suture, and pterygoid plates.
  - Within the nose, the fracture extends through the base of the perpendicular plate of the ethmoid air cells, the vomer, and both parts of the nasal septum.

COMPLICATIONS

- Le Fort type I fracture
  - Mobile palatomaxillary segment
  - Palatal mucosal laceration
  - Dislocation of maxillary teeth
  - Malocclusion

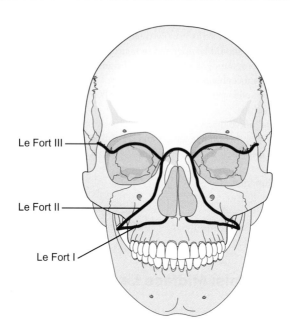

Classification of Le Fort fractures. Source: C. Edibam & H. Robinson, Chapter 78: Maxillofacial and upper-airway injuries, in A. D. Bersten & J. M. Handy (Eds.), *Oh's intensive care manual* (8th ed.), Elsevier, 2018

- Le Fort type II fracture
  - Injury to infraorbital nerve, resulting in reduced sensitivity in the frontal teeth, upper lip, cheek, and skin of the lateral nose
- Le Fort type III fracture
  - Oral and nasal bleeding
  - Malocclusion
  - Orbital edema
  - CSF rhinorrhea
  - V2 branch of trigeminal nerve injury
  - Olfactory nerve injury

TREATMENT

- Surgical treatment involves:
  - exposure.
    - Le Fort type I fracture
      - Gingivolabial incision
    - Le Fort II type fracture
      - Sublabial incision for the exposure of maxillary bone
      - Subciliary or transconjunctival incision for the exposure of the orbital rim
    - Le Fort type III fracture
      - Sublabial incision for the exposure of maxillary bone
      - Subciliary or transconjunctival incision for the exposure of the orbital rim

Lateral brow incision, glabellar fold incision, or bicorporal scalp flaps for additional exposure to the frontozygomatic buttress
- Fracture reduction
- Prior to fixation of the involved maxillary fractures, mandibular and cranial fractures should be stabilized.
- Maxillomandibular (MMF) fracture technique
  - Fixation with arch bar
  - Fixation with miniplates and screws
  - Hybrid of arch bar, miniplates, and screws

Must-Know Essentials: Nasal Bone Fracture

TYPES

- Isolated nasal bone fracture
- Nasal fracture with concomitant other facial fractures

COMPLICATIONS

- Epistaxis
- Cosmetic deformity
- Blockage of nasal passage with difficulty breathing
- Septal hematoma leading to:
  - septal necrosis resulting in septal perforation, severe nasal collapse, and facial deformity.
  - septal abscess.

TREATMENT

- Nondisplaced fracture
  - No treatment
- Displaced fracture
  - Reduction and splint

Must-Know Essentials: Frontal Fracture

TYPES

- Fracture may involve:
  - anterior wall.
  - posterior wall.
  - both anterior and posterior walls.

COMPLICATIONS

- Cosmetic deformity
- Dural tear causing CSF rhinorrhea
- Mucocele
- Intracranial infection
  - Meningitis
  - Meningoencephalitis
- Pneumocephalus
- Frontal sinusitis

TREATMENT

- Usually treated nonoperatively
- Indications for operative treatment
  - Cosmetic deformity
  - Meningitis
  - Sinus dysfunction, such as development of a mucocele

Must-Know Essentials: Nasoorbitoethmoidal (NOE) Fracture

ANATOMY OF NASOORBITOETHMOID COMPLEX

- Nasoorbitoethmoid (NOE) complex consists of:
  - Nasal bones
  - Frontal process of the maxilla
  - Nasal process of the frontal bone
  - Lacrimal bone
  - Lamina papyracea (medial wall of the orbit)
  - Ethmoid bone
  - Sphenoid bone
  - Nasal septum
- Medial canthal tendon (MCT)
  - Pivotal soft tissue in NOE area
  - Supports the canthus and enables proper apposition between the eyelid and the globe
  - Important for lacrimal pump
- Nasolacrimal duct (NLD)
  - Lies in the bone of the lateral nasal wall and extends to the nasal cavity through the inferior meatus under the inferior turbinate
- NOE structures separate the nasal and orbital cavities from cranial cavity.

ASSESSMENT

- NOE fracture can cause severe facial dysfunction and malformation.
- Detailed physical examination and imaging, including two-dimensional (2D) CT and three-dimensional (3D) CT, are essential for the evaluation.
- Manifestations
  - Ophthalmic
    - Diplopia
    - Telecanthus
      - Increase in intercanthal distance due to medial canthal tendon injury
      - Suggests displaced fracture of the medial wall of the orbit
    - Visual changes
    - Orbital injury leading to enophthalmos or exophthalmos
    - Epiphora due to lacrimal duct injury.
    - Shortened palpebral fissure due to medal canthal tendon malformation
  - Nasal
    - Retrusion of the nasal bridge
    - Anosmia due to injury of the cribriform plate
    - Septal hematoma or bony/cartilaginous deformity
    - CSF rhinorrhea due to fracture through the cribriform plate

CLASSIFICATION

- Based on the attachment of the medial canthal tendons to the medial orbital wall and central fracture fragment.
  - Type I injury: MCT attached to a single-segment central fracture fragment.
  - Type II injury: MCT attached to a comminuted central fragment
  - Type III injury: MCT separated from the comminuted central fragment

MANAGEMENT

- Goal of the management of NOE fractures
  - Restoration of facial appearance
  - Reconstruction of orbital wall to correct the telecanthus, enophthalmos, and epiphora
  - Management of NLD injury to prevent epiphora
  - Reattachment of the MCT
    - To prevent the telecanthus and shortened palpebral fissure
    - To improve the facial function and appearance
- Surgical procedure
  - Exposure
    - Coronal incision is commonly used to provide exposure of the NOE fractures.
    - Some fractures may require additional exposure.
      - Infraorbital incision
      - Sublabial incision
      - Subciliary incision
      - Transconjunctival and/or lateral rim incisions
  - Fixation of fractures
    - Type I injury
      - Fixation of the superior horizontal buttress, inferior horizontal buttress and vertical buttress with plate and screw fixation
      - Horizontal buttress consists of frontal bone, superior orbital rims, and inferior orbital rims
      - Medial vertical buttress consists of internal angular process of the frontal bone and the bilateral frontal processes of the maxilla
    - Type II injury
      - Medial orbital wall bony fragments restored with titanium microplates or absorbable mesh for the proper reduction of MCT
    - Type III injury
      - Requires more complex repair and reconstruction of the orbital wall and MCT

Must-Know Essentials: Orbital Blowout Fractures

FEATURES

- Fracture of one or more of the orbital walls with intact orbital rim
- Caused by a direct blow to the central orbit, resulting in sudden increase in intraorbital pressure
- Clinical manifestations
  - Enophthalmos due to increased orbital volume
  - Diplopia due to extraocular muscle entrapment
  - Orbital emphysema due to fracture into an adjacent paranasal sinus
  - Malar region numbness due to injury to the inferior orbital nerve

- Hypoglobus: inferior displacement of the globe in the orbit; may be associated with enophthalmos
- Intraorbital hemorrhage; may result in stretching or compression of the optic nerve due to increased intraocular pressure resulting in an acute ocular compartment syndrome
- Injury to globe of the eye
- Visual changes
- CT scan for detailed evaluation

TYPES OF BLOWOUT FRACTURE

- Inferior (floor)
  - Most common
  - Mostly situated posterior and medial to the infraorbital groove.
  - May be associated with prolapse of the orbital fat and inferior rectus muscle into the maxillary sinus
  - Associated with medial wall fracture in 50% of patients
- Medial wall (lamina papyracea)
  - Second most common injury type
  - May result in orbital fat and medial rectus muscle prolapse into the ethmoid air cells
- Superior (roof)
  - Pure superior blowout fractures without associated orbital rim fracture are uncommon.
  - Fractures may involve the sinus, the anterior cranial fossa, or both sinus and anterior cranial fossa.
  - Fractures communicating with the anterior cranial fossa are at risk for CSF leak and meningitis.
- Lateral wall
  - Pure lateral blowout fractures are rare due to bone being thick and bounded by muscles.
  - Usually associated with orbital rim or other significant craniofacial injuries.

MANAGEMENT

- Injury of the globe is the priority.
- Posttraumatic diplopia or extraocular muscle impairment may improve with nonoperative management.
- Indications for operative management
  - Significant enophthalmos
  - Significant diplopia
  - Muscle entrapment
  - Significant fractures
- Acute ocular compartment syndrome
  - A surgical emergency that requires decompression with lateral canthotomy and cantholysis within 1–2 hours to prevent ischemia of the optic nerve or retina
  - Features of acute ocular compartment syndrome
    - Ocular pain
    - Proptosis
    - Decreased vision
    - Diplopia

- Limited extraocular movements
- Ecchymosis around the eye
- Relative afferent pupillary defect (pupillary dilation with light) or dilated fixed pupil
- Increased intraocular pressure (IOP) >35–40 mm Hg
- Technique of lateral canthotomy or cantholysis
  - Lateral canthus tendon attaches the eyelids to the orbital rim, which prevents anterior displacement of the globe.
  - Lateral canthus tendon has a superior crus and an inferior crus.
  - Inject 1% lidocaine with epinephrine into the lateral canthal incision site.
  - Using a hemostat, crush the tissue from the lateral canthus to the rim of the orbit to minimize bleeding.
  - Canthotomy: After lifting the respective lower or upper eyelids, cut the inferior crus or the superior crus of the lateral canthus to the rim of the orbit using an iris surgical scissors pointing away from the globe.
  - Inferior canthotomy is preferred over the superior canthotomy. Most often, inferior canthotomy is sufficient for orbital decompression.
  - Cantholysis: Cut both superior and inferior crus of the lateral canthal ligament if IOP persists.
  - Place a dressing.

Must-Know Essentials: Zygomaticomaxillary Complex Fractures

FEATURES

- Zygomaticomaxillary complex (ZMC) fractures are also known as tripod, tetrapod, quad-ripod, malar, or trimalar fractures.
- Fractures include:
  - Zygomatic arch and or diastasis of the temporozygomatic suture
  - Inferior orbital rim, and anterior and posterior maxillary sinus walls and/or diastasis of zygomaticomaxillary suture
  - Lateral orbital rim and/or diastasis of the frontozygomatic suture
- Second most common facial bone fracture after nasal bone fracture
- Results from a direct blow to the malar eminence
- Requires clinical examination and CT scan for assessment
- Clinical manifestations
  - Malar depression
  - Enophthalmos
  - Malocclusion
  - Trismus and difficulty with mastication, due to impingement of the temporalis muscle
  - Hypoesthesia in the distribution of infraorbital nerve due to its injury at the infraorbital foramen
  - Visual changes

MANAGEMENT

- Closed or open reduction to preserve normal facial structure, sensory function, globe's position, and mastication function

Must-Know Essentials: Paranasal Sinus Fractures

FEATURES

- Paranasal sinuses
  - Maxillary sinus
  - Sphenoid sinus
  - Frontal sinus
  - Ethmoid sinus
- Types of fractures
  - Isolated
  - Associated with complex facial fracture
    - Le Fort types I and II fractures in maxillary sinus fracture
    - Le Fort types II and III fractures in ethmoid sinus fracture
    - NOE complex fracture with associated frontal and ethmoid sinus fractures
- Usually associated with brain injury
- CT findings
  - Blood in sinuses
  - Dislocated bone fragments
  - Air in soft tissues
  - Pneumocephalus
- Specific features of the maxillary sinus fracture
  - Most common paranasal sinus fracture
  - May be associated with Le Fort type I and II fractures
  - Sites of fracture
    - Blowout fracture: floor of orbit/roof of sinus
    - Inferior sinus wall: may be due to iatrogenic injury or displaced dental implant
  - Manifestations
    - Hypoesthesia of upper lip/dental arch
    - Diplopia
    - Complications
      - Oroantral fistula
      - Maxillary sinus infection
- Specific features of the ethmoidal sinus fracture
  - Features of the associated NOE complex fractures and frontal sinus fracture
  - Isolated fracture is rare.
  - Superior sinus wall (cribriform plate) is the common site of fracture.
  - Manifestations
    - Hyposmia
    - Anosmia
    - Complications
      - Olfactory nerve injury
      - Dacryocystitis
      - CSF rhinorrhea
      - Intracranial infection
- Specific features of the sphenoidal sinus fracture
  - Transsphenoidal fractures are usually seen in association with:
    - basilar skull fractures involving anterior cranial fossa or petrous temporal bones.
    - complex craniofacial fractures.
  - Isolated fracture is rare.

- Manifestations
  - CSF rhinorrhea
  - Visual disturbance
  - Complications
    - Optic/oculomotor nerve injury
    - Internal carotid artery injury

MANAGEMENT

- Prophylactic antibiotics are indicated in frontal, ethmoidal, and sphenoidal sinus fractures.
- Maxillary and ethmoid sinus fractures are usually treated nonoperatively.
- Surgical management
  - Frontal sinus fractures
    - CSF leak
    - Nasofrontal outflow tract injury
    - Associated depressed skull fractures
  - Maxillary sinus fracture
    - Isolated anterior wall of the maxillary sinus fracture

Must-Know Essentials: Mandibular Fractures

FEATURES

- Angle and body of the mandible are the most common sites of fracture.
- Manifestations
  - Pain
  - Tenderness and abnormal mobility of the mandible
  - Trismus
  - Malocclusion
  - Chin numbness (mental nerve injury)
  - Dental injury
- Imaging for further evaluation
  - High-resolution CT images
  - Panorex x-ray
    - Dentition-related injuries seen best on this view
  - MRI: useful for the evaluation of temporomandibular joint (TMJ) dysfunction and condyle displacement

TYPES OF FRACTURES

- Based on anatomical locations
  - Angle of the mandible: 20%–30%
  - Body: 20%–30%
  - Condyle or neck: 15%–36%
  - Parasymphyseal: 14%–15%
  - Ramus: 5%
  - Coronoid process: 1%–3%
  - Alveolar ridge: 2%

- Based on the number of fracture fragments
  - Unifocal fractures (Simple): 40%
  - Multifocal fractures (comminuted): 60%
- May be associated with condylar subluxation

MANAGEMENT

- Symphysis/parasymphysis fractures
  - Closed reduction and external fixation with intermaxillary fixation/maxillomandibular fixation (IMF/MMF) using arch bars
  - Internal fixation with an intraoral approach using plates and screws
- Body
  - Closed reduction and external fixation
  - Internal fixation with an intraoral or extraoral approach using plates and screws
- Angle
  - May cause injury to inferior alveolar nerve and artery
  - Risk of injury to the third molar or wisdom tooth
  - Internal fixation with an intraoral approach or an extraoral approach (for comminuted and complex fractures) using plates and screws
- Ramus
  - Open reduction and internal fixation with plates and screws
  - Exposure may require preauricular or submandibular incision based on the location of fracture.
  - Nondisplaced fractures treated with external fixation with IMF/MMF have a high failure rate.
- Coronoid fracture
  - Nonoperative management
    - Isolated fracture, and the patient can open and close the mouth without difficulty
  - Open reduction and internal fixation
    - If unable or difficult to open/close the mouth
- Condyle
  - Head of the condyle
    - Intracapsular head-of-the-condyle fracture has high risk of ankylosis of the TMJ.
    - Operative treatment options
      - Open reduction with external fixation using IMF/MMF
      - Open reduction with or without internal fixation
      - Endoscopic surgery
  - Extracapsular condylar neck (neck of the mandible)
    - Stabilization of maxilla is most important in the management of a fracture of the neck of the mandible.
    - Unstable maxilla
      - Stabilization of the maxilla first followed by management of the mandible
    - Stable maxilla and normal occlusion
      - Unilateral fracture: nonoperative management
      - Bilateral fracture: at least unilateral fixation with open approach
    - Stable maxilla with malocclusion
      - Unilateral: open reduction and MMF followed by TMJ rehabilitation
      - Bilateral: unilateral open approach with subsequent contralateral management based on the status of the occlusion

- Edentulous mandible fracture
  - Open reduction and internal fixation
- Complex mandibular fracture
  - Complex injuries, such as comminuted fractures, blast injuries, or multiple fractures may require:
    - exposure of the fractures with intraoral and extraoral approach.
    - bone graft to fill the bone defect.
    - external fixation for:
      severe comminution.
      infections.
      nonunions.
      significant bone or soft-tissue defects.

COMPLICATIONS

- Osteomyelitis
- Permanent malocclusion
- Nonunion
- Malunion

Spine Trauma

Cervical Spine Clearance

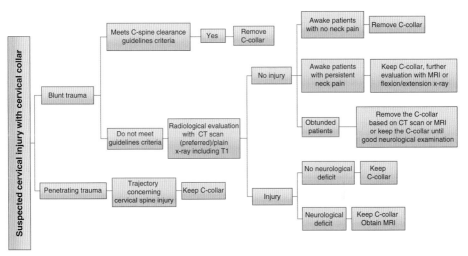

Algorithm: Cervical spine clearance

Must-Know Essentials: Cervical Spine Clearance

BACKGROUND

- Incidence of cervical spine injury in the adult trauma population is around 3.7%.
- Cervical spine injury with or without neurological deficit should be suspected in patients with multiple injuries.
- C-collar is recommended for the immobilization of the spine to prevent the worsening of neurological or spinal injury.
- C-collar should be removed as soon as possible after spinal injury is ruled out.
- Improper and prolonged use of a hard cervical collar results in multiple problems including:
  - airway obstruction.
  - reduced access for orotracheal intubation.
  - reduced access for central venous access.
  - increase in intracranial pressure (ICP) by affecting the venous return from the brain.
  - problems during surgical management of maxillofacial trauma.
  - increased ventilator days.
  - increased incidence of delirium.
  - increased incidence of pneumonia.
  - decubitus ulcer.

NEXUS CERVICAL SPINE CLEARANCE GUIDELINES

- National Emergency X-Radiography Utilization Study (NEXUS) criteria for cervical spine clearance in blunt trauma
- C-collar can be removed if the patient meets the following criteria:
  - Awake and alert, Glasgow Coma Scale (GCS) = 15, baseline mental status
  - No focal neurological deficit
  - No midline posterior cervical spine tenderness
  - No painful distracting injury
  - No evidence of intoxication (alcohol or drugs, including iatrogenic)
- NEXUS criteria have a 99.6% sensitivity and a 96.4% negative predictive value.
- Unlike the Canadian C-Spine Rule (CCR), NEXUS criteria do not have age cutoffs and are theoretically applicable to all patients >1 year of age.
- Cervical spine CT scan
  - Recommended as the first-line imaging modality in all blunt trauma patients who do not meet the NEXUS criteria
  - Should include the occiput to the first thoracic vertebrae
  - More cost effective, more time efficient, and a higher sensitivity for detection of cervical spine injuries than plain radiographs
  - Spinal cord injury without radiological abnormality (SCIWORA) is rare (0.08%) in cervical spine injuries but may be seen in both adults and children.

CANADIAN C-SPINE RULE FOR CERVICAL SPINE CLEARANCE

- C-collar can be removed without any radiological assessment if the following criteria are met:
- No high-risk factors, including:
  - age >65 years.
  - dangerous mechanism:
    - fall from >1 meter or 5 stairs.
    - axial load on the head.
    - major vehicle collision:
      - high speed (>100 km/hr).
      - rollover.
      - ejection.
    - motorized recreational vehicle collision.
    - bicycle collision.
  - paresthesia in extremities.
- Low-risk factors, including:
  - simple rear-end motor vehicle collision.
  - sitting in the emergency department.
  - ambulatory at any time.
  - delayed onset of neck pain.
  - no midline cervical tenderness.
- Patient safely able to actively rotate the neck (45 degrees left and right).
- Neck radiography should be performed if it does not meet the C-spine clearance criteria.
- In stable alert trauma patients:
  - CCR is superior to the NEXUS criteria with respect to sensitivity and specificity
  - CCR results in reduced rates of radiography.
- X-ray (flexion/extension) versus CT scan was decided based on clinical judgment.

EASTERN ASSOCIATION FOR THE SURGERY OF TRAUMA (EAST) GUIDELINES FOR CERVICAL SPINE CLEARANCE

- Patients with penetrating trauma to the brain
  - Immobilization in a cervical collar is unnecessary unless the trajectory suggests direct injury to the cervical spine.
- There is no indication for cervical spine imaging and the C-collar can be removed if the following criteria are met:
  - Awake, alert patient without neurologic deficit
  - No distracting injury
  - No neck pain
  - No cervical spine tenderness
  - Full range of motion of the cervical spine
- Imaging for cervical spine clearance
  - Indicated if patients do not meet the criteria for C-collar clearance
  - CT scan of the cervical spine
    - Should include the occiput to T1 with sagittal and coronal reconstructions
  - Plain radiographs do not provide any additional information and is not recommended.
  - MRI of the cervical spine
    - Recommended if there is a neurologic deficit attributable to a cervical spine injury
    - Most common injuries diagnosed with MRI
      - Disc herniation
      - Spinal stenosis
      - Cord edema
      - Cord contusion
      - Ligamentous injury
- Neurologically intact, awake, and alert patient with negative C-spine CT with neck pain
  - Continued cervical spine immobilization in a C-collar until a negative MRI or flexion/extension (F/E) x-ray of the C-spine
- Obtunded patient with a negative cervical spine CT with gross motor function in all four extremities
  - No consensus for appropriate clearance method
  - MRI is good for the evaluation of ligamentous injury.
  - Incidence of ligamentous injury in the setting of a negative CT is low (<5%).
  - Cervical collar can be removed after a negative high-quality C-spine CT scan result alone.

CHAPTER 15

Evaluation and Management of Cervical Spine Injuries

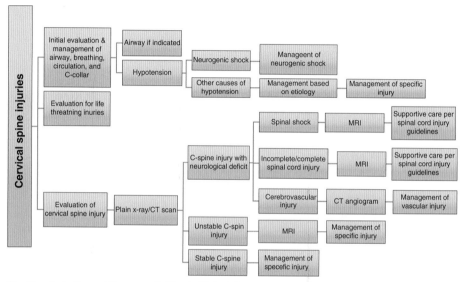

Algorithm: Evaluation and Management of Cervical Spine Injuries

Must-Know Essentials: Evaluation of Cervical Spine Injury

INITIAL EVALUATION

- Primary survey and resuscitation
  - Airway
  - Protect the C-spine
  - Breathing
  - Circulation
- Rule out life-threatening injuries.

EVALUATION OF FRACTURE

- Clinical
  - Neck pain
  - C-spine tenderness
- Imaging
  - Plain film
    - Anteroposterior (AP) view, lateral view (must include C7–T1), and open-mouth odontoid views are required for the evaluation.
    - Information from lateral view
      - Vertebral alignment for the diagnosis of subluxation
        - Pseudo-subluxation: physiological misalignment, normally seen in children
        - Displacement of >3 mm is considered pathological.
    - Diagnosis of cervical fractures based on soft-tissue swelling
      - Normal nasopharyngeal space in an adult at C1 level: 10 mm
      - Normal retropharyngeal space in an adult at C2–4 level: 5–7 mm
      - Normal retrotracheal space at C5–6 level: 22 mm (adults), 14 mm (children)
    - 20% of injuries can be missed in plain x-ray.
    - Flexion/Extension view is indicated to evaluate the stability of the injury.
    - Open-mouth view is good for the evaluation of odontoid fracture.
  - CT scan
    - Imaging of choice for the evaluation of details of the bony structures, fracture displacement, and disc herniation
    - Indications
      - Spine injury with neurological deficit
      - Fracture of the posterior element of the cervical canal
      - Subtle fractures for detailed information
      - Bony details in fractures
  - Magnetic resonance imaging (MRI)
    - Imaging of choice for the evaluation of soft tissue structures, disc herniation, and neural structures
    - Indications
      - Fracture with spinal canal involvement
      - Fracture with neurological deficits
      - Suspected ligamentous injuries and soft tissue injuries
      - Evaluation of intervertebral disc
      - Evaluation of epidural hematoma

EVALUATION OF COMPLICATIONS OF CERVICAL SPINE INJURY

- Respiratory failure
  - Phrenic nerve injury causing diaphragmatic palsy in C3–C5 spinal cord injury
  - Atlantooccipital dislocation causing brainstem injury and acute respiratory failure
- Neurogenic shock
  - Cervical and upper thoracic spinal cord injury due to loss of sympathetic tone
- Neurological deficit
  - Spinal shock
  - Spinal cord injury at C1–C8 results in complete or incomplete quadriplegia.
  - Nerve injury at neural foramina
- Blunt cerebral vascular injury (BCVI)
  - Injury to carotid and vertebral arteries

Must-Know Essentials: Cervical Spine Injury Pattern

MECHANISM AND CERVICAL SPINE INJURY PATTERN

- Flexion
  - Most common mechanism
  - Usually after MVC or diving injury
  - Injuries
    - Anterior atlantoaxial subluxation
    - Anterior subluxation (hyperflexion sprain)
    - Anterior wedge fracture
    - Clay shoveler's fracture
    - Flexion teardrop fracture
    - Bilateral facet dislocation
    - Hyperflexion fracture–dislocation
- Lateral flexion
  - C1 (atlas) lateral mass fracture
- Flexion/rotation
  - Unilateral facet dislocation
  - Rotatory atlantoaxial dislocation
- Extension
  - Hangman's fracture: symmetric fracture of bilateral pedicles (pars interarticularis) of C2 (axis) vertebra
  - Extension teardrop fracture
  - Posterior arch C1 fracture
  - Posterior atlantoaxial subluxation
- Extension/rotation
  - Articular pillar fracture
  - Floating pillar
- Axial loading/compression
  - Burst fracture
  - Jefferson fracture: burst fracture of the atlas (C1) with involvement of anterior and posterior arches
- Complex mechanism
  - Odontoid process fracture: hyperflexion or hyperextension with or without compression
  - Atlantooccipital dislocations due to shearing mechanism
- Direct injury: Penetrating injury

STABILITY OF CERVICAL SPINE INJURIES

- Structure of vertebra
  - Body with articular cartilage on superior and inferior surface
  - Vertebral canal between the body and the lamina
  - Arch that includes the pedicle and the lamina
  - Process that includes the spinous process and the transverse process
  - Foramina: vertebral, intervertebral, and transverse foramina
  - Ligaments (from anterior to posterior)
    - Anterior longitudinal ligament
    - Anterior atlantooccipital membrane
    - Apical ligament
    - Alar ligaments

- Cruciate ligaments of the atlas
- Posterior longitudinal ligament
- Tectorial membrane
- Ligamentum flavum
- Posterior atlantooccipital membrane
- Ligament nuchae
- Interspinous ligaments
- Intertransverse ligaments
- Supraspinous ligaments
- Stable fracture
  - No displacement of vertebral components with normal neck movements
  - Two intact vertical columns are essential for the stability of a cervical spine fracture.
    - Anterior column
      Vertebral body
      Disk spaces
      Anterior and posterior longitudinal ligaments
      Annulus fibrosus
    - Posterior column
      Pedicles
      Facets
      Apophyseal joints
      Laminar spinous processes
- Unstable fracture
  - Displacement of vertebral components during movements with risk of damage or further deterioration of neural tissues
  - Fractures with disruption of both anterior and posterior columns
  - Features of indicators of instability in imaging
    - Increased or reduced intervertebral disc space height
    - Increased interspinous distance
    - Widening of the facet joint
    - Vertebral body compression >25%
    - More than one vertebral column involvement
    - Injury to both anterior and posterior ligament complexes

COMMON UNSTABLE CERVICAL INJURIES

- Jefferson fracture: burst fracture of C1 vertebra
- Hangman's fracture: fracture of bilateral pars interarticularis with associated posterior longitudinal ligament causing subluxation of C2 on C3
- Types II and III fractures of the odontoid process of C2
- Atlantooccipital dissociation
- Bilateral cervical facet dislocation
- Flexion teardrop fracture

Must-Know Essentials: Specific Cervical Spine Fractures and Treatments

C1: JEFFERSON FRACTURE

- Burst fracture of atlas (C1) with involvement of anterior and posterior arches
- Each arch may be fractured at one or more places.

- Causes displacement of lateral masses
- Associated with transverse ligament tear
- Mechanism of injury: axial load, such as diving
- Retropulsion of bony fragment may cause spinal cord injury.
- Features in imaging
  - Displacement of lateral masses of C1 beyond the margins of body of C2 in CT scan
  - More than 5-mm increase in atlantodental interval suggests injury to the transverse atlantal ligament; may be seen in CT and odontoid view plain x-ray.
  - Prevertebral edema, ligament injury, or cord edema is best evaluated in MRI.
- Treatment
  - Stable fracture
    - Anterior 1/4, posterior 1/4, or posterior 1/2 fracture without transverse atlantal ligament injury
    - Nonoperative treatment with hard cervical collar immobilization (cervical orthosis)
  - Unstable fracture
    - Fracture with injury to transverse atlantal ligament
    - Treatment options
      - Halo immobilization
      - Posterior C1/2 lateral mass internal fixation
      - Transoral internal fixation

HANGMAN'S FRACTURE

- Symmetric fractures of bilateral pedicles (pars interarticularis) of C2 (axis) with extension across the posterior part of body
- May be associated posterior longitudinal ligament injury causing subluxation
- Mechanism of injury: hyperextension of neck (e.g., hanging, dashboard neck injury in MVC)
- Features in imaging
  - Prevertebral soft tissue swelling
  - Avulsion of anterior inferior corner of C2 associated with rupture of anterior longitudinal ligament
  - Anterior dislocation of C2 vertebral body
  - Bilateral C2 pars interarticularis fracture
  - Intact dens
- Classification (Levine and Edwards)
  - Type I
    - Fracture with <3 mm anteroposterior displacement
    - No angulation
    - Stable fracture
  - Type II
    - Fracture with >3 mm anteroposterior displacement
    - Significant angulation (>10 degree)
    - Disruption of posterior longitudinal ligament
    - Unstable fracture
    - Type IIa
      - Fracture line horizontal/oblique (instead of vertical).
      - No anteroposterior displacement
      - Significant angular deviation without anterior translation
      - Unstable fracture
  - Type III
    - Severe angulation and displacement and facet dislocation, unstable fracture

- Neurological injuries are uncommon due to wide spinal canal at this level.
- There is risk of vertebral artery injury if fracture line involves the transverse foramina.
- Treatment
  - Type I
    - Rigid C-collar (cervical orthosis) for 4–6 weeks
  - Type II
    - <5 mm anteroposterior displacement and Type IIA
      Closed reduction and halo immobilization for 8–12 weeks
    - >5 anteroposterior displacement
      Surgical stabilization
  - Type III
    - Reduction of facet dislocation followed by surgical stabilization
  - Surgical stabilization techniques
    - Anterior C2–C3 interbody fusion
    - Posterior C1–C3 fusion
    - Bilateral C2 pars screw osteosynthesis

FRACTURE OF C2 DENS (ODONTOID PROCESS)

- Most common fracture of the axis
- Incidence: 10%–15% of all cervical fractures
- Mechanism of injury: hyperflexion or hyperextension with or without compression
- Displacement of fracture may be anterior (hyperflexion) or posterior (hyperextension)
- High risk of neurological injury due to its proximity to the medulla oblongata and the mobility of the craniocervical junction
- May develop dysphagia due to association with a large retropharyngeal hematoma
- Classification (Anderson and D'Alonzo)
  - Type I
    - Avulsion of the odontoid tip by the alar ligaments
    - Very rare
  - Type II
    - Fracture at the base of the odontoid process
    - Most common type of odontoid fracture
    - High nonunion rate due to interruption of blood supply
    - Type IIA
      Horizontal fracture
      Nondisplaced/minimally displaced with no comminution
    - Type B
      Oblique fracture line anterosuperior to posteroinferior
    - Type C
      Reverse fracture line
      Fracture from anteroinferior to posterosuperior, or with significant comminution
      Treatment with posterior stabilization
  - Type III
    - Extends into the lateral mass
    - Has good healing potential
- Features of instability in odontoid fracture
  - Atlantodens interval (ADI) >10 mm
  - Increase in predental space >5 mm due to fracture of odontoid process or disruption of transverse ligament; distance increased

- Instability in flexion/extension x-ray
- Presence of neurological deficit
- Treatment
  - Nonoperative management
    - Type I: cervical orthosis (hard C-collar) for 6–8 weeks
    - Type IIA: halo for 6–12 weeks if no risk factors for nonunion
    - Type III: cervical orthosis (hard collar) or halo
      - No evidence to support halo over hard collar
      - Halo fixators are highly controversial as they are found to aggravate mortality and morbidity, especially in elderly patients.
    - Risk factors for the failure of nonsurgical treatment
      - Age >50 years
      - Type IIC fractures
      - Dens displacement >5 mm
      - Angulation of the fracture >10 degrees
      - Comminution on the base of the odontoid process
      - Tobacco use
      - Inability to achieve acceptable fracture alignment by nonoperative treatment
  - Operative management
    - Anterior odontoid osteosynthesis (odontoid screw)
      - Indications
        - Type IIA fracture with risk factors for nonunion and unacceptable alignment
        - Type B fracture with good bone density
      - Anterior odontoid osteosynthesis associated with high failure
      - Contraindications of odontoid screw
        - Osteoporosis
        - Severe ossification/arthrosis of the alar ligament
        - Fused anterior atlas ring to tip of odontoid
        - Nonreducible fracture
        - Severe kyphosis
    - Posterior C1–C2 fusion
      - Indications
        - Nonunion after nonoperative management of Type IIA and Type III fractures
        - Failed anterior odontoid osteosynthesis for Type IIA, and Type IIB fractures
        - Type IIC fractures
    - Transoral odontoidectomy
      - For severe posterior displacement of dens with spinal cord compression and neurologic deficits

BURST FRACTURE

- Fracture of C3–C7 due to axial compression
- Always involves the posterior vertebral body
- Spinal cord injury common due to displacement of posterior fragments
- Treated with rigid immobilization or fusion

CLAY SHOVELER'S FRACTURE

- Avulsion fracture of C6–T1 spinous process
- Mechanism: powerful hyperflexion usually combined with contraction of paraspinal muscles

- Usually treated nonoperatively
- May require excision of avulsion fragment for persistent pain

WEDGE FRACTURE

- Single column anterosuperior fracture of the vertebral body
- Mechanism: hyperflexion and compression
- Causes loss of height of anterior vertebral body
- Treatment
  - Nonoperative
    - Immobilization in a brace for 6–12 weeks for fractures with wedging <30%
  - Operative: restoration of vertebral height and spinal fusion
    - Indications
      Fracture affects adjacent vertebrae.
      Anterior wedging >30%–50%
      Severe kyphosis
      Bone fragment(s) in the spinal canal
      Spinal cord dysfunction

FLEXION TEARDROP FRACTURE

- Posterior ligament disruption with anterior compression fracture of the vertebral body
- Most common at mid/lower cervical spine, specifically at C4, C5, or C6
- Mechanism of injury: hyperflexion and compression injury, as seen in diving into shallow water or MVC
- An unstable fracture
- High risk of associated spinal cord injury
- Characteristic features in imaging
  - Teardrop avulsion fracture of the anterior vertebral body
  - Loss of anterior height of the vertebral body
  - Sagittal fracture through the vertebral body
  - Posterior vertebral body subluxation into the spinal canal
  - Spinal cord compression from vertebral body displacement
  - Fracture of the spinous process
- Treatment
  - Decompression and internal fixation

EXTENSION TEARDROP FRACTURE

- Avulsion of the anteroinferior corner of the vertebral body due to forced hyperextension of the neck
- Fractures are stable in flexion and unstable in extension due to disruption of anterior longitudinal ligament.
- Usually affects C2
- Considered less severe compared to flexion tear teardrop fracture
- Often managed nonoperatively with a cervical brace

ATLANTOOCCIPITAL DISLOCATION

- Uncommon fatal injury, usually due to flexion and shearing mechanism

- Mortality at the scene from respiratory arrest due to brainstem injury
- Patients who survive are quadriplegic and ventilatory dependent.

CERVICAL FACET DISLOCATION AND FRACTURE

- Mechanism
  - High-speed deceleration injury in MVC or motorcycle accident
  - Low-energy trauma, such as fall in elderly patients
- Injury pattern
  - Facet fracture
    - Commonly involves superior facets
    - May be unilateral or bilateral
    - Predisposes for facet dislocation
  - Unilateral facet dislocation
    - Associated with injury to nerve roots due to involvement of the neuroforamina from displaced inferior facet of the cephalad vertebrae
    - Mechanism of injury: flexion/rotation
    - Usually stable injury
    - Characteristic features
      - Anterior subluxation of the affected vertebral body by <50 %
      - Widening of the disc space
  - Bilateral facet dislocation
    - High risk of associated spinal cord injury
    - Mechanism of injury: hyperflexion and distraction
    - Unstable injury
    - Characteristic features
      - Anterior subluxation of the affected vertebral body by >50%
      - Disruption of posterior ligament complex and anterior longitudinal ligament
  - Degree of facet dislocation
    - Subluxation
      - Partial dislocation of facet joint
    - Perched facet
      - Inferior articular process of a vertebra overlying the ipsilateral superior articular process of the vertebra below
    - Locked facet
      - Inferior articular process of a vertebra slipping over the superior articular process of the vertebra below and becoming locked
      - Can be unilateral or bilateral
- Treatment of facet fracture
  - Nonoperative
    - External immobilization (halo vs hard orthosis) for 6–12 weeks, depending on degree of instability and age of patient
    - Indications
      - Unilateral nondisplaced facet fractures without radiographic instability
  - Operative
    - Single-level surgical stabilization with plates using anterior or posterior approach
    - Indications
      - Unstable facet fracture
      - Bilateral facet fracture
      - Unilateral fracture involving >40% of the lateral mass or an absolute height of >1 cm

- Treatment of facet dislocation
  - Reduction of dislocated facet
    - Emergency reduction of dislocation followed by surgical stabilization; indicated for the unilateral or bilateral facet dislocation with neurological deficit
    - Nonemergent closed reduction followed surgical stabilization; indicated for the unilateral/bilateral dislocation without spinal cord injury
    - Reduction can be performed by closed or open technique
    - Closed reduction should not be formed in patients with mental status changes
    - After reduction without neurological deficit, stabilization should be performed within 24 hours.
    - Unilateral dislocations are more difficult to reduce but more stable after reduction.
    - Bilateral dislocations are easier to reduce due to torn posterior longitudinal ligament but less stable after reduction.
  - Surgical stabilization
    - Anterior cervical discectomy and surgical stablilization (single level) with anterior plating: Indications
      - Large disc herniation following reduction with compression on the spinal cord or nerve roots
      - Failed closed reduction
    - Posterior reduction and surgical stabilization: Indications
      - No disc herniation
      - Bilateral or unilateral facet dislocations that are not reducible from the front or through closed reduction
    - Combined anterior decompression and posterior reduction/stabilization: Indications
      - Disc herniation
      - Failure to reduce dislocation through closed or open anterior technique

CHAPTER 16

Thoracic and Lumbar Spine Injuries

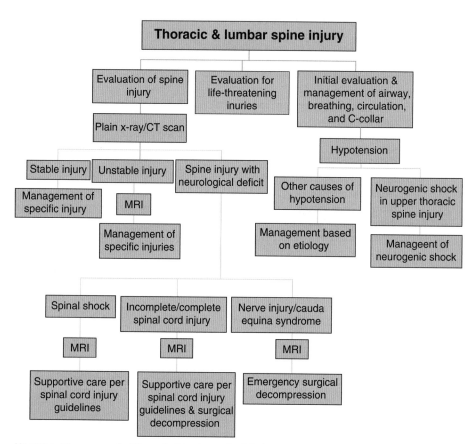

Algorithm: Management of thoracic & lumbar spine injuries

Must-Know Essentials: Evaluation of Thoracolumbar Spine Injuries

INITIAL EVALUATION

- Primary survey and resuscitation
  - Airway
  - Protect the C-spine
  - Protection of thoracolumbar spine in suspected injury

146

- Breathing
- Circulation
- Rule out life-threatening injuries.

EVALUATION OF FRACTURE

- Clinical
  - Back pain
  - Spine tenderness
  - Step-off deformity
  - Neurological evaluation
- Imaging
  - Plain film
    - Usually does not provide details of the fractures.
    - Anteroposterior (AP) view, lateral view may evaluate:
      vertical alignment of the vertebral body and pedicles.
      distance between the pedicles of each vertebra.
      subluxation.
      fractures.
      bone instability.
    - CT scan
      Imaging of choice for the evaluation of details of the bony structures, including vertebral bodies, pedicles, laminae, facets, transverse processes, and spinous processes
      Provides information on fractures displacement and disc herniation
  - Magnetic resonance imaging (MRI)
    - Imaging of choice for the evaluation of ligaments, disc herniation, and neural structures
    - Indications
      Fracture with spinal canal involvement
      Fracture with neurological deficits
      Suspected ligamentous injuries and soft tissue injuries
      Evaluation of intervertebral disc
      Evaluation of epidural hematoma (EDH)
      Evaluation of an occult fracture

EVALUATION OF COMPLICATIONS

- Neurogenic shock
  - Upper thoracic spinal cord injury due to loss of sympathetic tone
- Neurological deficit
  - Spinal shock
  - Spinal cord injury: complete or incomplete paraplegia due to injury above T10
  - Nerve injury due to involvement of neural foramina causing numbness, tingling, or weakness in the limbs
  - Injury to conus medullaris due to injury below L1
    - Most distal part of spinal cord is called the conus medullaris
    - Contains sacral nerves (S2–S5) and coccygeal nerves
    - Manifestations
      Severe back pain
      Sexual, bowel, and bladder dysfunction
      Weakness, numbness, or tingling in lower limbs

- Injury to cauda equina: due to injury below L1
  - Bundle of nerve fibers and nerve roots located at the lower end of the spinal cord
  - Contains lumbar (L2) through sacral (S5) nerves and coccygeal nerves
  - Located in the distal third of the lumbar vertebral canal; extends into the sacral canal
  - Manifestations
    - Severe back pain
    - Sexual, bowel, and bladder dysfunction
    - Weakness, numbness, or tingling in the lower limbs

Must-Know Essentials: Thoracolumbar Spine Injury Pattern

ETIOLOGY

- Usually due to high-energy and high-velocity blunt injuries
  - Motor vehicle collision (MVC) or motorcycle accident
  - Fall from a significant height
  - Sports accident
- Penetrating injury
  - Gunshot wound
- Lower-energy injury, such as twisting or ground-level fall in patients with osteoporosis

MECHANISM AND FRACTURE PATTERN

- Thoracic spine fractures
  - Fractures/dislocations are relatively uncommon in the thoracic and lumbar spine due to orientation of the facet joints.
  - Fracture subluxation of the thoracic spine commonly results in complete neurological deficits due to narrow thoracic spinal canal.
  - Significant force is required for thoracic spine injury because of its rigid structures and protection with thoracic cage.
- Thoracolumbar junction (T11–L1) fractures
  - Most common region of thoracolumbar fractures due to transition point of immobility of the thoracic spine compared with the lumbar spine
  - Usually unstable and results from a combination of acute hyperflexion and rotation mechanism of injury, such as a fall from a height and high-speed MVC
  - Approximately 27% patients may have associated neurological deficits
- Lumbar spine fractures
  - Cauda equina may be involved.
  - Complete neurological deficit is rare.
- Fracture pattern based on mechanism
  - Axial loading with flexion
    - Usually results from high-energy axial loading with flexion, such as falling from a height or MVC
    - Causes anterior wedge compression fracture
    - Mostly stable fracture
  - Vertical-axial compression
    - Usually caused by landing on the feet after falling from a significant height
    - Results in a burst fracture
    - Majority involve L1 but may affect T9-L5.
    - Burst fractures are usually unstable.

- Flexion-distraction
  - Flexion injury of the vertebral body and distraction-type injury of the posterior elements
  - Typically involves all three columns
  - Usually seen in an MVC patient with lap belt without a shoulder strap where the flexion fulcrum occurs anterior to the abdomen
  - Majority occur at the thoracolumbar junction.
  - Results in an unstable transverse fracture through the vertebral body and injury to posterior column known as Chance fracture
  - Associated with retroperitoneal and abdominal visceral injuries
- Hyperflexion, rotation, and shearing
  - Usually seen in high-energy acceleration/deceleration injuries, such as high-speed MVC.
  - Majority affect thoracolumbar junction (T11–L1), leading to unstable vertebral fracture with dislocation of facet joints and/or the intervertebral disc space.
  - High risk of injury to the spinal cord, conus medullaris, or cauda equina, depending on the location of the injury
- Translation-rotation
  - Severe torsional and shear injury due to high-energy mechanism
  - It causes:
    - horizontal displacement or rotation of one vertebral body with respect to another, leading to vertebral body subluxation/translation or rotation.
    - unilateral or bilateral perched or dislocated facet joints.
    - posterior ligament complex injury causing:
      - splaying of the spinous process with widening of the interspinous space.
      - avulsion fracture of the superior or inferior aspects of the contiguous spinous processes.
- Transverse process fractures
  - Mechanism of injury
    - Direct blunt trauma
    - Violent lateral flexion-extension force
    - Psoas muscle avulsion
  - Stable fractures
  - Common in lumbar vertebra
  - Usually multiple
  - Major force is required for these fractures
  - May have associated intraabdominal or thoracic injuries.

DENIS THREE-COLUMN CONCEPT OF THORACOLUMBAR FRACTURE STABILITY

- Stability of the thoracolumbar spine depends on the integrity of three parallel vertebral columns.
- Fractures are defined as unstable if injury involves two contiguous or all three columns.
- Three columns of the thoracolumbar spine
  - Anterior column
    - Anterior longitudinal ligament
    - Anterior two-thirds of the vertebral body
    - Anterior two-thirds of the intervertebral disc

- Middle column
  - Posterior one-third of the vertebral body
  - Posterior one-third of the intervertebral disc
  - Posterior longitudinal ligament
- Posterior column
  - Pedicles
  - Facet joints and articular processes
  - Posterior bony arch
  - Ligamentum flavum
  - Interspinous ligaments
  - Supraspinous ligaments

MCAFEE CLASSIFICATION OF THORACOLUMBAR SPINE FRACTURE BASED ON THREE-COLUMN CONCEPT

- Wedge compression
  - Isolated anterior column compression fracture
- Stable burst
  - Anterior and middle column compression with normal posterior column
- Unstable burst
  - Anterior and middle column compression with disrupted posterior column
- Flexion-distraction
  - Anterior column compression
  - Middle and posterior column: tensile failure
  - Axis of flexion: posterior to anterior longitudinal ligament
- Chance fractures
  - Pure bony injuries that extend all the way through the spinal column: from posterior to anterior through the spinous process, pedicles, and vertebral body, respectively
  - Axis of flexion: anterior to (infront of) anterior longitudinal ligament
- Translational fractures
  - Shear force to all three columns usually seen in thoracic spine fracture dislocations

THORACOLUMBAR INJURY CLASSIFICATION AND SEVERITY SCALE

- The Thoracolumbar Injury Classification and Severity (TLICS) scale is based on injury mechanism/fracture morphology, integrity of the posterior ligamentous complex, and the presence of neurological injury.
- TLICS scale
  - Injury mechanism/fracture morphology (based on CT scan):   Point
    - Compression   1
    - Burst   2
    - Translation/rotation   3
    - Distraction   4
  - Integrity of the posterior ligamentous complex (based on MRI):   Point
    - Intact   0
    - Suspected/indeterminate   2
    - Injured   3
  - Neurological status (physical examination):   Point
    - Intact   0
    - Nerve root   2

- Complete cord injury   2
- Incomplete cord injury   3
- Cauda equina   3

TREATMENT RECOMMENDATION OF THORACOLUMBAR INJURIES BASED ON TLICS SCALE

- Nonsurgical management: <4
- Indeterminate (both nonsurgical and surgical) managements are acceptable: 4
- Surgical management: >4

COMMON UNSTABLE THORACOLUMBAR FRACTURES

- Burst fractures
- Chance fractures
- Fracture-dislocations
- Computerized tomography (CT) features of unstable fractures
  - Widening of the interpedicular distance
  - Subluxations
  - Pattern of fracture such as Chance or burst fractures
  - Fractures of the posterior elements (pedicles, lamina, and spinous processes)
  - Involvement of spinal canal

Must-Know Essentials: Specific Thoracolumbar Spine Fractures

CHANCE FRACTURES

- Also called seatbelt fractures
- Usually due to flexion-distraction injury mechanism in patients involved in MVC
- Majority occur at the thoracolumbar junction.
- An unstable transverse fracture of the vertebral body with associated posterior column injury
- High risk of an associated retroperitoneal and abdominal visceral injuries, such as pancreas and duodenum
- Imaging
  - Vertical separation of the posterior elements displacing the spinous processes or spinous process fracture fragments of the vertebral body
  - Transverse fractures across the transverse processes, laminae, and articular processes
  - Widening of the interpedicular distance
  - Widening of the facet joints
  - Widening of the interspinous spaces

BURST FRACTURES

- Usually due to vertical-axial compression mechanism, such as landing on the feet after falling from a significant height

- Majority involve L1 but may affect T9–L5.
- Due to disruption of a vertebral body endplate with involvement of anterior and posterior columns
- Unstable fracture with retropulsion of posterior column bone fragment into the spinal canal
- Imaging
  - Loss of vertebral height
  - Compression of both anterior and posterior portion of the vertebral body
  - Widening of interpedicular distance
  - Retropulsion of bony fragment into the spinal canal

WEDGE (COMPRESSION) FRACTURES

- Fracture of anterior vertebral body due to axial loading with flexion mechanism in patients falling from a height or MVC
- Stable fracture due to involvement of only anterior column
- Most common thoracolumbar fracture
- Imaging
  - Cortical disruption with impaction of one end plate without the involvement of the posterior wall

THORACOLUMBAR FRACTURES AND DISLOCATIONS

- Mechanism of injury
  - Hyperflexion, rotation, and shearing injury due to high-energy acceleration/deceleration MVC
  - Severe torsional and shear injury in high-energy MVC
- Majority involve thoracolumbar junction (T11–L1)
- Unstable injury
- High risk of injury to the spinal cord, conus medullaris, or cauda equina, depending on the location of the injury
- Imaging
  - CT and MRI are essential for detailed evaluation of these injuries.
  - Hyperflexion, rotation, and shearing injury may show:
    - vertebral body fracture.
    - dislocation of facet joints.
  - Severe torsional and shear injury may show:
    - horizontal displacement or rotation of one vertebral body, causing vertebral body sub-luxation/translation or rotation.
    - horizontal displacement or rotation of one vertebral body with respect to another, leading to vertebral body subluxation /translation or rotation.
    - unilateral or bilateral perched or dislocated facet joints.
    - widening of the interspinous space.
    - avulsion fracture of the superior or inferior aspects of the contiguous spinous processes.
  - Spinal canal involvement with evidence of spinal cord/cauda equina/conus medullaris injury depending on the location of injury
- Treatment: posterior spinal fusion

Must-Know Essentials: Management of Thoracolumbar Injuries

SUPPORTIVE CARE

- Spinal precautions
  - Limit the flexion, extension, rotation, and twisting of the spine to prevent exacerbation of the spinal cord injury.
- Patients with spinal cord injury
  - Prevention of hypoxia
  - Treatment of hypotension
  - Use of vasopressor to maintain mean arterial pressure (MAP) >85 mm Hg for 7 days to improve neurological outcome.

MANAGEMENT OF INJURIES

- Nonoperative management
  - Immobilization using thoracolumbar orthosis for approximately 6–12 weeks
    - Indicated for stable fractures such as:
      most of the anterior wedge compression fractures.
      stable burst fracture.
      fractures without neurological deficits with stable posterior elements.
  - Transverse process fractures
    - Usually treated with pain medication
    - May require bracing for comfort
- Operative management
  - Indications
    - Early surgical decompression and stabilization are recommended for adults with:
      complete acute spinal cord injury (SCI) regardless of the level.
      traumatic central cord syndrome.
      incomplete SCI.
      surgical intervention within 8 hours is ideal; if not possible, it should be performed within 24 hours of the injury.
      early decompression (<8 hours) improves neurological outcome, especially in patients with complete SCI.
      Surgical Timing in Acute Spinal Cord Injury Study (STASCIS) score showing at least 2 grade improvements in the American Spinal Injury Association (ASIA) Impairment score at 6 months after early (<24 hours) compared to late (>24 hours) decompression after cervical SCI.
    - unstable spine fractures based on Denis three-column concept without neurological injury.
    - fracture with TLICS score of >4.
    - significant comminution (multiple bone fragments).
    - severe loss of vertebral body height.
    - excessive forward bending or angulation at the injury site.
    - Chance fracture.
    - fracture-dislocations.

- Approach for surgical intervention depends on the location of the injury.
  - Anterior approach: indications
    - Anterior column fractures
  - Posterior approach: indications
    - Most patients with thoracolumbar fracture dislocation
    - Unstable fracture patterns
    - Disrupted posterior osteoligamentous complex
- Operative procedures
  - Decompression of the spinal canal with laminectomy
  - Reduction of the fracture for fracture dislocation
  - Stabilization of the fracture

CHAPTER 17

Evaluation and Management of Spinal Cord Injury

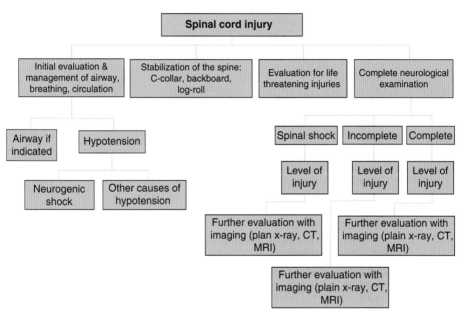

Algorithm: Evaluation of spinal cord injuries

Must-Know Essentials: Etiology and Mechanism of Spinal Cord Injury

INCIDENCE OF SPINAL CORD INJURY (SCI)

- Cervical 50%
- Thoracic 35%
- Lumbar 11%

ETIOLOGY

- Trauma accounts for more than 90% of spinal cord injuries.
- Causes include:
  - motor vehicle collision (MVC).
  - fall.

- sports injuries.
- penetrating injuries.

MECHANISM OF SCI

- Primary injury (immediate)
  - Spinal cord transection from:
    - fracture.
    - dislocation.
    - penetrating injury.
  - Spinal cord compression from:
    - epidural hematoma (EDH).
    - acute disc herniation.
  - Spinal cord infarction
    - Injury to spinal artery
- Secondary injury
  - Acute phase (<48 hours)—multiple factors, including:
    - direct cellular damage.
    - hypotension.
    - hypoxia.
    - ischemia.
    - cellular edema, inflammation, and cell necrosis due to:
      - calcium influx: free calcium-dependent excitotoxicity.
      - glutamate excitotoxicity.
      - ionic imbalance.
      - ATP depletion.
      - proinflammatory cytokine release by neutrophils and lymphocytes.
      - free radical formation.
      - lipid peroxidation.
  - Subacute phase (<14 days)—mechanism includes:
    - apoptosis.
    - demyelination of surviving axons.
    - Wallerian degeneration.
    - axonal dieback.
    - matrix remodeling.
    - evolution of a glial scar around the injury site.
  - Chronic phase (6 months)
    - Formation of a cystic cavity
    - Progressive axonal dieback
    - Maturation of the glial scar

Must-Know Essentials: Basic Spinal Cord Anatomy
SPINAL COLUMN

- The vertebral column consists of 7 cervical vertebrae, 12 thoracic vertebrae, 5 lumbar vertebrae, 5 fused sacral vertebrae, and a variable number (3–5) of coccygeal vertebrae.
- The spinal cord originates at the lower end of the medulla oblongata at the foramen magnum and ends near the L1-L2 bony level as the conus medullaris.
- The cauda equina starts below the level of the conus medullaris.

BLOOD SUPPLY TO THE SPINAL CORD

- The anterior spinal artery from the vertebral artery supplies the entire length of the anterior two-thirds of the spinal cord.
- Two posterior spinal arteries from the vertebral artery supply the entire length of the posterior one-third of the spinal cord.
- Segmental arteries to the spinal cord directly from the aorta.
- Artery of Adamkiewicz
  - Branches from left posterior intercostal artery between T8-L1
  - Enters the spinal canal in the lower thoracic region but sends branches as far cephalad as T4
  - Much of the midthoracic area is a watershed area of the arterial supply and vulnerable to ischemic injury.

SPINAL CORD PATHWAYS

- Pyramidal tracts (corticospinal tract)
  - Descending tracts from cerebral cortex to alpha motor neuron in the ventral horn of the spinal cord
  - Controls the motor function
  - Lateral corticospinal tract
    - Descends after decussating at medulla as lateral corticospinal tract
    - Upper extremity fibers are situated in the inner side and lower extremity fibers in the outer side of the spinal cord.
  - Anterior corticospinal tract
    - 10% of the uncrossed pyramidal tract from the cerebral cortex
- Spinothalamic tract
  - Ascending pathways for contralateral temperature, pain, and crude touch.
  - Lateral spinothalamic tract
    - Decussate at segmental level or shortly above their segments
  - Anterior spinothalamic tract
    - Located anteriorly within the spinal cord
    - Primarily responsible for transmitting coarse touch and pressure
  - Posterior column (fasciculus gracile and fasciculus cuneata)
    - Decussation at medulla
    - Ipsilateral in the spinal cord
    - Conveys ipsilateral fine touch, vibration, pressure sensation

ESSENTIAL MYOTOMES

- Myotomes are used to evaluate the level of motor functions.
- Key spinal myotomes
  - C5: Elbow flexors (biceps)
  - C6: Wrist extensors
  - C7: Elbow extensors (triceps)
  - C8: Finger flexors
  - T1: Finger abductors
  - L2: Hip flexors
  - L3: Knee extensors
  - L4: Ankle dorsiflexion

- L5: Long toe extensors
- S1: Ankle planter flexors

ESSENTIAL DERMATOMES

- Dermatomes are used to evaluate the level of sensory segment.
- Key spinal sensory dermatomes
  - C5: Area over deltoid
  - C6: Thumb
  - C7: Middle finger
  - C8: Little finger
  - T4: Nipple
  - T8: Xiphisternum
  - T10: umbilicus
  - T12: Symphysis pubis
  - L4: Medial aspect of calf
  - L5: Web space between first and second toes
  - S1: Lateral border of the foot
  - S3: Ischial tuberosity area
  - S5: Perineal area

Must-Know Essentials: Manifestations of Spinal Cord Injury

SPINAL SHOCK

- Acute concussive injury of the spinal cord leading to loss of all sensorimotor functions below the level of injury
- Clinical features
  - Bilateral flaccid paralysis depending on the level of injury
    - Decreased muscle tone
    - Decreased muscle power
    - Hyporeflexia or areflexia
  - Bilateral loss of sensation (temperature and pain)
  - Autonomic dysfunction because of interruption of sympathetic innervation causing
    - Orthostatic hypotension
    - Relative bradycardia from unopposed vagal stimulation
    - Warm extremities
    - Loss of bladder control: urinary retention, incontinence
    - Loss of bowel control: paralytic ileus
    - Impaired breathing
  - Bulbocavernosus reflex
    - Polysynaptic reflex involving sacral (S2-S4) segment of spinal cord
    - Involves internal/external anal sphincter contraction in response to squeezing the glans penis/clitoris or tugging on an indwelling Foley catheter
    - Absent in spinal shock
    - Early return of bulbocavernosus reflex after recovery from the spinal shock
    - Present in complete SCI

- Absent motor and sensory function after the return of bulbocavernosus reflex indicates complete SCI.
- Priapism in male patients
- May recover partially or completely after a few days to weeks

INCOMPLETE SPINAL CORD INJURIES

- Sacral sparing
  - Suggests incomplete injury with better prognosis for functional recovery
  - Characteristics
    - Presence of S4–S5 dermatome light-touch sensation
    - Presence of S4–5 dermatome pinprick sensation
    - Presence of anal sensation (S3-S5)
    - Voluntary anal sphincter contraction (S3-S5)
    - Great toe flexion (S1)
- Central cord syndrome
  - Most common incomplete spinal cord syndrome
  - Commonly seen in elderly patients with degenerative disease of the cervical spine after hyperextension injury such as MVC with whiplash injury, and after a fall
  - Injury of the central area of the spinal cord involving bilateral central corticospinal tracts and lateral spinothalamic tracts
  - Presentation
    - Bilateral motor paralysis in upper and lower extremities
    - Disproportionately greater motor impairment in upper extremities compared to lower extremities
    - Distal weakness more than proximal weakness
    - Variable degree of sensory loss in upper and lower extremities
    - Bladder dysfunction and urinary retention
- Brown-Sequard syndrome
  - Occurs after a hemisection of the spinal cord due to penetrating trauma
  - May be seen in unilateral cord compression in disc herniation, EDH, and crush injuries
  - Presentation
    - Ipsilateral motor paralysis below the level of injury
    - Ipsilateral loss of posterior column sensation (vibration, tactile discrimination, and joint position)
    - Contralateral loss of pain and temperature sensations one or two levels below the level of the injury
    - May have autonomic fiber injury leading to dysfunction of bowel and bladder
- Anterior cord syndrome
  - Injury in the anterior of the spinal cord leading to dysfunction of anterior corticospinal and spinothalamic tracts.
  - Etiology
    - Hyperflexion injury
    - Penetrating injury
  - Presentation
    - Bilateral spastic motor paralysis (paraplegia/quadriplegia) below the level of injury
    - Dissociated sensory loss
      Bilateral loss of pain and temperature sensation
      Preserved posterior column (pressure, position, and deep pressure) function

- Autonomic dysfunction below the injury
  - Bladder dysfunction
  - Bowel dysfunction
  - Sexual function
- Posterior cord syndrome
  - Injury of the posterior spinal cord affecting posterior column (fine touch, vibration, pressure, and proprioception)
  - Results from:
    - penetrating injury.
    - posterior spinal artery occlusion.
  - Characterized by ipsilateral loss of posterior column sensation below the level of injury
- Conus medullaris syndrome
  - Can be caused by severe trauma to the lower back, resulting in injury to the conus medullaris
  - Clinical presentations
    - Bilateral lower extremity weakness
    - Abnormal sensation in the lower back
    - Bowel and bladder dysfunction
    - Sexual dysfunction
    - Usually absent radicular pain
  - Cauda equina syndrome has almost similar presentations along with severe radicular pain.
- Cauda equina syndrome
  - Can be caused by severe trauma to the lower back, resulting in injury to the conus medullaris
  - Manifestation
    - Severe radicular low back pain
    - Saddle anesthesia
    - Weakness in one or both legs
    - Bowel or bladder dysfunction
    - Sexual dysfunction
  - Early decompression recommended to prevent permanent paralysis

COMPLETE SPINAL CORD INJURY

- Complete loss of motor and sensory function below the level of the injury
- No sacral sparing or islands of sparing
- Spinal shock may mimic a complete cord injury.
- Clinical features
  - Spastic paralysis with increased muscle tone and clonus
  - Hyperreflexia
  - Sensory loss below the level of injury
  - Spared sensation above the level of injury
  - Upward plantar reflex (Babinski reflex)
  - Positive bulbocavernosus reflex
  - Autonomic dysfunction
    - Spastic bladder: involuntary contraction of bladder with urinary incontinence, overflow incontinence
    - Sexual dysfunction
    - Loss of bowel control: paralytic ileus

- Impaired breathing
- Orthostatic hypotension and bradycardia

Must-Know Essentials: Evaluation and Management of Spinal Cord Injuries

INITIAL EVALUATION

- Airway, Breathing, Circulation
  - Emergent airway, breathing, and circulation are priority to prevent hypoxia and hypotension.
  - Hypoxia and hypotension can cause secondary, and deteriorating, SCI.
  - Diaphragm is innervated by the phrenic nerve, which originates from the cervical spinal cord at C3-C5.
  - High cervical cord injury paralyzes the diaphragm, leading to respiratory failure.
  - Hypotension in patients with SCI
    - Hemorrhagic shock from associated injuries
    - Neurogenic shock
      Characterized by hypotension with bradycardia
      Seen in cervical and upper thoracic SCI due to loss of sympathetic tone
    - Spinal shock: due to associated autonomic dysfunction
- Stabilization of spine
  - Prevents worsening of neurological or spinal injury
  - Methods for stabilization
    - Rigid cervical collar
    - Backboard
    - Log roll

NEUROLOGICAL EVALUATION

- Level of injury
  - Quadriplegia: spinal cord injury involving the cervical (C1-C8) segments due to injury above the first thoracic vertebra
  - Paraplegia: spinal cord injury involving thoracic and lumbar (T1- L5) segments due to injury from the base of the neck down to the sacral spine
- Extent of spinal cord injury (SCI)
  - Spinal shock
  - Complete spinal cord injury
  - Incomplete spinal cord injury
  - Sacral sparing
  - Central cord syndrome
  - Brown–Sequard syndrome
  - Anterior cord syndrome
  - Posterior cord syndrome
  - Conus medullaris syndrome
  - Cauda equina syndrome
- American Spinal Injury Association (ASIA) Score evaluation
  - Commonly used scoring system for spinal cord injury
  - Defines the extent and severity of the spinal cord injury

- It should be completed within 72 hours after the initial injury
- Based on the sensory function (scored from 0–2) and motor function (scored from 0 to 5)
  - Motor scoring
    - Grade 0: Total paralysis
    - Grade 1: Palpable or visible contraction
    - Grade 2: Active movement, gravity eliminated
    - Grade 3: Active movement against gravity
    - Grade 4: Active movement against some resistance
    - Grade 5: Normal, corrected for pain or disuse
  - Sensory grading
    - Grade 0: Absent sensation
    - Grade 1: Altered
    - Grade 2: Normal sensation
- ASIA Impairment Scale (AIS) evaluation
  - A = Complete: No motor or sensory function including sacral segments (S4-S5) below the level of injury
  - B = Incomplete: Some sensory function preserved, including sacral segments (S4-S5) but no motor function below the level of injury
  - C = Incomplete: Motor function preserved below the neurological level, and muscle grade less than 3 (no movements against gravity) for more than half of the key muscles below the neurological level
  - D = Incomplete: Motor function preserved below the neurological level, and a muscle grade of 3 or more (can move against the gravity) for at least half of the key muscles below the neurological level
  - E = Normal: Motor and sensory functions are normal.

IMAGING

- Complete evaluation of cervical/thoracic/lumbar by plain film/computerized tomography (CT)/MRI
- CT superior to plain films for diagnosing fractures
- MRI good for detailed information on ligaments, discs, EDH, and spinal cord pathology
- SCIWORA (spinal cord injury without radiographic abnormality) syndrome
  - Rare; more common in children but can be seen in adults

CARDIOPULMONARY MANAGEMENT

- Treatment of hypotension (SBP <90 mm Hg) prevents secondary injury and improves outcome after SCI.
- Cervical or high thoracic lesions can result in neurogenic shock characterized by hypotension and bradycardia.
- Other causes of hypotension must be differentiated from neurogenic shock in the management of SCI.
- Vasopressors
  - Recommended for neurogenic shock
  - To maintain mean arterial pressure (MAP) >85 mm Hg

- Norepinephrine, which has chronotropic, inotropic, and vasoconstrictor effects, is preferred.
- MAP >85 mm Hg for 7 days in patients with SCI improves neurological outcome.

NONSURGICAL MANAGEMENT

- Spine immobilization
  - Cervical spine immobilization
    - C-collar
    - Brace
    - Cervical traction
    - Halo-vest
  - Thoracolumbar immobilization
    - Brace

SURGICAL MANAGEMENT

- Early surgical decompression and stabilization are recommended for adults with:
  - complete acute spinal cord injury (SCI) regardless of the level.
  - traumatic central cord syndrome.
  - incomplete SCI.
- Surgical intervention within 8 hours is ideal; if that is not possible, it should be performed within 24 hours of the injury.
- Early decompression (<8 hours) improves neurological outcome (ASIA score), especially in patients with complete SCI.
- Surgical Timing in Acute Spinal Cord Injury Study (STASCIS) showed at least two grade improvements in the ASIA impairment scale at 6 months after early (<24 hours) compared to late (>24 hours) decompression after cervical SCI.

PREVENTION AND MANAGEMENT OF COMPLICATIONS

- SCI are associated with a high risk for complications.
- Prevention and management of the following complications are important:
  - Bradycardia: C1-C4 quadriplegia involving phrenic nerve
  - Pneumonia: in patients with thoracic and cervical cord injuries due to inability to clear respiratory secretions
  - Deep vein thrombosis: due to venous stasis secondary to paralysis
  - Pressure ulcers: due to pressure on insensate skin
  - Autonomic hyperreflexia (mass reflex)
    - Due to hollow organ over distention such as urinary bladder from urinary retention, and rectum from fecal impaction
    - Manifestations
      Severe hypertension
      Diaphoresis
      Pallor
      May develop seizures
- Urinary tract infection (UTI): due to chronic indwelling Foley catheter

REHABILITATION

- Physical therapy
- Occupational therapy

RECOVERY AFTER SCI

- Most of the functional recovery occurs during the first 3 months and in most cases reaches a plateau by 9 months.
- Spontaneous sensory recovery usually follows the motor recovery.
- Limited recovery after complete SCI
- Good neurological improvement after incomplete paraplegia and quadriplegia.
- Poor prognosis after autonomic injury
- Central cord syndrome
  - May show neurological improvement with nonoperative management with cervical spine immobilization
  - Improvement is first seen in the lower extremities; bladder and upper extremities are last to recover.
  - Surgical decompression and stabilization improve neurological outcome.
- Anterior cord syndrome: unlikely to recover

Neck Trauma

CHAPTER 18

Evaluation and Management of Blunt Neck Trauma

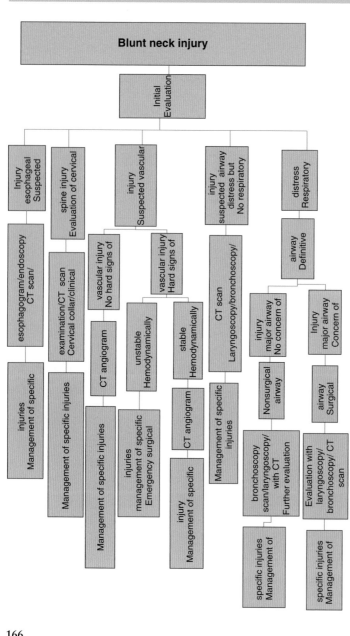

Algorithm: Blunt neck injury evaluation & management

Must-Know Essentials: Evaluation of Blunt Neck Injury

MECHANISM OF BLUNT NECK INJURIES

- Motor vehicle collision (MVC)
  - Most common cause
  - Injuries may result from:
    - steering wheel.
    - dashboard.
    - shearing force from shoulder belt.
- Hanging leading to neck strangulation
- Punching in the neck
- Chiropractic excessive manipulation leading to carotid or vertebral arterial injury

COMMON BLUNT NECK INJURIES

- Laryngotracheal injury
- Cervical spine injury with or without spinal cord injury (SCI)
- Pharyngoesophageal injury
- Blunt cerebrovascular injury
- Brachial plexus injury
- Apex of the lung injury

INITIAL EVALUATION

- Assessment of the airway
  - Definitive airway for respiratory distress
  - Causes of respiratory distress
    - Tracheal injury
    - Laryngeal injury
    - Neck hematoma
    - Tracheal or laryngeal edema
  - Surgical airway: tracheostomy
    - If suspected or confirmed airway injury
  - Nonsurgical airway: Endotracheal (ET) intubation
    - If no concern of airway injury
    - Laryngeal injury where trachea or larynx is tenuously attached can result in complete loss of the airway if the larynx detaches and dislodges into the chest during ET intubation.
- Protection of the C-spine
- Assessment for impaired breathing
  - Impaired breathing in blunt neck trauma may be due to:
    - associated hemothorax or pneumothorax in Zone I neck injury.
    - tracheobronchial obstruction from foreign body.
    - pulmonary edema in patients with strangulation.
- Assessment of the circulation
  - Hemodynamic instability
  - Hard signs of vascular injury
    - Carotid bruit
    - Expanding/pulsating hematoma

- Absent pulse
- Neurological deficit
■ Assessment for neurological deficit
- Associated cervical spine injury may cause SCI or brachial plexus injury leading to neurological deficit.
- Blunt cerebrovascular injury may result in cerebral ischemia leading to neurological deficit.

MANIFESTATION OF SPECIFIC NECK INJURIES

■ Laryngeal or tracheal injury
  - Hoarseness of voice
  - Pain on palpation or with coughing or swallowing
  - Dyspnea
  - Hemoptysis
  - Stridor
  - Subcutaneous emphysema and/or crepitus
  - Distortion of the normal anatomic appearance
■ Tracheobronchial or apical pleural or lung injury
  - Respiratory distress
  - Hoarseness or dysphonia
  - Subcutaneous emphysema
  - Respiratory distress
  - Hemoptysis
  - Tension pneumothorax
    - Decreased breath sounds
    - Hyperresonance to percussion
    - Hypotension
    - Hypoxia
■ Carotid artery injury
  - Decreased level of consciousness
  - Contralateral hemiparesis
  - Pulsatile neck hematoma
  - Dyspnea secondary to compression of the trachea
  - Bruit
  - Pulse deficit
■ Jugular vein injury
  - Hematoma
  - Hypotension
■ Esophageal and pharyngeal injury
  - Dysphagia
  - Blood in saliva
  - Blood in nasogastric aspirate
  - Pain and tenderness in the neck
  - Crepitus

IMAGING IN BLUNT NECK TRAUMA

■ Chest X -ray may reveal:
  - cervical emphysema.
  - pneumothorax.

- pneumomediastinum.
- hemothorax.
- Computerized tomography (CT) of the neck for evaluation of:
  - Cervical spine injury
  - Airway injury
  - Findings suggestive of laryngotracheal injury
    - Cervical emphysema
    - Separation in the tracheobronchial air column
    - Displacement of trachea
- CT of the chest
  - Zone I injury may demonstrate:
    - hemothorax.
    - pneumothorax.
    - widened mediastinum.
    - mediastinal emphysema.
    - apical pleural hematoma.
    - great vessel injuries.
    - mediastinal hematoma.
- CT angiography: Chest
  - Evaluation of aortic injury in Zone I blunt trauma
- CT angiography of the neck:
  - Evaluation of the suspected cervical vascular injury or for the screening of cervical vascular injury if indicated.
- Contrast esophagogram
  - Evaluation of cervical esophageal injury
  - Water-soluble iodinated contrast should be used for preliminary detection of perforation.
  - Barium-contrast esophagogram is recommended if high index of suspicion for injury with negative water-soluble contrast esophagogram.
  - Nontransmural esophageal injuries are not detected on an esophagogram.
  - Does not rule out a pharyngoesophageal leak

ENDOSCOPY

- Bronchoscopy
  - For definitive diagnosis of suspected airway injury
  - Fiberoptic bronchoscopy can be used even in patients with cervical spine injuries.
- Laryngoscopy
  - Provides information about the location and extent of injury
  - Rigid endoscopes are superior to flexible scopes.
- Esophagoscopy
  - Role of esophagoscopy in blunt injury is inconclusive.
  - It is contraindicated in patients with small mucosal or submucosal tears seen in CT scan or esophagogram. It may exacerbate the injury or cause perforation.
  - It may be performed in patients with high index of suspicion of injury despite negative CT scans and esophagograms.
  - It is not indicated as the initial diagnostic tool.
  - Flexible endoscopy and contrast esophagography are complementary and together give the highest diagnostic yield.

Must-Know Essentials: Tracheobronchial Injury

BACKGROUND

- Low incidence of tracheal injury after a blunt trauma compared to penetrating trauma
- Most blunt trauma involves the distal intrathoracic trachea and right mainstem bronchus.
- Mechanism of injury
  - Direct neck trauma causing impact against the vertebral bodies
  - MVC with sudden hyperextension injury
    - Neck hitting the steering wheel or dashboard
    - Traction and distraction injury causing laryngotracheal separation
    - Seat belt injury causing compressive and rotational impact to the neck

EVALUATION

- Patients may die immediately after the injury due to asphyxia.
- Patients may present with manifestations as described earlier
- Frequently associated with head, facial, or cervical spine injuries
- May cause vocal cord dysfunction due to associated recurrent laryngeal nerve injury
- Persistent pneumothorax or air leak may suggest intrathoracic tracheal or bronchial injury.

MANAGEMENT

- Establish a definitive nonsurgical (endotracheal tube [ETT]) or surgical (tracheostomy) airway, depending on the extent of injury.
- Nonoperative
  - Indications
    - Linear laceration involving less than one-third of the diameter of the airway
    - Mucosal tracheal injuries
  - ETT intubation with cuff inflated distal to the injury
- Operative
  - Indications
    - Tracheal injury with subcutaneous or mediastinal emphysema
    - Associated with esophageal injury
    - Open tracheal injury
  - Surgical exposure
    - Low collar incision
      - For the exposure of proximal half of the trachea
    - Left lateral neck incision along the anterior border of the sternocleidomastoid
      - For the exposure of proximal half of the trachea with associated cervical esophageal injury
    - Low collar incision with sternotomy
      - For the exposure to the middle or lower third of the trachea
    - Low collar incision with right thoracotomy
      - For the exposure to distal third of the trachea, carina, and right mainstem bronchus
    - Left thoracotomy
      - For the exposure to the left mainstem bronchus

- Steps of the proximal tracheal injury repair
  - Incision: Make a curvilinear incision two fingerbreadths above the sternal notch extending to the medial borders of the sternocleidomastoid muscles.
  - Divide the platysma muscle.
  - May ligate the anterior jugular veins bilaterally
  - Create subplatysmal flaps to expose the strap muscles (sternohyoid, sternothyroid, and thyrohyoid).
  - Split the strap muscle in the avascular midline plane to expose the trachea.
  - Divide the thyroid isthmus using electrocautery or suture ligation.
  - Protect the esophagus during dissection of the posterior surface of the membranous trachea.
  - Expose the lateral surface of the trachea by retracting the structures in the carotid sheath (common carotid artery, internal jugular vein, and the vagus nerve) and the thyroid lobes.
  - Protect the recurrent laryngeal nerves in the tracheoesophageal groove.
  - Debride the devitalized tissue and cartilage.
  - Repair the trachea.
    Small injury: Repair with absorbable interrupted 3-0 polydioxanone sutures (PDS).
    Larger injury:
      Mobilize the trachea with blunt dissection of anterior avascular pretracheal area or suprahyoid laryngeal release.
      Perform primary anastomosis with absorbable interrupted 3-0 PDS.
    Buttress the suture line with the adjacent strap muscle flap in complex repair.

Must-Know Essentials: Laryngeal Injury

BACKGROUND

- MVC is the most common cause of blunt laryngeal trauma.
- Other causes include:
  - assaults.
  - sports injuries.

CLINICAL PRESENTATIONS

- Pain or tenderness over the larynx
- Hoarseness
- Dysphagia
- Respiratory distress
- Stridor
  - Inspiratory stridor due to supraglottic obstruction from edema or a hematoma
  - Expiratory stridor due to subglottic injury
  - Biphasic stridor (inspiratory and expiratory) due to injury at the level of the glottis
- Hemoptysis
- Subcutaneous emphysema
- Loss of normal thyroid prominence
- Deviation of larynx

EVALUATION

- Airway is the priority in laryngeal injury.
- ET intubation
  - Indications
    - Laryngeal injury with stridor
    - Severe respiratory distress
    - Subcutaneous emphysema
    - Neck hematoma
  - It should be performed in the operating room with surgical support for tracheostomy for failed intubation.
- Tracheostomy
  - Indications
  - Failed intubation
  - Complex laryngeal injury
- Chest x-ray to evaluate for pneumothorax
- Computed tomography (CT) neck and chest to evaluate for:
  - laryngeal fractures.
  - vascular injuries.
  - esophageal injuries.
- Fiberoptic laryngoscopy
  - Should be performed for the initial evaluation of all laryngeal injuries
  - Secured airway is essential before the procedure.
- Rigid laryngoscopy
  - Should be performed for detailed evaluation after flexible fiberoptic laryngoscopy in patients with laryngeal injuries
- Bronchoscopy to evaluate trachea and bronchus
- Esophagoscopy to evaluate esophagus

SCHAEFER-FUHRMAN CLASSIFICATION OF LARYNGEAL INJURY

- Group I injury
  - Minor endolaryngeal hematomas or lacerations without detectable fractures
- Group II injury
  - More severe edema, hematoma, minor mucosal disruption without exposed cartilage, or nondisplaced fractures
- Group III injury
  - Massive edema, large mucosal lacerations, exposed cartilage, displaced fractures, or vocal cord immobility
- Group IV injury
  - Same as group III, but more severe, with disruption of anterior larynx, unstable fractures, two or more fracture lines, or severe mucosal injuries
- Group V injury
  - A life-threatening laryngeal injury; complete laryngotracheal separation due to injury at the level of the cricoid cartilage, either at the cricothyroid membrane or cricotracheal junction

MANAGEMENT

- Group I injury
  - Definitive airway is not indicated.
  - Observe for airway and respiratory distress.
  - Adjunctive measures
    - Elevation of head of bed helps to improve laryngeal edema.
    - Systemic corticosteroids: Supporting data are minimal, but steroids may help to reduce edema in the early hours after injury.
    - Anti-reflux medication
    - Voice rest
    - Air humidification
- Group II injury
  - Nondisplaced laryngeal fractures are treated nonoperatively.
  - A tracheotomy may be required if deterioration in breathing is due to an expanding hematoma or worsening edema.
  - Adjunctive measures as in group I injury
- Group III injury
  - Tracheotomy
  - Displaced thyroid and cricoid cartilage fractures require reduction and fixation with non-absorbable 3-0 polypropylene suture to stabilize the laryngeal framework.
  - Displaced cartilage fracture with endolaryngeal soft-tissue injury requires reduction and fixation of the fractures with nonabsorbable suture first, followed by repair of endolaryngeal soft tissue with 5-0 absorbable suture.
  - The endolarynx is generally best approached through a midline thyrotomy, along with a transverse incision through the cricothyroid membrane.
  - Repair of the vocal cord
    - Even minor lacerations of the true vocal cord margin or anterior commissure require repair.
    - Injury of the anterior attachment of the true vocal cord requires reattachment to the external perichondrium.
- Group IV injury
  - Tracheotomy
  - Head and neck surgical consultation
  - Exploration and surgical repair of the injury; may require stent placement
- Group V injury
  - Tracheostomy
  - Evaluation and treatment for pneumothorax as it is common in laryngotracheal separation injury
  - Head and neck surgical consultation
  - Repair should be performed with nonabsorbable 3-0 polypropylene sutures with the knots placed extraluminally.
  - Most laryngotracheal separations are associated with bilateral vocal cord paralysis due to recurrent laryngeal nerve injury.
    - Nerve injury may be due to stretching or tearing of the recurrent laryngeal nerves or may be due to compression near the cricoarytenoid joint.
    - The injured nerve should be repaired if possible.
    - If primary nerve repair is impossible, the ansa cervicalis may be redirected and sutured to the distal stump of the recurrent laryngeal nerve to improve vocal cord function.

Must-Know Essentials: Cervical Esophageal Injury

BACKGROUND

- Most common esophageal injury.
- Penetrating injury is more common than blunt injury.
- Blunt injury is more common in the abdominal/distal esophagus.
- MVC is the most common cause of blunt injury.
- Penetrating injuries are due to gunshot and stab wounds.
- Cervical esophageal injuries have the lowest morbidity and mortality.

ANATOMY OF THE ESOPHAGUS

- Esophagus begins at pharyngoesophageal junction, at the level of the cricoid cartilage and C6 vertebra.
- Pharyngoesophageal junction is approximately 15 cm from the incisor teeth.
- Esophagus is approximately 25 cm long and terminates in the stomach at the level of T11-T12 vertebra.
- Esophagus descends through the superior and posterior mediastinum and terminates in the cardia of the stomach.
- In the left posterior chest, the esophagus is situated on the right side of the descending thoracic aorta, then it crosses the aorta anteriorly before terminating in the cardia of the stomach on the left side of the abdominal aorta.
- Three anatomical regions of the esophagus include: cervical, thoracic, and intraabdominal.
- Layers of the esophagus: mucosa, submucosa, muscularis propria, and adventitia.
- The muscularis propria is critical for esophageal structure and function. It is composed of two layers: inner circular layer and outer longitudinal layer.
- Relations of the cervical esophagus
  - Anterior: trachea
  - Posterior: cervical spine
  - Lateral: carotid sheath containing common carotid artery, internal jugular vein, and vagus nerve bilaterally
- Arterial supply
  - Cervical esophagus
    - Inferior thyroid artery
  - Thoracic esophagus
    - Branches of the thoracic aorta
    - Branches of the bronchial arteries
  - Abdominal esophagus
    - Left gastric artery
    - Inferior phrenic artery
- Venous drainage
  - Cervical esophagus
    - Inferior thyroid vein
  - Thoracic esophagus
    - Azygous vein
    - Hemizygous vein
    - Bronchial veins
  - Abdominal esophagus
    - Coronary veins

MANIFESTATIONS

- Dysphagia
- Blood in saliva
- Blood in nasogastric aspirate
- Pain and tenderness in the neck
- Subcutaneous emphysema

EVALUATION

- Chest x-ray
  - May show mediastinal air and subcutaneous emphysema
- CT Chest
  - Gas and fluid around the esophagus
  - Esophageal wall thickening
  - Mediastinal air and subcutaneous emphysema.
- Esophagogram
  - Water-soluble contrast is commonly used for the detection of perforation.
  - Barium contrast is used if the initial esophagogram is negative, but suspicion for the presence of injury remains high.
  - The false negative rate of esophagograms is approximately 10%.
- Esophagoscopy
  - The role of esophagoscopy in nonpenetrating injury is inconclusive.
  - Contraindicated with small mucosal or submucosal tears seen in CT scan because it may exacerbate the injury or may lead to perforation
  - Recommended in patients with associated laryngeal and tracheal injuries
  - Recommended in patients with strong suspicion of injury despite negative CT scans and esophagograms

AMERICAN ASSOCIATION FOR THE SURGERY OF TRAUMA (AAST) GRADING OF ESOPHAGEAL INJURY

- Grade I
  - Contusion/hematoma, partial-thickness tear
- Grade II
  - Laceration <50% circumference
- Grade III
  - Laceration >50% circumference
- Grade IV
  - < 2 cm disruption of tissue or vasculature
- Grade V
  - >2 cm disruption of tissue or vasculature

MANAGEMENT

- Nonoperative treatment
  - Grade I blunt cervical injury with contusion/hematoma, partial-thickness tear
  - Grade II blunt trauma
    - Very small perforation with contained leak
    - Minimal symptoms
    - Hemodynamically stable

- Supportive care
  - Nothing by mouth (NPO)
  - Careful insertion of nasogastric tube
  - Broad-spectrum antibiotics
  - Fluid resuscitation
- Repeat esophagogram after a few days to reassess for the leak before starting an enteral diet
- May require:
  - drainage of the collection in the neck by interventional radiology.
  - gastrostomy tube placement.
- Operative management
  - Surgery is recommended in most esophageal injuries with perforation
  - The degree of inflammation in surrounding tissues, rather than the time of the initial injury, determines the choice of primary repair versus drainage.
  - Lack of a serosal layer makes any esophageal repair more tenuous with high risk of breakdown.
  - Surgical steps of repair
    - Place the patient in the supine position with the neck extended and turned to the right side.
    - If possible, carefully place a nasogastric tube.
    - Make a longitudinal left neck incision along the anterior border of the sternocleido-mastoid muscle.
    - Divide the omohyoid muscle.
    - Open the investing fascia.
    - Retract the sternocleidomastoid muscle laterally.
    - Bluntly spread the areolar tissues.
    - Retract the carotid sheath laterally.
    - Dissect the esophagus between the vertebral body posteriorly, trachea anteriorly, and carotid sheath laterally.
    - Limit the mobilization of the esophagus to prevent segmental ischemia.
    - Protect the left recurrent laryngeal nerve, which is located posterior to the trachea in the tracheoesophageal groove.
    - Use a nasogastric tube helps to identify the esophagus.
    - Place a Penrose drain encircling the esophagus.
    - Identify the injury.
    - Debride the nonviable tissue.
    - Extend the muscular defect to identify the mucosal injury.
    - Repair the injury in two layers:
      - Inner mucosal layer with running 3/0 PDS absorbable suture
      - Outer muscular layer with interrupted 3/0 silk nonabsorbable suture
      - Buttress the repair with the sternocleidomastoid muscle. Other muscles, such as the platysma, omohyoid, and strap muscles, can also be used as an alternative.
    - Place a Jackson-Pratt (JP) drain at the site of the repair.
    - Close the incision in layers.
    - If the patient is stable:
      - Perform a gastrostomy for decompression.
      - Perform a jejunostomy for feeding.
- Damage control procedures
  - Recommended in patients where primary repair is not possible:
    - Significant inflammation in the surrounding tissue due to delay in diagnosis
    - Extensive injury in unstable patients

- Irrigation and placement of a drain
- Esophageal diversion
    - Diverting cervical esophagostomy
        Place a 16-French Levin tube and advance it into the stomach, or place a T-tube directly through the injury.
        Secure the tube to the skin.
        Place a JP drain at the injury site and secure it to the skin.
        Close the skin or place a wound vac.
    - Esophageal exclusion with diversion
        Perform a cervical esophagostomy or T-tube diversion proximal to the excluded esophagus.
        Close the distal esophagus at the gastroesophageal (GE) junction with absorbable sutures or a stapling device through a laparotomy.
- Place a gastrostomy tube for decompression.
- Place a jejunostomy tube for feeding.

Must-Know Essentials: Blunt Cerebral Vascular Injury

BACKGROUND

- Incidence of blunt cerebral vascular injury (BCVI) after neck trauma in the United States
    - 0.1% in patients with symptomatic cerebral ischemia
    - 1%–2 % in asymptomatic patients after screening for BCVI
- BCVI may cause dissection, thrombosis, occlusion, or pseudoaneurysm of the carotid and vertebral cerebral vessels, resulting in cerebral ischemia leading to stroke or transient ischemic attacks.
- Mechanism of injury
    - Cervical hyperextension and rotation, hyperflexion injury
    - Direct blow to cervical spine
- High-risk factors for BCVI, as in the Denver and the Memphis screening criteria
- Delayed diagnosis is associated with high morbidity and mortality.

SCREENING CRITERIA FOR BCVI

- Modified Memphis Screening Criteria
    - Base of skull fracture with involvement of carotid canal
    - Base of skull fracture with involvement of petrous temporal bone
    - Cervical spine fracture
    - Neurological examination finding not explained by neuroimaging
    - Horner syndrome: due to disruption of oculosympathetic pathway. Features include:
        - ipsilateral enophthalmos.
        - pupillary miosis.
        - anhidrosis.
    - Partial drooping of upper eyelid (partial ptosis)
    - Le Fort type II or III fracture pattern (unilateral or bilateral)
    - Neck soft-tissue injury (seatbelt injury, hanging, hematoma)
- Expanded Denver Screening Criteria
    - Signs/symptoms of BCVI
        - Arterial hemorrhage from neck/nose/mouth
        - Cervical bruit in patients <50 years

- Expanding cervical hematoma
- Focal neurological deficit: transient ischemic attack (TIA), hemiparesis, vertebrobasilar symptoms, Horner syndrome
- Neurological examination incongruous with head CT findings
- Stroke on secondary CT scan or MRI scan
- Risk factors for BCVI (high-energy transfer mechanism with:
- midface fracture: Le Fort type II or III fracture.
- mandible fracture.
- complex skull fracture/basilar skull fracture/occipital condyle fracture
- Severe traumatic brain Injury (TBI) with Glasgow Coma Scale (GCS) <6
- Cervical spine fracture, subluxation, or ligament injury at any level
- Near hanging with anoxic brain injury
- Seat-belt abrasion with significant swelling, pain, or altered mental status
- TBI with thoracic injury
- Scalp degloving
- Thoracic vascular injury
- Upper ribs fracture

SCREENING MODALITY FOR BCVI

- Level I: No level I recommendation
- Four-vessel cerebral angiography (FVCA)
  - Remains the gold standard
  - Higher risk of procedure-related complication such as stroke, pseudoaneurysm, and hematoma at the site of vessel puncture
- Duplex ultrasound: not adequate for screening
- Computed tomographic angiography (CTA)
  - Four (or less)-slice multidetector is neither sensitive nor specific enough for the screening.
  - Eight (or greater)-slice multidetector has a detection rate of BCVI comparable to FVCA.
  - Recommended for screening of BCVI
- Magnetic Resonance Angiography (MRA)
  - Sensitivity and specificity are comparable to CTA.

BIFFL SCALE FOR GRADING BCVI

- Grade I
  - Luminal irregularity or dissection with <25% luminal narrowing
- Grade II
  - Dissection or intramural hematoma with ≥25% luminal narrowing
  - Intraluminal thrombosis
  - Raised intimal flap
- Grade III
  - Pseudoaneurysm
- Grade IV
  - Occlusion
- Grade V
  - Transection with free extravasation

TREATMENT OF BCVI

- Incidence of stroke after BCVI
  - Up to 50% after carotid artery injury
  - Between 20%–25% after vertebral artery injury
- Stroke rates directly correlate with increasing grades of injury.
- Early antithrombotic therapy in asymptomatic patients with BCVI reduces or nearly eliminates BCVI-related strokes.
- Anticoagulation and antiplatelet agents are equally effective to prevent stroke in BCVI.
- Heparin
  - Preferred in patients with increased risk of bleeding
  - Unfractionated heparin dose: 15 units/kg/hour without a loading dose with a goal partial thromboplastin time (PTT) between 40 and 50 seconds in patients with risk of bleeding
  - Subcutaneous low-molecular-weight heparin (LMWH; fractionated heparin) may be used as an alternative at an antithrombotic dose (1 mg/kg body weight) daily.
- Antiplatelets
  - Clopidogrel (Plavix) 75 mg daily or aspirin 325 mg daily: Both are equally effective.
  - May be used in patients where heparin is contraindicated
  - Not recommended in injured patients with high risk of bleeding
- Treatment based on the grading
  - Grade I and II injuries
    - Usually heal completely
    - May develop a pseudoaneurysm
    - Treated with antithrombotic medications
    - Follow-up angiogram after 7 days and 30 days
    - Management of persistent narrowing in asymptomatic patients after 3–6 months is controversial.
    - Persistent narrowing in symptomatic patients after 3–6 months may be treated with continued antithrombotic medications or endovascular intervention with antithrombotic medications.
  - Grade III injuries
    - Rarely resolves
    - May develop thrombosis and cerebral embolism
    - Treated with surgery or endovascular stents
    - Surgery is strongly recommended for larger pseudoaneurysms (>4 cm)
    - Post-stent antithrombotic medications (antiplatelet or anticoagulation)
    - Follow-up angiogram after 7 days and 30 days
  - Grade IV
    - May recanalize, can cause cerebral embolic events
    - Treatment
      - Thrombectomy recommended in surgically accessible areas
      - Endovascular stents in inaccessible areas.
      - Double platelets after surgery and stents recommended
    - Follow-up angiogram after 7 days and 30 days

- Grade V
  - Open vascular reconstruction if surgically accessible
  - Endovascular stent in surgically inaccessible areas
  - Postoperative anticoagulation or antiplatelet
  - Follow-up angiogram after 7 days and 30 days

CHAPTER 19

Evaluation and Management of Penetrating Neck Injuries

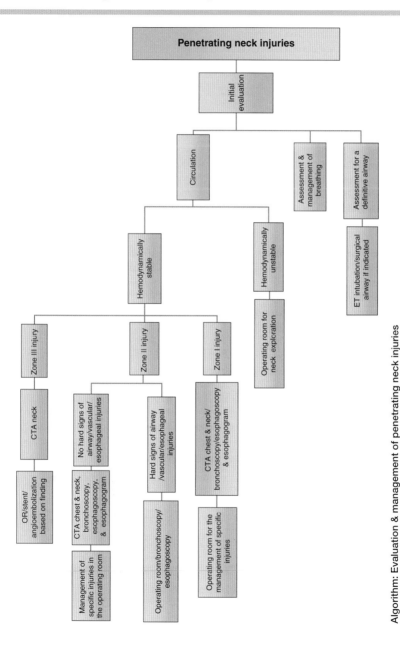

Algorithm: Evaluation & management of penetrating neck injuries

Must-Know Essentials: Anatomical Zones of Penetrating Neck Injuries

ZONE 1

- Extends between the clavicle and sternal notch inferiorly to a horizontal plane passing through the cricoid cartilage superiorly
- Structures
  - Proximal common carotid arteries
  - Vertebral and subclavian arteries
  - Subclavian, innominate, and jugular veins
  - Trachea
  - Recurrent laryngeal nerves
  - Vagus nerves
  - Brachial plexus
  - Esophagus
  - Thoracic duct (left-sided injury)
  - Thymus
  - Thyroid gland
  - Parathyroid gland
  - Spinal cord

ZONE 2

- Extends between a horizontal plane passing through the cricoid cartilage inferiorly to a horizontal plane passing through the angle of the mandible superiorly
- Structures
  - Common carotid artery
  - Internal and external carotid arteries
  - Jugular and vertebral veins
  - Pharynx
  - Larynx
  - Recurrent laryngeal nerves
  - Vagus nerve
  - Spinal cord

ZONE 3

- Extends between the horizontal plane passing through the angle of the mandible inferiorly to the base of the skull superiorly
- Structures
  - Extracranial internal carotid arteries
  - Vertebral arteries
  - Jugular veins
  - Cranial nerves IX–XII
  - Sympathetic trunk
  - Spinal cord

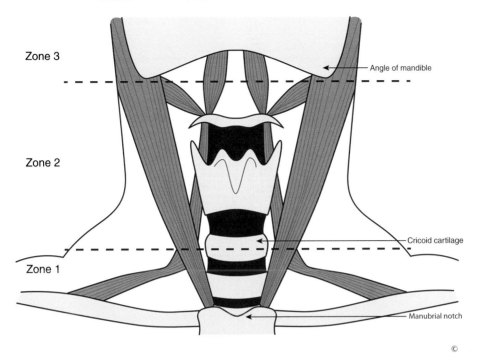

Coronal view: Anatomical zones of injury

LARYNX AND TRACHEA

- The larynx and the trachea are the most anterior structures in the neck.
- Larynx
  - Three paired cartilages
    - Arytenoid
    - Corniculate
    - Cuneiform
  - Three unpaired cartilages
    - Thyroid
    - Cricoid
    - Epiglottis
  - Thyrohyoid membrane: fibrous tissue that connects thyroid cartilage to the hyoid bone
  - Cricothyroid membrane: membranous tissue that connects the cricoid cartilage to the thyroid cartilage
  - Trachea begins at the cricoid cartilage.
- Trachea
  - Extends from the cricoid cartilage to the carina, which corresponds to C6–T5
  - Approximately10–12 cm long
  - 1.5–2.5 cm in transverse diameter
  - Extends into the superior mediastinum and divides into right and left branches at the carina, which corresponds to the fifth thoracic vertebrae level and sternal angle

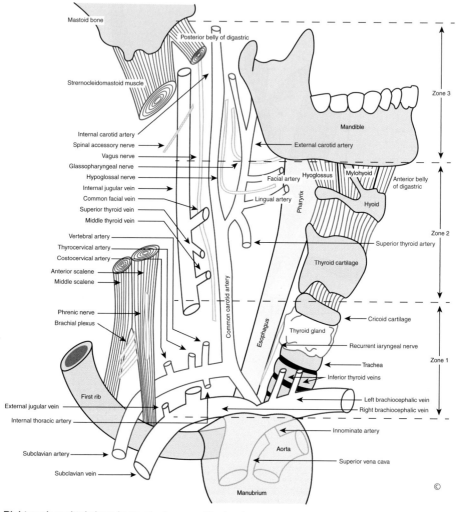

Right neck sagittal view: Anatomical zones with structures

- Has 16 to 20 C-shaped incomplete cartilaginous rings on the anterolateral surface.
- Posterior wall composed of muscle and fibrous tissue
- Relations of the trachea
  - Anterior
    - Platysma
    - Paired strap muscles: sternohyoid, sternothyroid, and thyrohyoid
    - Thyroid isthmus
- Lateral
  - Sternocleidomastoid muscle
  - Carotid sheath containing common carotid artery, internal jugular vein, and vagus nerve
  - Thyroid lobes
  - Recurrent laryngeal nerves lie in the tracheoesophageal groove.

- Posterior
  - The esophagus is posterior to the trachea.

ARTERIES IN THE NECK

- Subclavian artery
  - Right subclavian originates from the innominate (brachiocephalic) artery on the left.
  - Left subclavian artery originates from the aortic arch.
  - Courses laterally, passing between the anterior and middle scalene muscles
  - Three parts
    - First part: from the origin to the medial border of the anterior scalene muscle, deep to the sternocleidomastoid and strap muscles
    - Second part: posterior to the anterior scalene muscle and superficial to the upper and middle trunks of the brachial plexus
    - Third part: lateral to the anterior scalene muscle and superficial to the lower trunk of the brachial plexus
  - Continues as axillary artery at the level of the inferior border of the middle third of the clavicle
  - Branches of subclavian artery
    - First part
      - Vertebral artery
      - Internal thoracic artery (internal mammary artery)
      - Thyrocervical trunk and branches
        - Inferior thyroid artery
        - Ascending cervical artery
        - Suprascapular artery
    - Second part
      - Costocervical trunk and branches
        - Deep cervical artery
        - Superior (supreme) intercostal artery
    - Third part
      - Dorsal scapular artery
        - May arise from the first or second part of the cervical artery
- Common carotid artery
  - Right common carotid artery is a branch from the innominate (Brachiocephalic) artery. Brachiocephalic artery is also called brachiocephalic trunk.
  - Left common carotid artery originates directly from the aortic arch in the superior mediastinum.
  - Common carotid artery divides into internal and external carotid arteries at the level of the superior border of the thyroid cartilage.
- Internal carotid artery
  - Does not have any extracranial branches
  - Enters the carotid canal behind the styloid process
- External carotid artery
  - Lies medial to the internal carotid artery
  - Branches
    - Superior thyroid artery: first branch near the carotid bifurcation
    - Lingual artery
  - Ascending pharyngeal artery
  - Facial artery

- Occipital artery
- Posterior auricular artery
- Superficial temporal artery: terminal branch
- Maxillary artery: terminal branch
- Terminates in the parotid gland and divides into the superficial temporal and maxillary arteries
- Carotid sheath: contents
  - Common and internal carotid arteries medially
  - Internal jugular vein laterally
  - Vagus nerve posteriorly between the arteries and the vein
- Vertebral artery
  - First cephalad branch from the first part of the subclavian artery.
  - Enters the foramen transversarium of C6 at the cricoid level and continues in the vertebral canal up to the C1 level
  - Enters the base of the skull through the foramen magnum
  - Joins the opposite vertebral artery to form the basilar artery
- Important relations
  - Hypoglossal nerve (cranial nerve XII): crosses superficially to the external carotid arteries at the level of the angle of mandible.
  - Glossopharyngeal nerve (cranial nerve IX): located in front of the internal carotid artery above the hypoglossal nerve
  - Posterior belly of digastric muscle: crosses the external carotid artery at the level of the angle of the mandible
  - Facial vein: crosses the carotid sheath superficially to enter the internal jugular vein at the level of the carotid bifurcation

VEINS IN THE NECK

- External jugular veins
  - Formed by retromandibular vein and posterior auricular vein
  - Start at the level of the angle of the mouth in the parotid gland, run along the posterior border of the sternocleidomastoid muscle, and join the subclavian vein
- Internal jugular veins
  - Begin at the sigmoid sinus and enter the neck through the jugular foramen at the base of the skull
  - Join the subclavian veins and form brachiocephalic veins
  - Branches
    - Facial veins
    - Lingual veins
    - Pharyngeal veins
    - Superior and middle thyroid veins
  - The left thoracic duct drains at the junction of the left subclavian vein and the internal jugular vein.
  - In the carotid sheath, the internal jugular vein lies lateral and superficial to the common carotid artery and the vagus nerve.
  - The facial veins cross the carotid sheaths superficially to enter the internal jugular veins at the level of the carotid bifurcation.
- Subclavian veins
  - Continuation of the axillary vein at the level of the outer border of the first rib
  - Situated anterior to the anterior scalene muscles
  - Connect to the internal jugular veins at the medial border of the anterior scalene muscles

- Brachiocephalic veins
  - Formed from the union of the subclavian veins with the internal jugular veins
  - The left and right brachiocephalic veins join to form the superior vena cava.
  - The thoracic duct drains into the left subclavian vein at its junction with the left internal jugular vein.
  - The right lymphatic duct (right thoracic duct) drains into the junction of the right subclavian vein and right internal jugular vein.

NERVES IN THE NECK

- Vagus nerves
  - Situated in the carotid sheaths posterior to the common carotids medially and internal jugular veins laterally
  - Right vagus nerve
    - Located on the anterior surface of the first part of the right subclavian artery medial to the internal mammary (internal thoracic) artery
  - Left vagus nerve
    - Located between the left common carotid and the subclavian arteries medial to the internal mammary (internal thoracic) artery
- Recurrent laryngeal nerve
  - Right recurrent laryngeal nerve
    - Branches from the right vagus nerve as it crosses the right subclavian artery
    - Loops behind the right subclavian artery and ascends posterior to the carotid artery into the tracheoesophageal groove
  - Left recurrent laryngeal nerve
    - Branches from the left vagus nerve at it crosses the aortic arch
    - Loops around the aortic arch and ascends into the tracheoesophageal groove
- Phrenic nerves
  - Located on the anterior surface of the anterior scalene muscles
  - Situated lateral to the internal mammary (internal thoracic) arteries
- Brachial plexus
  - Located between the anterior and middle scalene muscles

CERVICAL ESOPHAGUS

- Begins at the pharyngoesophageal junction, which corresponds to the level of the cricoid cartilage, and the sixth cervical vertebral body
- On esophagoscopy, the pharyngoesophageal junction is approximately 15 cm from the incisor teeth.
- The esophagus is approximately 25 cm long and terminates in the stomach at the level of T11–12.
- Descends through the superior and posterior mediastinum and terminates in the cardia of the stomach
- Divided into three main anatomical regions: cervical, thoracic, and intraabdominal esophagus
- Layers of the esophagus: mucosa, submucosa, muscularis propria, and adventitia
- Muscularis propria is critical to esophageal structure and function. It is composed of two layers: inner circular layer and outer longitudinal layer.
- Relations of the cervical esophagus
  - Anterior: Trachea
  - Posterior: Cervical spine

- Lateral: Carotid sheath containing common carotid artery, internal jugular vein, and vagus nerve bilaterally
- Arterial supply: Inferior thyroid artery
- Venous drainage: Inferior thyroid vein.

Must-Know Essentials: Evaluation and Management of Penetrating Neck Injuries

INITIAL EVALUATION AND MANAGEMENT

- Commonly due to gunshot and stab wounds
- Transcervical gunshot wounds result in more severe injuries.
- Injuries depend on the involved anatomical neck zones.
- Airway
  - Causes of respiratory distress
    - Airway injuries
    - Vascular injuries with hematomata leading to airway obstruction
    - Spinal cord injuries
  - Management
    - Definitive airway for respiratory distress
      - ET intubation
      - Surgical airway: tracheostomy/cricothyroidotomy
    - If suspected or confirmed of airway injury
    - Definitive airway, which include ET intubation or surgical airway (tracheostomy/cricothyroidotomy)
- Breathing
  - Causes of impaired breathing
    - Spinal cord injury involving C4–C5 levels, leading to diaphragmatic paralysis
    - Pneumothorax or hemothorax in lower neck injuries
  - Management
    - Intubation and ventilatory support in spinal cord injury (SCI)
    - Chest tube thoracostomy for pneumothorax or hemothorax
- Circulation
  - Causes of hypotension
    - Vascular injury with active bleeding
    - Neurogenic shock due to spinal cord injury
    - Air embolism due to major venous injury
  - Management
    - Control of bleeding
      - Direct pressure on the bleeding wound
      - Placement of a Foley catheter into the wound and inflation of the balloon catheter with sterile water
    - In suspected air embolism, placement of the patient in the Trendelenburg position with occlusion of the wound with a dressing
    - In patient with suspected subclavian venous injury, placement of IV access in the arm opposite the side of the neck injury
    - Resuscitation with crystalloids and blood transfusion

EVALUATION FOR SPECIFIC INJURIES

- Considered in hemodynamically stable asymptomatic patients or patients without hard signs of injuries

- Zone I injury
  - Physical examination
    - Highly sensitive (95%) for detecting arterial vascular injury
    - Low sensitivity for venous injuries
    - Low sensitivity for aerodigestive tract injuries
  - CT angiogram of the chest and neck
    - Evaluation of vascular and initial evaluation of aerodigestive injuries
  - Esophagography/esophagoscopy
    - Detailed evaluation of esophageal injury
    - Both esophagography and esophagoscopy are equally effective for the evaluation of esophageal injury.
- Zone II injury
  - Mandatory neck exploration of Zone II injuries has a high negative exploration rate.
  - Selective operative management after evaluation is recommended to minimize unnecessary operation (Eastern Association for the Surgery of Trauma [EAST] Level I recommendation).
  - Computed tomographic angiography (CTA) of the neck for the evaluation of vascular and initial evaluation of aerodigestive injury
  - Bronchoscopy for the detailed evaluation of the airway injury
  - Esophagography/esophagoscopy
    - Detailed evaluation of esophageal injury
    - Detailed evaluation of esophageal injury
    - Both esophagography and esophagoscopy are equally effective for the evaluation of esophageal injury.
- Zone III injury
  - CTA of the neck and head to evaluate for vascular and initial evaluation of aerodigestive injuries
  - Aerodigestive or pharyngeal injuries
    - Contrast swallow studies are less sensitive.
    - Flexible nasoendoscopy or video endoscopy is recommended for detailed evaluation.

INDICATIONS FOR SURGICAL INTERVENTION

- Hemodynamically unstable patients
- Hemodynamically patients with hard signs of injury
  - Compromised airway
  - Respiratory distress
    - Hoarseness
    - Hemoptysis
    - Air bubbling through the wound
    - Massive subcutaneous emphysema
  - Vascular injury
    - Expanding hematoma
    - Pulsatile active bleeding
    - Bruit/thrill
    - Neurological deficit from cerebrovascular injury
    - Shock
  - Digestive tract injury
    - Hematemesis
    - Dysphagia

- Hemodynamically stable patients
  - Zone I injury
    - Positive arterial or aerodigestive injury after evaluation
    - Endovascular covered stents may be considered as indicated
  - Zone II injury
    - Mandatory operative neck exploration with intraoperative evaluation of trachea and esophagus with bronchoscopy and esophagoscopy can be considered.
    - Mandatory neck exploration has a high negative exploration rate.
    - Selective operative management if positive arterial or aerodigestive injury after evaluation
  - Zone III injury
    - Positive vascular and aerodigestive injuries after evolution
    - Some vascular injuries may require interventional radiology for angioembolization.

SURGICAL EXPOSURE IN PENETRATING NECK INJURIES

- Zone I injuries
  - Collar incision
    - Preferred incision for central injuries
    - Used for repair of the central airway injury
    - Skin wound can be incorporated into the incision.
    - Can be extended to either side of the neck
    - Can be joined with sternocleidomastoid incision
    - Can be extended down for median sternotomy
  - Sternocleidomastoid incision
    - Most of the structures including the carotid arteries, the jugular vein, the vertebral artery, and the cervical aerodigestive tract can be exposed with this incision.
    - Can be extended down for median sternotomy for access to the thoracic inlet and up to the mastoid process to expose the vertebral artery and the distal internal carotid artery
    - Can be joined with a collar incision for the complete exposure of all neck structures
  - Clavicular incision
    - For the exposure of subclavian vascular injuries
    - May require excision of the clavicle
    - May be combined with median sternotomy for exposure of the proximal subclavian vessels
- Zone II injuries
  - Transverse collar incision
    - Good for transcervical injuries
  - Collar incision
  - Collar incision with extension to sternocleidomastoid incision
  - Sternocleidomastoid incision
  - Median sternotomy may be required with any of the above incisions for proximal control of the vessels.
- Zone III injuries
  - Difficult exposure for distal vascular control
  - Sternocleidomastoid incision
  - Exposure of the distal internal carotid artery usually requires extension of the incision around the ear with subluxation of the mandible.

COLLAR INCISION

- Steps
  - Place the head in the midline position.
  - Extend the extension using shoulder rolls if no there is no concern of C-spine injury.
  - Prepare the neck, chest, and both sides of the groin.
  - Make a curvilinear incision two fingerbreadths above the sternal notch extending to the medial borders of the sternocleidomastoid muscles.
  - If possible, incorporate any existing wound in the incision.
  - Divide the platysma muscle.
  - May ligate the anterior jugular veins bilaterally.
  - Create subplatysmal flaps to expose the strap muscles (sternohyoid, sternothyroid, and thyrohyoid).
  - Split the strap muscle in the avascular midline plane to expose the trachea.
  - Divide the thyroid isthmus using electrocautery or suture ligation.
  - Identify the structures.
    - Posterior membranous trachea lies on the anterior surface of esophagus.
    - Expose the lateral surfaces of the trachea and esophagus by retracting the structures in the carotid sheath (common carotid artery, internal jugular vein, and vagus nerve) and the thyroid lobes.
    - Protect the recurrent laryngeal nerves, which lie in the tracheoesophageal groove.
  - Identify the injuries.

STERNOCLEIDOMASTOID INCISION

- Steps
  - Extend the neck with shoulder roll and rotate the head to the opposite side.
  - Prepare the neck, chest, and both sides of the groin.
  - Make a skin incision along the anterior border of the anterior sternocleidomastoid muscle, extending just below the mastoid process proximally to the sternal notch distally.
  - Curve the proximal incision posteriorly to avoid injury to the marginal mandibular branch of the facial nerve.
  - Divide the platysma muscle in the line of incision to expose the anterior border of the sternocleidomastoid muscle.
  - Identify the middle cervical fascia (areolar tissue) and retract the sternocleidomastoid muscle laterally.
  - Identify and protect the accessory (cranial nerve XI) nerve at the upper part of the incision as it enters the sternocleidomastoid muscle.
  - If desired, divide the omohyoid muscle for better exposure of the proximal carotid sheath.
  - If desired, ligate and divide the common facial vein to expose the carotid bifurcation.
  - Ligate and divide a few small branches of the external carotid artery.
  - Incise the carotid sheath longitudinally and identify the carotid artery, internal jugular vein, and vagus nerve.
  - Manipulation of the carotid body at the carotid bifurcation may cause hypotension and bradycardia; prevent that with injection of 1% lidocaine in the carotid body.
  - Identify and protect the ansa cervicalis and the hypoglossal nerve at the carotid bifurcation.
  - Identify the injuries.

- Exposure of the distal internal carotid artery and proximal common carotid artery for the control of vessels may be required.
- Exposure of the distal internal carotid artery
  - Perform subluxation of the mandible.
  - Extend the incision posteriorly around the ear.
  - Divide the posterior belly of the digastric, stylohyoid, stylopharyngeus, and styloglossus muscles.
  - Remove the styloid process.
  - Avoid injury to the glossopharyngeal nerve (cranial nerve IX) deep to the posterior digastric muscle during division of the posterior belly of the digastric and stylohyoid muscles.
- Perform a median sternotomy for exposure of the proximal common carotid artery and the proximal internal jugular vein.

CLAVICULAR INCISION

- Steps
  - Extend the neck with a shoulder roll and rotate the head to the opposite side.
  - Prepare the neck, chest, and both sides of the groin.
  - Make an incision starting at the sternoclavicular junction and extend it over the medial half of the clavicle.
  - Curve the incision downward into the deltopectoral groove in the middle of the clavicle.
  - Detach the muscles (platysma and clavicular head of the sternocleidomastoid, pectoralis major, and subclavius) attached to the medial half of the clavicle.
  - With a Gigli saw, divide the clavicle close to the sternoclavicular junction or excise the medial half of the clavicle for the exposure of the subclavian vessels.
  - The subclavian veins are the most superficial structures posterior to the clavicle.
  - The subclavian arteries are posterior to the anterior scalene muscles. Divide the strap muscles and the anterior scalene muscle to expose the first and second parts of the subclavian artery.
  - Identify and protect the phrenic nerve as it lies anterior to the anterior scalene muscle.
  - During right subclavian artery dissection, protect the right recurrent laryngeal nerve.
  - Identify and protect the left thoracic duct during left subclavian vein dissection, as it connects with the vein at the junction of the left subclavian vein and the left internal jugular vein.
  - If needed, perform a median sternotomy for proximal control of the subclavian vessels.

American Association for the Surgery of Trauma (AAST) Grading of Vascular Neck Injury

GRADE I

- Injury to thyroid vein
- Injury to facial vein
- Injury to external jugular vein
- Injury to unnamed arterial/venous branches

GRADE II

- Injury to external carotid arterial branches
- Injury to thyrocervical trunk or primary branches

- Injury to internal jugular vein
- Injury to external carotid artery

GRADE III

- Injury to subclavian vein
- Injury to vertebral artery
- Injury to common carotid artery

GRADE IV

- Injury to subclavian artery

GRADE V

- Injury to internal carotid artery (extracranial)

(NOTE: Increase one grade for multiple Grade III or IV injuries involving more than 50% vessel circumference. Decrease one grade for less than 25% vessel circumference disruption for Grade IV or V).

MANAGEMENT OF CAROTID ARTERY INJURY

- Carotid artery injury can result in significant neurological deficit.
- Early revascularization (within 4-6 hours) is recommended.
- Common and internal carotid artery injuries
  - Ligation may be considered in delayed presentation (>6 hours) in comatose patient with uncontrolled bleeding. Delayed revascularization may convert an ischemic stroke into hemorrhagic stroke.
- Damage control: Temporary shunt followed by delayed reconstruction
- Small injuries: Repair the injury with 5-0 polypropylene nonabsorbable suture.
  - Complex injuries
    - Intraoperative prophylactic shunt to prevent ischemic stroke
    - Repair with patch angioplasty using a vein patch (saphenous vein or external jugular vein) or synthetic material (Dacron, polytetrafluoroethylene [PTFE], bovine pericardium).
    - Repair with an interposition graft using a reverse saphenous vein or prosthetic material (Dacron, PTFE).
- The external carotid artery and its branches can be ligated.
- Endovascular stent graft
  - May be considered in a hemodynamically stable patient with Zone I and Zone II carotid artery injuries

MANAGEMENT OF SUBCLAVIAN ARTERY INJURY

- Procedures
  - Damage control: Temporary shunt followed by delayed reconstruction in hemodynamically unstable patient
  - Small injuries: Repair with 5-0 polypropylene nonabsorbable suture
  - Complex laceration: Reconstruction with 6-mm or 8-mm PTFE or saphenous vein graft
  - Endovascular stent graft: May be considered in a hemodynamically stable patient

MANAGEMENT OF VERTEBRAL ARTERY INJURIES

- A rare injury
- Exposure of the vertebral artery is difficult.
- Damage control
  - Pack the wound with local hemostatic agents if vertebral artery injury is suspected during neck exploration for trauma, followed by postoperative angioembolization.
  - Ligate the origin of the artery with uncontrolled bleeding.
- Hemodynamically stable patient
  - Angioembolization is the treatment of choice.

MANAGEMENT OF SUBCLAVIAN VEIN INJURIES

- Damage control: Ligate the vein in unstable patients. It is well tolerated.
- Repair
  - If there is no concern of significant stenosis (>50%) in stable patients, use 5-0 polypropylene.
  - Stenosis increases the risk of thrombosis and pulmonary embolism.

MANAGEMENT OF INTERNAL JUGULAR VEIN INJURIES

- Unilateral injury
  - Damage control: Ligate the vein in unstable patients. It is well tolerated.
  - Repair
    - If there is no concern of significant stenosis (>50%) in stable patients, use 5-0 polypropylene sutures.
    - Buttress the repair with the strap muscles if there are associated tracheal or esophageal injuries.
- Bilateral injuries
  - Consider repair of the vein on at least one side.

MANAGEMENT OF CERVICAL ESOPHAGEAL INJURIES

- Described in Chapter 18.

MANAGEMENT OF LARYNGEAL AND TRACHEAL INJURIES

- Described in Chapter 18.

Chest Trauma

CHAPTER 20

Emergency Thoracotomies

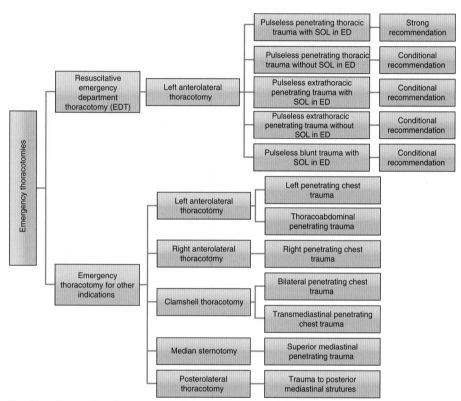

Algorithm: Approaches for emergency thoracotomies

Must-Know Essentials: Anatomy of the Chest

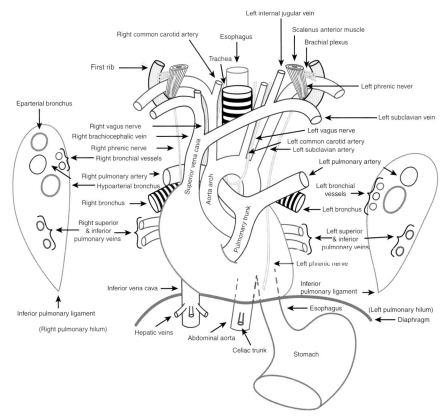

Thoracic anatomy: Anterior-posterior view

THORACIC MEDIASTINAL STRUCTURES (SEE ILLUSTRATIONS)

- Ascending aorta
    - Two main coronary arteries originate from the root of the ascending aorta.
        - The left main coronary artery branches into the left anterior descending artery (LAD) and the circumflex artery to supply the left heart.
        - The right coronary artery branches into the right posterior descending artery and acute marginal arteries to supply the right heart, sinoatrial (SA) node, and atrioventricular (AV) node.
- Aortic arch and its branches
    - Innominate (brachiocephalic) artery: first branch of the aortic arch
    - Left common carotid artery
    - Left subclavian artery
- Thoracic (descending) aorta
    - Begins just distal to the left subclavian artery on the left side of T4 vertebra and continues as the abdominal aorta at the level of T12 vertebra.

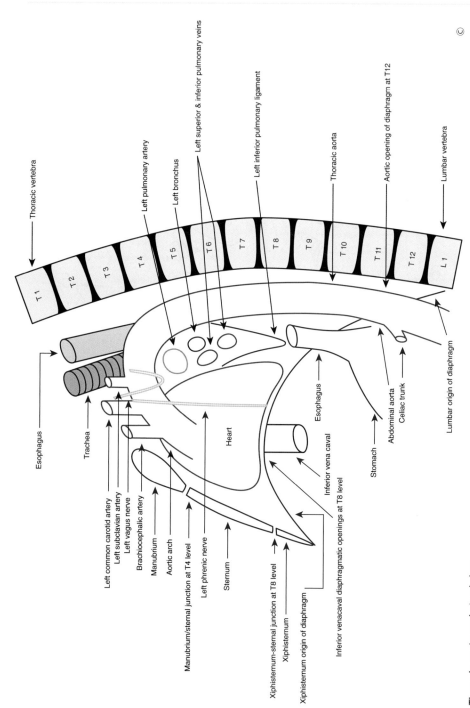

Thoracic anatomy: Lateral view

- Enters the abdominal cavity through the aortic opening of the diaphragm
- Branches
  - Bronchial arteries: one on each side to supply the lungs
  - Mediastinal arteries: multiples branch to supply mediastinal lymph nodes and areolar tissues
  - Pericardial arteries
  - Esophageal arteries: four or five branches from the anterior surface of the thoracic aorta
  - Superior phrenic arteries
  - Posterior intercostal arteries
    - First and second posterior intercostal arteries: branches from superior intercostal artery branch of costocervical trunk of the subclavian artery
    - Lower nine posterior intercostal arteries: branches from posterior thoracic aorta
  - Anterior intercostal arteries
    - Upper five or six anterior intercostal arteries: branches from the internal thoracic artery
    - Remaining anterior intercostal arteries: branches from the musculophrenic branch of internal thoracic artery
- Internal mammary (internal thoracic) artery
  - Branch from the subclavian artery
  - Vagus nerves are located medial, and phrenic nerves are lateral to the internal mammary artery.
  - Terminal branches
    - Musculophrenic artery
    - Epigastric artery
- Brachiocephalic vein
  - Left brachiocephalic vein
    - Most superficial structure in the superior mediastinum posterior to the manubrium
    - Covered with the remnant of thymus and mediastinal fat
    - Aortic arch, innominate artery, left common carotid artery, and left subclavian artery are posterior and inferior to the left brachiocephalic vein.
  - Right brachiocephalic vein joins the left brachiocephalic vein to form the superior vena cava at the right parasternal level in the second intercostal space.
- Superior vena cava
  - Situated lateral to the ascending aorta
  - Distal part covered with pericardium
- Thoracic part of trachea
  - Situated in the superior mediastinum
  - Trachea divides into right and left bronchus at carina, which corresponds to the level of T5 vertebra and sternal angle.
  - Right bronchus
    - Shorter and vertical compared to the left bronchus and divides into the upper, middle, and lower lung lobes bronchi.
  - Left bronchus
    - Divides into the left upper and lower lung lobes bronchi
- Thoracic esophagus
  - Located on the right side of the thoracic aorta in the upper chest, then courses anterior to the thoracic aorta at the level of the diaphragm, and then enters the abdomen on the left side of the abdominal aorta at the level of T12 vertebra.
- Azygos vein
  - Situated in the right posterior chest
  - A continuation of the right ascending lumbar vein
  - Drains in the superior vena cava

- Accessory hemiazygos vein
  - Situated posterior and lateral to the descending thoracic aorta in the left chest
  - Connects the azygos vein in the right chest
- Hemiazygos vein
  - Continuation of the left ascending lumbar vein
  - Connects the azygos vein in the right posterior chest
- Heart and pericardium
  - The pericardium covers the part of the ascending aorta, pulmonary artery, pulmonary veins, distal superior vena cava, and distal inferior vena cava.
  - The left phrenic nerve descends on the lateral surface of the pericardium near the apex.
  - The right phrenic nerve is situated lateral to the inferior vena cava.
- Pulmonary artery trunk
  - Originates from the right ventricle and branches into the right and left pulmonary arteries
  - The right pulmonary artery is situated posterior to the aorta and superior vena cava.
  - The left pulmonary artery is situated anterior to the left mainstem bronchus.
- Pulmonary veins
  - There are four pulmonary veins: two on the left side, two on the right side.
  - The pulmonary veins drain oxygenated blood from the lung to the left atrium.
- Pulmonary hilum
  - Right hilum
    - Contains right epiarterial bronchus, right hypoarterial bronchus, right pulmonary artery, two right pulmonary veins, right bronchial artery, and right bronchial vein
    - Bronchus is located posteriorly.
    - Pulmonary artery is located anteriorly and superiorly.
    - Pulmonary veins are located anteriorly and inferiorly.
  - Left hilum
    - Contains left bronchus, left pulmonary artery, two left pulmonary veins, left bronchial arteries, and left bronchial vein
    - Bronchus is located posteriorly.
    - Pulmonary artery is located anteriorly and superiorly.
    - Pulmonary veins are located anteriorly and inferiorly.
  - Covered superiorly, anteriorly, and posteriorly by pleura
  - At the inferior border of the hilum, the pleura forms the inferior pulmonary ligament that connects the lower lobe of the lung to the diaphragm.
  - The inferior pulmonary veins are in close relation with the inferior pulmonary ligament, and it is the most inferior structures at the pulmonary hilum.
- Thoracic duct: located in the right posterior chest medial to the azygos vein
- Vagus nerve
  - Left vagus nerve
    - Located between the left subclavian and left common carotid artery and descends on the anterior surface of the aortic arch
    - The left recurrent laryngeal nerve branch of the left vagus nerve loops around the aortic arch and travels in the tracheoesophageal groove.
  - Right vagus nerve
    - Located on the anterior surface of the right subclavian artery
    - The right recurrent laryngeal nerve loops around the subclavian artery and travels posteriorly to the common carotid artery in the tracheoesophageal groove.

Must-Know Essentials: Emergency Thoracotomy

INDICATIONS

- Resuscitative emergency department thoracotomy (EDT)
- Penetrating or open chest trauma
- Hemothorax with an initial chest tube output of 1000–1500 mL
- Cardiac tamponade
- Penetrating cardiac injury
- Tracheobronchial injury
- Major vessel injuries

Must-Know Essentials: Resuscitative Emergency Department Thoracotomy (EDT)

BACKGROUND

- The majority of patients who survive an EDT for penetrating injury are neurologically intact.
- Survival following EDT for a stab wound is substantially greater than for a gunshot wound.
- Patients with blunt injuries who survive after EDT have poor neurologic outcome.
- Survival following cardiac arrest secondary to trauma is universally poor.
- Patients who had thoracotomy performed within 5 minutes of losing vital signs following penetrating trauma, the chance of survival is variable.
- EDT may be justifiable when vital signs are lost and there is immediate access to surgical intervention.
- Increased thoracotomy survival rates are associated with signs of life in the emergency department (ED).

RECOMMENDATIONS FOR EMERGENCY DEPARTMENT THORACOTOMY (EAST GUIDELINES 2015)

- Strong recommendation: Definite benefit after EDT
  - Pulseless patients in the ED with signs of life after penetrating thoracic trauma
- Conditional recommendation: Patients may benefit after EDT
  - Pulseless patients in the ED without signs of life after penetrating thoracic trauma
  - Pulseless patients in the ED with signs of life after penetrating extrathoracic trauma
    - All extrathoracic injury locations such as the neck, abdomen, and extremities may not have equivalent salvage rates after EDT.
    - Does not apply to patients with isolated cranial trauma
  - Pulseless patients in the ED without signs of life after penetrating extrathoracic trauma
    - All extrathoracic injury locations, such as the neck, abdomen, and extremities, may not have equivalent salvage rates after EDT.
    - Does not apply to patients with isolated cranial injuries
  - Pulseless patients in the ED with signs of life after blunt trauma
- No recommendation
  - Pulseless patients in the ED without signs of life after blunt trauma

SIGNS OF LIFE (SOL)

- Presence of pupillary response
- Presence of spontaneous breathing
- Cardiac electrical activities
- Presence of carotid pulse
- Measurable or palpable blood pressure
- Presence of spontaneous extremity movement

CONDITIONAL RECOMMENDATION CRITERIA FOR EMERGENCY DEPARTMENT THORACOTOMY

- Penetrating trauma patients
  - Cardiac arrest with <10 min CPR on arrival in ED
  - Pulseless electrical activity (PEA)
  - Witnessed cardiac activity prehospital or in ED
  - Precordial wound in a patient with prehospital cardiac arrest
  - Possible indication in penetrating abdominal injury with at least one field SOL and <15 minutes CPR.
  - Penetrating nonthoracic injury (abdominal, peripheral) with traumatic arrest and previously witnessed cardiac activity (prehospital or in hospital)
- Blunt trauma
  - Loss of signs of life within 5 minutes of arrival in the ED
  - Persistent hypotension (SBP <70 mm Hg) despite resuscitation
  - Witnessed cardiac activity prehospital or in the ED
  - Rapid exsanguination from the chest tube (>1500 mL of blood return)
  - Profound hypotension (<70 mm Hg) in a patient with a truncal wound who is unconscious or for whom an operating room is unavailable

SURGICAL STEPS FOR LEFT ANTEROLATERAL RESUSCITATIVE EMERGENCY DEPARTMENT THORACOTOMY

- Place the patient in supine position with both arms abducted at right angles or elevated over the head.
- Prep and drape the patient in sterile fashion from neck to groin.
- Incision: Make a skin incision in the left fourth or fifth intercostal space (below the nipple or in the inframammary fold) from sternal border to the midaxillary line following the intercostal space with slightly upward curve.
- Divide the pectoral fascia and pectoral muscles anteriorly and the serratus anterior muscle laterally.
- Make an incision with scalpel in the intercostal muscle closer to the upper border of the rib to enter the pleural space and divide the entire length of the intercostal muscles with a Mayo scissors.
- Place a Finochietto rib spreader into the incision with the handle toward the axilla.
- Mobilize the lung by cutting the inferior pulmonary ligament by pulling the lower lobe of the lung cranially, putting the inferior pulmonary ligament under tension. Risk of injury to the inferior pulmonary vein leading to massive bleeding.
- Perform the damage control procedures and resuscitation.
- Transfer the patient to the operating room after return of the spontaneous circulation for further management of the injuries.

DAMAGE CONTROL PROCEDURES AFTER EMERGENCY DEPARTMENT THORACOTOMY

- Pericardiotomy and release of cardiac tamponade
  - Lift the pericardium with a pickup, and use scissors to open the pericardium at least 1 cm anterior to, and parallel to, the left phrenic nerve. Avoid injury to the left phrenic nerve.
  - Evacuate any blood and blood clot.
  - Inspect the heart for any injury.
- Transthoracic cross-clamping of the descending thoracic aorta
  - It helps to:
    - maximize cerebral and coronary blood flow.
    - control infradiaphragmatic exsanguination.
  - Steps
    - Divide the inferior pulmonary ligament by retracting the lung anteriorly and superiorly.
    - With scissors, open the pleura overlying the aorta.
    - Dissect the thoracic aorta anteriorly and posteriorly and place a vascular clamp on the aorta.
  - Complications
    - Avulsion of the intercostal arteries during dissection of the aorta resulting in significant bleeding
    - The esophagus anterior to the aorta may get injured during dissection. Palpation of a previously placed nasogastric tube may help in rapid identification of the esophagus.
    - Injury to the inferior pulmonary vein during division of the inferior pulmonary ligament can result into massive bleeding.
- Open cardiac massage
  - Maximizes cerebral and coronary blood flow
  - Two-handed technique
    - Place one hand flat under the posterior surface and other hand on the anterior surface of the heart.
    - Squeeze the heart from the apex upward at a rate of approximately 100 beats per minute.
    - Avoid using fingertips for the compression to prevent myocardial injury.
- Control of bleeding cardiac wounds
  - Temporary bleeding control techniques
    - Digital occlusion.
    - Occlusion of the laceration with inflated balloon of a Foley catheter.
    - Use a skin stapler to control bleeding myocardial wounds.
    - Use a Satinsky clamp for atrial wounds.
  - In fibrillating heart with laceration
    - Use 2-0 or 3-0 nonabsorbable polypropylene interrupted vertical mattress or figure-of-eight closure sutures to control the bleeding.
    - Use a horizontal mattress if the injury is close to the coronary vessels.
  - It is difficult to control bleeding in a posterior cardiac injury due to location.
  - Manipulation can cause arrhythmias.
- Control of exsanguinating hemorrhage from pulmonary lacerations
  - For a central laceration, methods of bleeding control include:
    - cross-clamp the pulmonary hilum using a Satinsky clamp.
    - perform a hilar twist to control hemorrhage.
      - Divide the inferior pulmonary ligament.
      - Twist the whole lung 180 degrees at the hilum.

- Peripheral laceration
- Pack the wound with lap pads or gauze.
- Control of air embolism
  - Coronary arteries air embolism
    - Air can enter into the pulmonary veins in severe lung trauma causing coronary artery embolism.
    - Cross-clamp the pulmonary hilum using a Satinsky clamp.
  - Coronary venous air embolism
    - Injuries to the low-pressure cardiac chambers can result in air embolism in the coronary veins.
    - Air bubbles can be seen in the coronary veins.
    - Aspirate the right ventricle.

Must-Know Essentials: Approaches for Operating Room Emergency Thoracotomies

ANTEROLATERAL THORACOTOMY

- Indications for left anterolateral thoracotomy
  - Resuscitative EDT
  - Penetrating injury left chest
    - High-energy injuries
    - Low-energy injuries with hemodynamic instability
  - Blunt injury to the left chest
    - Hemodynamic instability
    - Right hemothorax with chest tube: Persistent significant bleeding with hemodynamic instability
  - Left supraclavicular penetrating injury
  - Cross-clamping of the aorta in the operating room
  - Injury to the posterior surface of the heart
- Indications for right anterolateral thoracotomy
  - Penetrating injury right chest
    - High-energy injuries
    - Low-energy injuries with hemodynamic instability
  - Blunt injury to the right chest
    - Hemodynamic instability
    - Right hemothorax with chest tube: Persistent significant bleeding with hemodynamic instability
  - Right supraclavicular penetrating injury
- Surgical steps
  - The side of the thoracotomy depends on the indications.
  - The patient is placed in the supine position.
  - Steps are the same as in the left anterolateral EDT.

CLAMSHELL THORACOTOMY

- Indications
  - Bilateral penetrating chest injuries
  - Exposure of the:

- Anterior aspect of the heart.
- Superior mediastinal vessels.
- Both lungs after a left anterolateral thoracotomy.
- Transmediastinal injury
- For cardiac massage after right anterolateral thoracotomy
- For cross-clamping the descending thoracic aorta after a right anterolateral thoracotomy.
- Surgical steps
  - After a left or right anterolateral thoracotomy, extend the thoracotomy to the other side in the same intercostal space by dividing the sternum transversely using a bone cutter, heavy scissors, or a Gigli saw.
  - During the division of the sternum, both internal mammary arteries are transected; ligate the internal mammary arteries on both sides.

MEDIAN STERNOTOMY

- Indications
  - Exposure of anterior mediastinal structures
    - Vascular injury
    - Trachea injury
    - Left main bronchus injury
    - Heart injury
  - Bilateral lung injuries
  - Exposure of the innominate artery and its branches in thoracic outlet penetrating injury
- Surgical steps
  - Make an incision over the center of the sternum from the suprasternal notch to the xiphoid.
  - Using electric cautery, divide the attachment of the interclavicular ligament at the suprasternal notch.
  - Using blunt dissection, clear the posterior wall of the suprasternal notch and the manubrium.
  - Using a pneumatic saw or Lebsche knife, divide the sternum in the middle.
  - Place a Finochietto retractor in the upper part of the incision to expose the heart and mediastinal structure.
  - Additional steps, if needed
    - Extend the incision into the neck along the right sternocleidomastoid for exposure of the innominate artery and the right common carotid arteries.
    - Extend the incision into the neck along the left sternocleidomastoid for exposure of the left common carotid artery.
    - Extend the incision along the superior or inferior aspect of the clavicle on the side of the injury, and divide the clavicle to expose the subclavian artery.
- Limitation
  - Restricted access to the to the periphery of the lungs
  - Posterior mediastinum is inaccessible.

TRAPDOOR INCISION

- Indication: Exposure of the left subclavian artery in penetrating trauma
- Steps
  - Left anterolateral thoracotomy
  - Median sternotomy

- Left clavicular incision
- Clavicle may be divided near the sternum and retracted for better exposure of the proximal subclavian artery.
- Associated with significant postoperative bleeding and respiratory complications

POSTEROLATERAL THORACOTOMY

- Indications
  - Right upper posterolateral thoracotomy through fourth or fifth intercostal space for:
    - right pulmonary hilum injury.
    - right pulmonary lacerations.
    - upper and middle thoracic esophageal injury.
    - posterior low-energy penetrating right chest injury.
  - Left upper posterolateral thoracotomy through fourth or fifth intercostal space for:
    - left pulmonary hilum injury.
    - left pulmonary lacerations.
    - descending thoracic aortic injury.
    - posterior low-energy penetrating left chest injury.
  - Left lower posterolateral thoracotomy through sixth or seventh intercostal space for:
    - distal third thoracic esophageal injury.
- Surgical steps
  - Place the patient in left or right lateral decubitus position depending on the side of the thoracotomy.
  - Incision: Select the site of incision based on the injury.
  - Make a curvilinear incision in the selected intercostal space from anterior axillary line extending posteriorly two fingerbreadths below the tip of the scapula to midway between the spine and the medial border of the scapula.
  - Divide the serratus anterior, latissimus dorsi, and trapezius muscles using electrocautery.
  - Enter the pleural cavity by cutting the intercostal muscle along the superior border of the rib to prevent neurovascular bundle.

EXPOSURE FOR THORACOABDOMINAL INJURY

- Definition of thoracoabdominal injury
  - Anteriorly: Area between the bilateral fourth intercoastal space (nipple level) superiorly and bilateral costal margins inferiorly
  - Lateral: Area between the sixth intercostal space superiorly and costal margins inferiorly
  - Posterior: Area between eighth intercostal space (angle of the scapula superiorly to costal margins inferiorly)
- Criteria for access of the chest and abdomen
  - Unstable patient
    - Left anterolateral thoracotomy through fourth or fifth intercostal space followed by an exploratory laparotomy
  - Stable patient
    - Exploratory laparotomy first, followed by anterolateral thoracotomy on the side of the injury
  - Penetrating anterior thoracoabdominal injury
    - Median sternotomy
    - May extend the sternotomy incision into the abdomen, neck, or along the clavicle

Closure of Thoracotomy After Emergency Thoracotomy

TEMPORARY STERNOTOMY OR THORACOTOMY CLOSURE

- Indications
  - Persistent bleeding lung wounds requiring gauze and lap pads packing for bleeding control
  - High risk for postoperative cardiac arrest that may require immediate access to the heart for cardiac massage
  - After the damage control procedures
- Techniques
  - Place chest tubes in:
    - posterior recesses.
    - mediastinum.
  - Close the chest using one of the following:
    - Plastic bag
    - Wound vacuum
    - Towel clips

DELAYED DEFINITIVE CHEST CLOSURE

- Perform the definitive closure of the chest after resuscitation and normalization of the physiologic parameters including hypothermia, acidosis, and coagulopathy.
- Closure of median sternotomy
  - Check hemostasis along the divided bone edges. Obtain hemostasis with electrocautery and bone wax.
  - Check under the sternum for bleeding from the internal mammary arteries.
  - Place chest tubes drain under the sternum and chest cavities.
  - Close the sternum with steel wires.
  - Close the presternal fascia with heavy absorbable sutures.
  - Close the skin with staples.
- Closure of posterolateral thoracotomy
  - Place a chest tube at the midaxillary line and bring it out through a separate skin incision.
  - Close the chest wall in layers.
    - Close the intercostal space with interrupted figure-of-eight absorbable #1 Polydioxanone suture or Polyglactin sutures.
    - Reapproximate the divided muscles with interrupted or running absorbable # 1 Polydioxanone or Polyglactin sutures.
    - Close the fascia with running absorbable 3-0 Polydioxanone or Polyglactin sutures.
    - Close the skin with staples.

Must-Know Essentials: Complications of Emergency Thoracotomy

SOURCES OF INTRAOPERATIVE BLEEDING

- Internal mammary artery injury
- Intercostal vessels injury
- Injury to pulmonary veins during division of inferior pulmonary ligament for the mobilization of the lower lobe of the lung

CARDIAC COMPLICATIONS

- Cardiac arrhythmias
- Injury to coronary arteries
- Acute right heart failure after hilar clamp placement

PHRENIC NERVE INJURY

- During pericardiotomy

ESOPHAGEAL INJURY

- During aortic cross-clamping of the thoracic aorta

COMPLICATIONS FROM AORTIC CROSS-CLAMPING

- Ischemia to distal organs
- Spinal cord ischemia
- Renal failure

PULMONARY COMPLICATIONS

- Pneumonia
- Acute respiratory distress syndrome (ARDS)
- Empyema

CHAPTER 21

Evaluation and Management of Severe Thoracic Injuries

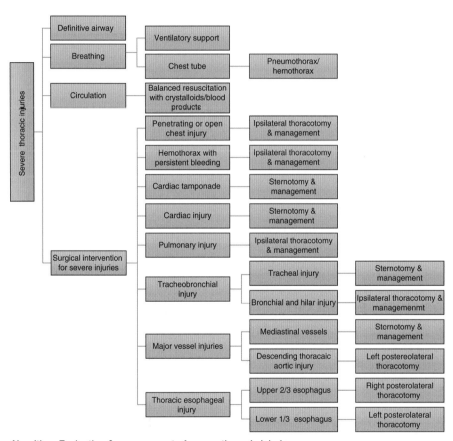

Algorithm: Evaluation & management of severe thoracic injuries

Must-Know Essentials: Evaluation of Thoracic Injuries

INITIAL EVALUATION AND MANAGEMENT

- Airway
  - Assessment for definitive airway.
  - Endotracheal (ET) intubation/surgical airway if indicated

- Breathing and Ventilation
  - Chest tube thoracostomy if indicated
  - Mechanical ventilators if indicated
- Circulation
  - Venous access or intraosseous access
  - Infusion of Crystalloid solution
  - Assessment for massive transfusion protocol

IMAGING

- Chest x-rays may reveal:
  - pneumothorax.
  - hemothorax.
  - pneumomediastinum.
    - Causes
      - Pharyngeal injury
      - Tracheal and bronchial injury
      - Esophageal injury
  - mediastinal hematoma.
    - Causes
      - Mediastinal vascular injuries
      - Sternal fracture
- Bedside ultrasound
  - Evaluation of hemopericardium
  - Evaluation of pneumothorax
- Computerized tomography (CT) scan
  - Detailed evaluation of thoracic injuries in stable patients
- Computed tomographic angiography (CTA) chest
  - Detailed evaluation of vascular injuries in stable patients

ESOPHAGEAL ENDOSCOPY

- For the evaluation of esophageal injury if indicated

BRONCHOSCOPY

- For the evaluation of tracheobronchial injury if indicated

Must-Know Essentials: Life-Threatening Chest Injuries
MECHANISMS OF THORACIC INJURIES

- Penetrating injury
- Blunt injury
- Crush injury
- Deceleration injury
- Blast injury

TWELVE LIFE-THREATENING CHEST INJURIES: THE DEADLY DOZEN

- Six lethal injuries
  - Acute airway obstruction including airway rupture
  - Tension pneumothorax
  - Open pneumothorax
  - Flail chest
  - Massive hemothorax
  - Cardiac tamponade
- Six hidden injuries (easily missed, potentially life-threatening)
  - Tracheobronchial injury
  - Aortic injury
  - Myocardial contusion
  - Pulmonary contusion
  - Diaphragmatic rupture
  - Esophageal rupture

Must-Know Essentials: Chest Wall Injuries

AAST GRADING OF CHEST WALL INJURIES

- Grade I
  - Chest wall contusion of any size
  - Laceration of skin and subcutaneous tissue of any size
  - Closed fractures of <3 ribs
  - Closed nondisplaced clavicle fracture
- Grade II
  - Laceration of skin, subcutaneous tissue, and muscle
  - Closed fractures of >3 adjacent ribs
  - Open and displaced clavicle fracture
  - Closed, nondisplaced sternal fracture
  - Closed or open scapular body fracture
- Grade III
  - Full-thickness laceration, including pleural penetration
  - Open or displaced sternal fracture
  - Flail sternum
  - Unilateral flail segment (<3 ribs)
- Grade IV
  - Avulsion of chest wall tissue with underlying ribs fracture
  - Unilateral flail segment (>3 ribs)
- Grade V
  - Bilateral flail chest (>3 ribs on both sides)

RIB FRACTURES

- Most common thoracic injuries in blunt trauma
- Severe force required for fractures of ribs 1–3 and sternal fractures

- Complications of ribs fracture
  - Associated injuries
    - Fractures of ribs 1–3 have high association with:
      - subclavian artery and vein injury.
      - brachial plexus injury.
    - Fractures of ribs 4–9 have high association with:
      - pulmonary contusion.
      - pneumothorax.
    - Fractures of ribs 10–12 have high association with abdominal injuries such as spleen, kidneys, and liver.
  - Pulmonary lacerations complicated with:
    - hemothorax.
    - pneumothorax.
  - Pulmonary hematoma
  - Hypoxia due to:
    - pulmonary contusion.
    - atelectasis.
  - Pneumonia
  - Impaired ventilation due to:
    - splinting from pain.
    - flail chest.
      - Two or more fractures per rib involving two or more adjacent ribs
      - Paradoxical breathing due to discontinuity of flail chest wall segment with the rest of the thoracic cage
      - Paradoxical breathing is characterized by inward chest wall movement during inspiration and outward chest wall movement during expiration.
      - Posterior chest wall flail is usually stable due to overlying muscles and the scapula and does not cause severe ventilation problems.
      - Anterior and lateral flail segments are usually associated with impaired ventilation.
      - Frequently associated with pulmonary contusions
- Treatment of rib fractures
  - Nonoperative treatment
    - Pain management modalities
      - Oral medications: narcotics/nonnarcotics
      - Parenteral narcotics
      - Patient-controlled analgesia (PCA) pump using narcotics
      - Intercostal nerve blocks
      - Continuous epidural anesthesia
    - Deep breathing exercises
  - Operative treatment: Internal fixation of ribs
    - Benefits
      - Restores chest wall dynamics
      - Decreases pain
      - Decreases incidence of pneumonia
      - Decreases incidence of tracheostomy
      - Decreases need for mechanical ventilation
    - Indications
      - Strongly recommended
        - ≥5 ribs flail chest on ventilatory support
        - Symptomatic nonunion

Severe displacement found during thoracotomy for other indications

May consider

≥3 ribs flail chest without mechanical ventilation

≥3 ribs with severely displaced fractures

≥3 ribs with mild to moderate displacement and 50% reduction of expected forced vital capacity despite optimal pain management

Pain not relieved with medical treatment with associated respiratory compromise (e.g., deficiency in pulmonary function tests)

Chest wall deformity

Thoracotomy for other indications, such as lung laceration or open pneumothorax

- Most commonly ribs 4–10 are fixed because these are the most mobile ribs and produce significant pain.
- For patients with multiple fractured ribs, severely displaced and accessible ribs should be fixed.
- Fixation of fractures of ribs 1–3 is not recommended as these ribs are difficult to access and no benefit has been shown.
- Contraindications

  Absolute: Contaminated field

  Relative

    Severe lung contusion requiring prolonged mechanical ventilation

    High cervical spine injury requiring mechanical ventilation

    Severe traumatic brain injury (TBI)

    Unstable spine fractures
- Surgical steps:

  Position of the patient

    Supine for anterior ribs fracture

    Lateral decubitus for lateral or posterior ribs fracture

  Access the fracture with:

    muscle sparing anterior, posterior or posterolateral approach.

    muscle splitting or cutting limited-exposure approach.

  Plates and fixation devices

    Synthes plates

    RibLoc U-shaped plates

    Intramedullary devices

    Absorbable plates

STERNAL FRACTURES

- Most sternal fractures involve the upper or middle part of the sternum.
- May have associated:
- pulmonary injuries.
- myocardial injuries.
- thoracic spine fractures.
- sternoclavicular dislocations:
  - Anterior dislocations

    More common

    Mostly treated non operatively
  - Posterior dislocations

    Associated with:

      injury to mediastinal blood vessels.

injury to trachea.
injury to esophagus.
Usually require closed or surgical reduction

Must-Know Essentials: Lung Injuries

AAST GRADING OF LUNG INJURIES

- Grade I
  - Lung contusion, unilateral <1 lobe
- Grade II
  - Lung contusion, unilateral single lobe
- Grade III
  - Simple pneumothorax
  - Persistent (>72 hours) air leak from distal airway
  - Lung contusion, unilateral >1 lobe
- Grade IV
  - Nonexpanding intraparenchymal hematoma
  - Major (segmental or lobar) air leak
- Grade V
  - Hilar vessel disruption
- Grade VI
  - Total uncontained transection of pulmonary hilum

Advance one grade for bilateral injuries up to Grade III.

TENSION PNEUMOTHORAX

- Air enters the pleural space and is captured during the process of exhalation.
- Causes collapse of the ipsilateral lung with subsequent compression of the mediastinum and the contralateral lung
- Clinical signs
  - Respiratory distress
  - Shock
  - Distended jugular veins
  - Tissue emphysema
  - Unilateral decrease in breath sounds
  - Hyperresonance
- Treatment
  - Surgical emergency: Immediate needle thoracostomy followed by chest tube placement (tube thoracostomy)

TENSION HEMOTHORAX

- Results from bleeding after blunt or penetrating trauma
- Sources of bleeding
  - Intercostal arteries
  - Internal mammary arteries
  - Lung parenchymal laceration
  - Cardiac injury
  - Hilar and great vessels injury

- Causes ipsilateral lung compression and subsequent displacement of the mediastinum and compression of contralateral lung
- Clinical signs
  - Respiratory distress
  - Shock
  - Distended jugular veins
  - Unilateral decrease in breath sounds
- Treatment
  - Chest tube placement (tube thoracostomy)
  - Thoracotomy: Indications
    - Continued bleeding per chest tube with hemodynamic instability
    - Chest tube with >1500 mL bleeding within 24 hours

PULMONARY CONTUSIONS

- Common after blunt chest trauma
- May be associated with penetrating chest or explosion injuries
- Commonly associated with rib fractures and a flail chest
- Pathophysiology
  - Usually evolve 24–48 hours after injury
  - Decreased lung compliance
  - Ventilation-perfusion mismatch
  - Intrapulmonary shunting
  - Severe inflammation may cause acute respiratory distress syndrome (ARDS).
- Presentation
  - May be asymptomatic
  - Difficulty in breathing
  - Hypoxia and hypercapnia
- Evaluated with chest x-ray (CXR) and CT scans
- Treatment
  - Most pulmonary contusions heal with supportive care within 5–7 days.
  - May require ventilatory support

PULMONARY LACERATIONS

- Pulmonary laceration may result from:
  - blunt injury.
  - penetrating injury.
  - blast injury.
- Presentations
  - Hemorrhagic shock
  - Hemothorax
  - Pneumothorax
  - Air embolism
- Management of pulmonary lacerations
  - Hemodynamically stable patient with small lacerations
    - Chest tube for hemothorax and pneumothorax
    - Majority of the bleeding after lung laceration stops spontaneously because of low-pressure vasculature and rich in thromboplastin

- Central laceration
  - Pneumonectomy if associated with extensive hilar vascular injury
    - Perform total pneumonectomy (en masse pneumonectomy) using a transverse anastamosis (TA) stapler at the hilum.
    - Reinforce the divided stump with nonabsorbable sutures, then buttress the stump with pericardial fat, pleura, or intercostal muscle flap.
  - Nonanatomical lobectomy
    - Divide the inferior pulmonary ligament.
    - Using a TA stapler, resect the lung.
    - Before release of the clamp, hold the divided lung with an Allis clamp to prevent the retraction of the stump, then perform pneumorrhaphy of the divided lung edge with running nonabsorbable sutures to reinforce the staple line.
- Isolated deep penetrating lobar lacerations
  - Pulmonary tractotomy
    - Perform with a linear stapler followed by pneumorrhaphy with running absorbable sutures in penetrating deep lacerations.
    - Tissue glue may be used along the staple line.
    - Closure of exit and entry wound is not recommended. It may result in:
      - air embolism.
      - intraparenchymal bleeding.
      - hemorrhage in the bronchial tree, including bleeding to the other lung.
  - Wedge resection
    - Perform a nonanatomical resection for a large peripheral injury using stapler or clamps
    - Place sutures or apply tissue glue at the resection edge for persistent bleeding or air leak.
  - Superficial lacerations
    - Pneumorrhaphy using absorbable sutures
    - Suture ligation of bleeders and air leaks

AIR EMBOLISM

- Etiology
  - Closure of entry and exit wounds of a penetrating lung injury
  - Hilar injury involving the bronchial tree and portal veins
  - Blast lung injury
- May involve coronary artery or coronary vein
- Coronary arterial embolism
  - Develops in severe lung trauma when air can access the pulmonary veins
  - Rare
- Coronary venous embolism
  - Develop after injuries to the low-pressure cardiac chambers
- Presentations
  - May be asymptomatic
  - Severe chest pain
  - Cardiac arrhythmia
  - Hypotension
  - Cardiac arrest
  - Stroke

- Management
  - Majority of the patients with minor embolism do not require any specific treatment.
  - Supportive care for symptomatic patients
    - Patient should be placed in Trendelenburg position.
    - 100% oxygen
    - Hyperbaric treatment if available
  - Massive embolism with hemodynamic instability
    - Vasopressor agents
    - Treatment of cardiac arrhythmias
    - Emergent thoracotomy
      Elevation of the apex of the heart and aspiration of both ventricles in coronary venous embolism
      Clamp the pulmonary hilum using a Satinsky clamp to control bronchovenous communication in coronary arterial embolism.

Must-Know Essentials: Diaphragm Injuries

ANATOMY OF THE DIAPHRAGM

- Two parts
  - Central tendinous part
  - Peripheral muscular part
- Attachment
  - Anterior: Xiphisternum
  - Lateral: Lower six ribs
  - Posterior: Lumbar vertebra (L1, L2)
- Three openings
  - Aortic opening
    - Aorta
    - Azygos vein
    - Thoracic duct
  - Esophageal opening
    - Esophagus
    - Vagus nerve
  - Opening for the inferior vena cava
- Innervation: Phrenic nerve (C3–C5 nerve roots)
- Arterial supply: Phrenic arteries from the aorta
- Venous drainage: Directly to the inferior vena cava (IVC)

ETIOLOGY OF INJURY

- May result from blunt or penetrating trauma of the chest
- Left diaphragm injuries are 3–4 times more common than right-sided injuries.

EVALUATION

- Diaphragmatic injuries are usually missed during primary evaluation.
- Majority of diaphragmatic injuries are diagnosed late.
- Asymptomatic patients with high index of suspicion should be evaluated with diagnostic laparoscopy.
- CT chest/abdomen

AAST GRADING OF DIAPHRAGM INJURIES

- Grade I
  - Contusion of diaphragm
- Grade II
  - Laceration <2 cm
- Grade III
  - Laceration 2–10 cm
- Grade IV
  - Laceration >10 cm with tissue loss <25 cm^2
- Grade V
  - Laceration with tissue loss >25 cm^2

Advance one grade for bilateral injuries up to grade III.
- Surgical repair
  - Approach
    - Transabdominal open or laparoscopic
    - Transthoracic in chronic injury
  - Perform the repair with interrupted figure-of-eight nonabsorbable #1 polypropylene or Ethibond sutures.
  - Peripheral injuries usually will require fixation of the diaphragm to the ribs.
  - Place a chest tube thoracostomy.

BACKGROUND

- Gunshot wounds account for 70%–80% of esophageal injuries.
- Blunt trauma, such as a motor vehicle collision (MVC), usually results in injury to the distal abdominal esophagus.
- Overall, cervical esophageal injuries are the most common.
- Associated with significant morbidities and morbidities

ANATOMY

- Approximately 25 cm long, extending from the pharyngoesophageal junction at the level of the cricoid cartilage and C6 and terminating in the stomach at the T11-T12 level
- Descends through the superior and posterior mediastinum and terminates at the cardia of the stomach
- In the left posterior chest, the esophagus is situated on the right side of the descending thoracic aorta, then crosses the aorta anteriorly before terminating in the cardia of the stomach on the left side of the abdominal aorta.
- Divided into three main anatomical regions: cervical, thoracic, and intraabdominal esophagus
- Layers of the esophagus: mucosa, submucosa, muscularis propria, and adventitia
- Muscularis propria is critical to esophageal structure and function. It is composed of two layers: an inner circular layer and an outer longitudinal layer.
- Arterial supply
  - Cervical esophagus
    - Inferior thyroid artery
  - Thoracic esophagus
    - Branches of the thoracic aorta

- Branches of bronchial arteries
- Abdominal esophagus
  - Left gastric artery
  - Inferior phrenic artery
- Venous drainage
  - Cervical esophagus
    - Inferior thyroid vein
  - Thoracic esophagus
    - Azygous vein
  - Hemizygous vein
    - Bronchial veins
  - Abdominal esophagus
    - Coronary veins

MANIFESTATIONS

- Acute chest pain
- Dyspnea
- Dysphagia
- Hemoptysis
- Hematemesis
- Subcutaneous emphysema in the chest

EVALUATION

- Early diagnosis of esophageal injury is associated with improved morbidity and mortality.
- Diagnostic tests
  - Chest x-ray findings suggestive for esophageal injury include:
    - mediastinal air.
    - mediastinal widening.
    - pleural effusion, unilateral or bilateral.
    - subcutaneous emphysema.
  - CT of chest and abdomen findings suggestive for esophageal injury include:
    - gas and fluid around the esophagus.
    - esophageal wall thickening.
    - esophageal mucosal thickening.
    - air or air-fluid collection in the mediastinum.
    - pleural effusion, unilateral or bilateral.
    - pneumocardium.
    - pneumoperitoneum.
  - Esophagogram
    - Water-soluble contrast should be used for preliminary detection of perforation.
    - Barium contrast esophagogram is recommended for high index of suspicion for injury with negative water-soluble contrast esophagogram.
    - Nontransmural esophageal injuries are not detected with an esophagogram.
    - 10% false negative rate
  - Flexible esophagoscopy
    - Very useful for direct visualization of the injury in penetrating trauma
    - Its role in blunt esophageal injury is inconclusive.

- Contraindicated in patients with small mucosal or submucosal tears seen in CT scan or esophagogram. It may exacerbate the injury or cause perforation.
- May be performed in patients with continued suspicion of injury despite negative CT scans and esophagograms

AAST GRADING OF ESOPHAGEAL INJURIES

- Grade I
  - Contusion/hematoma, partial-thickness tear
- Grade II
  - Laceration <50% circumference
- Grade III
  - Laceration >50% circumference
- Grade IV
  - Less than 2-cm disruption of tissue or vasculature
- Grade V
  - More than 2-cm disruption of tissue or vasculature

Advance one grade for multiple lesions up to Grade III.

MANAGEMENT

- Nonoperative treatment
  - May be considered in patients with blunt esophageal injury with the following:
    - Small perforation with contained leak
    - Minimal symptoms
    - Hemodynamically stable
    - No clinical evidence of mediastinitis and sepsis
    - Severe comorbidities
  - Supportive care
    - Nothing by mouth (NPO)
    - Careful insertion of nasogastric tube
    - Broad-spectrum antibiotics
    - Fluid resuscitation
  - May require additional procedures
    - Drainage of the collection in the chest under interventional radiology guidance
    - Chest tube placement
    - Gastrostomy tube placement
    - Feeding jejunostomy
  - Repeat esophagogram after a few days to reassess the leak before starting an enteral diet.
- Operative management
  - Recommended for most esophageal injuries
  - General principles of surgical management
    - Exposure of the injury depending on the location
    - Debridement of nonviable tissue
    - Extension of muscular defect to identify the mucosal injury
    - Limited mobilization of the esophagus to prevent segmental ischemia
    - Tension-free repair in two layers
      - Inner mucosal layer with running 3-0 polydioxanone absorbable sutures (PDS)
      - Outer muscular layer with interrupted 3-0 silk nonabsorbable sutures
    - Buttress of the repair with local tissue/muscle flaps

- Drainage tube placement at the repair site
- If possible:
  - Gastrostomy tube decompression
  - Jejunostomy for feeding
- Steps
  - Place the patient in lateral decubitus position.
    - Left lateral decubitus: right side up for the right posterolateral thoracotomy
    - Right lateral decubitus: left side up for the left posterolateral thoracotomy
  - Place a nasogastric tube if possible.
  - Perform posterolateral thoracotomy.
    - Right posterolateral thoracotomy through fifth or sixth intercostal space for proximal and midthoracic esophageal injury
    - Left posterolateral thoracotomy through seventh or eighth intercostal space for distal thoracic esophageal injury
  - Exposure of the esophagus after right thoracotomy
    - Divide the inferior pulmonary ligament and retract the right lung anteriorly to expose the esophagus.
    - Palpate the nasogastric tube to confirm the esophagus.
    - Identify and protect the azygos vein, which courses across the esophagus.
    - If required, may ligate and divide the azygos vein for exposure of the esophagus.
  - Exposure of the esophagus after left thoracotomy
    - Divide the inferior pulmonary ligament and retract the left lung anteriorly to expose the esophagus.
    - The esophagus is located to the right and anterior of the thoracic aorta.
    - Palpate the nasogastric tube to conform the esophagus.
  - After exposure of the esophagus, incise the pleura overlying the esophagus.
  - Mobilize the esophagus and place a Penrose drain.
  - Repair the esophageal injury using the principles previously described.
  - Buttress the repair with a muscle flap. Choices of tissue include:
    - intercostal muscle: simple and most reliable.
    - latissimus dorsi muscle: use in the unstable patient is limited because it takes time to harvest the muscle.
    - pedicle diaphragm.
    - pericardium or pleura: secondary choices because they are more fragile and comparatively less vascular.
  - Place drains in the mediastinum.
  - Place a chest tube.
  - Close the thoracotomy incision.
  - Consider:
    - Feeding jejunostomy for nutrition.
    - Gastrostomy tube for decompression.
- Damage control procedures
  - Recommended for injuries where primary repair is not possible, such as:
    - significant inflammation in the surrounding tissue due to delay in diagnosis.
    - extensive injury in unstable patients.
  - Procedures
    - Irrigation and placement of mediastinal drain and a chest tube
    - Esophageal diversion
      - Diverting cervical esophagostomy

- Make an incision in the cervical esophagus, place a 16-French Levin tube, and advanced it into the stomach.
- Secure the tube to the skin.
- Place a mediastinal drain.
- Place a chest tube.
- T-tube diversion
  - Place a T-tube directly through the injury.
  - Place a mediastinal tube.
  - Place a chest tube.
- Esophageal exclusion with diversion
  - Close the esophagus distal to the injury with absorbable sutures or a stapling device.
  - Perform a cervical esophagostomy or T-tube diversion proximal to the excluded esophagus.
  - Diversion helps to prevent the risk of "blind loop" syndrome from bacterial stasis and overgrowth within the excluded esophagus.
  - The esophagus usually gets recanalized in 2–3 weeks.
- Esophageal resection with diversion and delayed reconstruction
  - Esophagectomy is rarely required.
  - Used when diversion and/or exclusion is not possible or failed
  - Also performed for extensive soft-tissue loss or delayed diagnosis
- Once patient is stable
  - Gastrostomy tube for decompression.
  - Jejunostomy tube for feeding.
- Delayed reconstruction of esophagus
- Ivor Lewis technique (gastric pull-up) is preferred.
- Reconstruction with colonic interposition (usually transverse colon)
- Reconstruction with Roux-en-Y jejunal limb

COMPLICATIONS OF ESOPHAGEAL INJURIES

- Thoracic esophageal injuries have the highest morbidity and mortality due to the high risk of mediastinitis and sepsis.
- Complications
- Empyema
- Pneumonia
- Mediastinitis leading to sepsis
- Postoperative complications
  - Postoperative leak: Lack of a serosal layer makes esophageal repairs more tenuous and prone for leak.
  - Tracheoesophageal fistula
  - Esophageal structure
  - Esophageal diverticulum
  - Abscess
  - Wound infection

Must-Know Essentials: Cardiac Injuries
BACKGROUND

- Seen in both blunt and penetrating traumas
- Injury may involve pericardium, cardiac muscle, coronary vessels, and valves.

PERICARDIAL INJURY PATTERNS

- Pneumopericardium
- Hemopericardium
- Cardiac tamponade
  - Features:
    - Beck's triad: hypotension, muffled heart sounds, distended neck veins
    - Pulsus paradoxus: a drop of >10 mm Hg in systolic blood pressure (SBP) during inspiration
    - Echocardiography is the diagnostic. Findings include:
      - dilated IVC with minimal changes during breathing.
      - right atrial collapse during systole.
      - enlarged pericardium.
    - Focused Assessment with Sonography in Trauma (FAST)
      - Pericardial blood
      - Right ventricular collapse during ventricular diastole
      - Dilated inferior IVC
- Pericardial laceration
  - Usually due to penetrating injury
  - May also result from high-energy blunt trauma or acute increase in intraabdominal pressure
  - Features of blunt pericardial laceration
    - Laceration usually runs parallel to the phrenic nerve.
    - May involve both diaphragmatic and pleural surfaces of the pericardium
    - May develop cardiac herniation into the thoracic or abdominal cavity
    - Cardiac herniation may cause torsion of great vessels leadig to sudden death due to cardiac arrest.

BLUNT CARDIAC INJURY PATTERNS

- Blunt cardiac injuries are commonly associated with:
  - sternal fractures.
  - parasternal rib fractures.
  - diaphragm injury.
  - pneumothorax.
  - hemothorax.
  - pulmonary contusion.
- Myocardial contusion
  - Most common cardiac injury
  - Generally asymptomatic
  - May show EKG changes or elevated cardiac enzymes
  - Severe myocardial contusion may be associated with left anterior descending coronary artery injury causing:
    - myocardial infarction.
    - arrhythmias.
    - ventricular failure.
    - cardiac aneurysm.
    - delayed ventricular rupture.
- Ventricular rupture
  - Uncommon, often fatal

- Frequently involves the right ventricle
- Presents with severe hypotension and cardiac tamponade
- Coronary artery injury
  - Rare injury
  - Severe cardiac contusion may cause left anterior descending artery thrombosis resulting in:
    - myocardial infarction.
    - ventricular aneurysm.
    - ventricular rupture.
- Valve injury
  - Rare
  - Commonly involves aortic valve
  - May present with:
    - left ventricular dysfunction.
    - cardiogenic shock
    - pulmonary edema.
- Other rare injuries
  - Chordae tendineae injury
  - Papillary muscle rupture
  - Cardiac avulsion from the great vessels usually due to severe torsion.

EVALUATION

- Majority of patients remain asymptomatic.
- Patients with a high index of suspicion should be evaluated for cardiac injuries.
- Severe injuries may lead to exsanguination, pericardial tamponade, or death.
- CXR may show evidence of cardiac injuries:
  - Cardiomegaly due to hemopericardium
  - Displacement of the cardiac silhouette due to herniation
  - Pneumopericardium
- Electrocardiogram (EKG)
  - May show rhythm disorder, conduction disturbances, and ischemic changes
- Cardiac enzymes
  - Troponin may be elevated in blunt injury.
- Echocardiography
  - Can detect segmental wall abnormalities or valvular dysfunction
  - Transesophageal echo is more sensitive than transthoracic echo.

AAST GRADING OF CARDIAC INJURIES

- Grade I
  - Blunt cardiac injury with minor EKG abnormality (nonspecific ST of T-wave changes, premature atrial or ventricular contractions, or persistent sinus tachycardia
  - Blunt or penetrating pericardial wound without cardiac injury, tamponade, or cardiac herniation
- Grade II
  - Blunt cardiac injury with heart block or ischemic changes without cardiac failure
  - Penetrating tangential cardiac wound, up to but not extending through endocardium, without tamponade
- Grade III

- Blunt cardiac injury with sustained or multifocal ventricular contractions
- Blunt or penetrating cardiac injury with septal rupture, pulmonary or tricuspid incompetence, papillary muscle dysfunction, or distal coronary artery occlusion without cardiac failure
- Blunt pericardial laceration with cardiac herniation
- Blunt cardiac injury with cardiac failure
- Penetrating tangential myocardial wound, up to but not through endocardium, with tamponade
- Grade IV
  - Blunt or penetrating cardiac injury with septal rupture, pulmonary or tricuspid incompetence, papillary muscle dysfunction, or distal coronary artery occlusion producing cardiac failure
  - Blunt or penetrating cardiac injury with aortic or mitral incompetence
  - Blunt or penetrating cardiac injury of the right ventricle, right or left atrium
- Grade V
  - Blunt or penetrating cardiac injury with proximal coronary artery occlusion
  - Blunt or penetrating left ventricular perforation
  - Stellate injuries, less that 50% tissue loss of the right ventricle, right or left atrium
- Grade VI
  - Blunt avulsion of the heart
  - Penetrating wound producing more than 50% tissue loss of a chamber

Advance one grade for multiple wounds to a single chamber or multiple chamber involvement.

TREATMENT OF CARDIAC INJURIES

- Sternotomy
- Pericardiotomy for cardiac tamponade
  - Lift the pericardium with a pickup, and using scissors open the pericardium at least 1 cm anterior to, and parallel to, the left phrenic nerve.
  - Protect and avoid injury to left phrenic nerve.
  - Evacuate any blood and blood clot.
  - Inspect the heart for laceration.
  - Repair the pericardium with continuous 2-0 or 3-0 nonabsorbable polypropylene sutures leaving a small opening at the base for the drainage.
  - Do not close the pericardium if there is significant cardiac enlargement.
  - Place mediastinal drains.
- Cardiac laceration
  - Temporary control of bleeding
    - Perform digital occlusion at the laceration and suture the bleeder.
    - May perform occlusion of laceration with inflated balloon of Foley catheter
    - Use skin stapler for myocardial wounds.
    - Use Satinsky clamp for atrial wounds.
  - Repair of cardiac wounds
    - Bleeding in a posterior cardiac injury is difficult to control due to its location.
    - Manipulation can cause arrhythmias.
    - Grasp the heart by lifting the apex of the heart with a Duval clamp or with lap pads.
    - Repair the laceration with interrupted vertical mattress or figure-of-eight technique with or without pledgets using 2-0 nonabsorbable sutures.
  - Use the horizontal mattress if the injury is near the coronary vessels.

- Coronary arteries injury
  - The distal arteries may be ligated. The procedure is usually tolerated well.
  - Repair the partial injury to the major coronary artery if possible.
  - Ligation of the major coronary artery may lead to development of arrhythmia or cardiac arrest.

EASTERN ASSOCIATION FOR THE SURGERY OF TRAUMA (EAST) GUIDELINES FOR THE MANAGEMENT OF MYOCARDIAL CONTUSIONS

- Level I recommendations
  - Admission EKG should be obtained in all patients in whom blunt cardiac injury is suspected.
- Level II recommendations
  - If the admission EKG is abnormal, the patient should be admitted for continuous EKG monitoring for 24–48 hours. If it is normal, further pursuit of diagnosis should be abandoned.
  - If the patient is hemodynamically unstable, an imaging study, such as transthoracic echocardiography (TTE) or transesophageal echocardiography (TEE), should be obtained.
  - Nuclear medicine scans add little compared to echocardiography and are not useful if echocardiography has been performed.
- Level III recommendations:
  - Elderly patients with known cardiac disease, unstable patients, and those with abnormal admission EKGs can be safely operated on provided that they are closely monitored.
  - The presence of a sternal fracture does not predict the presence of blunt cardiac injury and does not necessarily indicate that monitoring should be performed.
  - Neither creatine phosphokinase (CPK) analysis nor measurement of circulating cardiac troponin T are useful in predicting which patients have or will have complications related to blunt cardiac injury.

Must-Know Essentials: Thoracic Vascular Injuries

AAST GRADING OF THORACIC VASCULAR INJURIES

- Grade I
  - Injury to intercostal artery/vein
  - Injury to internal mammary artery/vein
  - Injury to bronchial artery/vein
  - Injury to esophageal artery/vein
  - Injury to hemiazygos vein
  - Injury to unnamed artery/vein
- Grade II
  - Injury to azygos vein
  - Injury to internal jugular vein
  - Injury to subclavian vein
  - Injury to innominate vein
- Grade III
  - Injury to carotid artery
  - Injury to innominate artery

- Injury to subclavian artery
- Grade IV
  - Injury to descending thoracic aorta
  - Injury to intrathoracic inferior vena cava
  - Injury to pulmonary vein, primary intraparenchymal branch
- Grade V
  - Injury to thoracic aorta (ascending and arch)
  - Injury to superior vena cava
  - Injury to pulmonary vein, main trunk
  - Injury to pulmonary artery, main trunk
- Grade VI
  - Uncontained total transection of thoracic aorta or pulmonary hilum.

Increase one grade for multiple Grade III or IV injuries if >50 % circumference; decrease one grade for Grade IV injuries if <25 % circumference.

EXPOSURE OF HEART AND MEDIASTINAL VESSELS FOR INJURIES

- Perform a sternotomy for mediastinal vascular injuries.
- Open the pericardium, and protect the left phrenic nerve while making the pericardial incision.
- Examine the heart.
- Identify the left brachiocephalic vein, which is the most superficial vascular structure in the superior mediastinum and its connection with the right brachiocephalic vein.
- Identify the structures posterior and inferior to the left brachiocephalic vein, which include:
  - aortic arch.
  - innominate artery
  - left common carotid artery
  - left subclavian artery, situated just posterior and inferior to the left brachiocephalic vein
- May ligate and divide the left brachiocephalic vein for better exposure of the aortic arch and its branches.
- Identify and protect the left vagus nerve, which is located between the left subclavian artery and left common carotid artery, and the left recurrent laryngeal nerve, which loops the aortic arch.
- Identify the right vagus nerve, which is located anterior to the right subclavian artery; the right recurrent laryngeal nerve loops the right subclavian artery.

TREATMENT OF MEDIASTINAL VASCULAR INJURIES

- Brachiocephalic venous injury
  - Hemodynamically unstable patients
    - Ligate the vein. It is a damage control procedure and usually tolerated well.
    - May result in edema of the arm
  - Hemodynamically stable patients
    - Venorrhaphy: Repair the injury using 4-0 polypropylene sutures if there is no concern of stenosis.
    - Repair the injury using a prosthetic graft.
- Superior vena cava injury

- Ligation is incompatible with life.
- Small injury: Repair with 4-0 polypropylene sutures.
- Large injury: Reconstruct with a synthetic graft.
- Intraoperative air embolism is common and it is a lethal complication.
- Innominate artery injury
  - Obtain the proximal control after opening the pericardium.
  - Obtain distal control by clamping the distal innominate or right subclavian artery and the right common carotid.
  - Small injury: Repair with 4-0 polypropylene continuous sutures.
  - Complex injury—choices include:
    - perform an aorta to distal innominate artery bypass.
      - Side of the ascending aorta to the end of the distal innominate artery bypass with synthetic (8-mm Dacron) graft
    - Interposition synthetic (Dacron) graft
    - Damage control procedure: Shunt is usually unsuccessful.
- Proximal common carotid artery
  - Small injury: Repair with 4-0 polypropylene sutures.
  - Shunt: Damage control in hemodynamically unstable patients, followed by reconstruction with synthetic or saphenous vein graft
- Proximal subclavian artery injury
  - Damage control procedures
    - Shunt for distal injury
    - Difficult in very proximal injury
    - Ligation is not an option due to risk of limb ischemia.
  - Small injury: Repair with 4-0 polypropylene sutures.
  - Complex injury
    - Reconstruction with size 6-8 mm polytetrafluoroethylene (PTFE) graft.
- Descending thoracic aortic injury
  - Perform left posterolateral thoracotomy through the fourth or fifth intercostal space.
  - Expose the descending thoracic aorta by retracting the lung anteriorly after mobilizing the inferior pulmonary ligament.
  - Obtain proximal control of the aorta between the left subclavian and left common carotid arteries.
    - Protect the left vagus nerve and recurrent laryngeal nerve.
    - Perform finger dissection, place an umbilical tape around the aorta, and place a vascular clamp.
  - Control the proximal left subclavian artery with a Rummel tourniquet or a vascular clamp.
  - Locate the site for distal control after identifying the injury.
  - Distal control
    - Make an incision in the pleura.
    - Perform a limited finger dissection around the thoracic aorta to avoid injury to the posterior intercostal artery.
    - Protect the esophagus.
    - Place an umbilical tape and apply a vascular clamp.
  - Repair the laceration.
    - Small injury: Repair with continuous 4-0 polypropylene sutures.
    - Complex injury: Repair with interposition synthetic graft.

- Pulmonary artery or pulmonary venous injury
  - Damage control procedures
    - Staple the hilar structures using a TA stapler at the hilum to control the vascular and bronchial injuries.
  - Perform a hilar twist to control the hemorrhage.
    - Pulmonary resection (lobectomy or pneumonectomy)

BLUNT TRAUMATIC AORTIC INJURIES

- Seen after severe deceleration blunt chest trauma
- Injury frequently involves the aortic isthmus followed by the aortic root and the diaphragmatic aorta.
- The majority of the patients die at the scene of the accident.
- The patient may present with pseudoaneurysm due to intimomedial tears and aortic dissection.
- Types of aortic dissection
  - Type A (ascending aorta) dissection
    - May cause:
      - pericardial bleeding.
      - coronary artery laceration.
      - aortic valve rupture.
    - Treated with surgical repair
  - Type B (descending aorta) dissection
    - Managed nonoperatively
    - Repair with endovascular stent graft for aneurysm 6.0 cm in diameter.

Abdominal Trauma

Evaluation and Management of Hemodynamically Unstable Abdominal Penetrating/Blunt Trauma

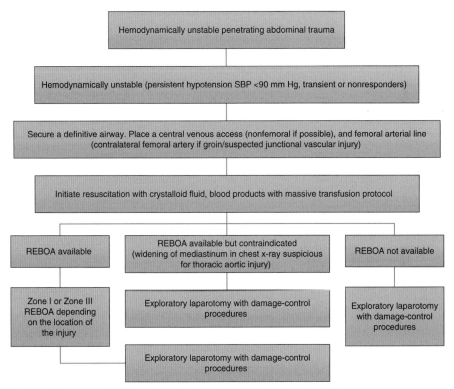

Algorithm: Management of hemodynamically unstable penetrating abdominal trauma

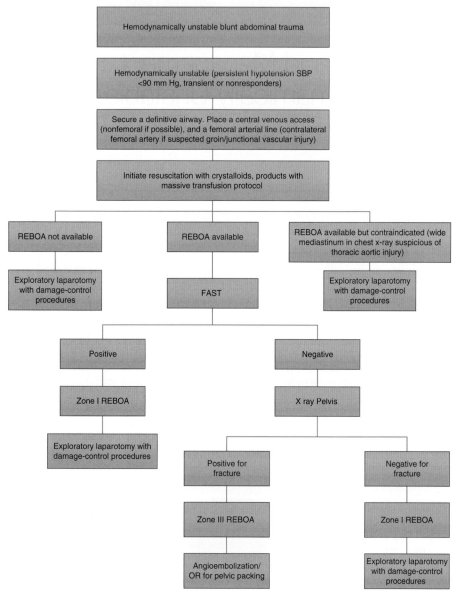

Algorithm: Management of hemodynamically unstable blunt abdominal trauma

Must-Know Essentials: Initial Evaluation and Management

UNSTABLE PATIENT

- Persistent hypotension: Systolic blood pressure (SBP) <90 mm Hg
- Transient or no response in blood pressure with crystalloid infusion

INITIAL MANAGEMENT

- Assessment of the airway
  - Secure a definitive airway.
  - Protect the cervical spine.
- Assessment of breathing and management as indicated
- Assessment of circulation
  - IV access, central venous access if possible
  - Arterial line if possible
  - Resuscitation with crystalloid solution infusion
  - Initiation of massive transfusion protocol
- Assessment for the neurological deficit

Must-Know Essentials: Resuscitative Endovascular Balloon Occlusion of Aorta (REBOA) (also see Chapter 9)

DEFINITION OF REBOA

- Involves placement of an endovascular balloon in the aorta to control hemorrhage

ZONES OF REBOA

- The aorta is divided into three separate zones for the purposes of REBOA balloon deployment.
  - Zone I
    - Extends from the origin of the left subclavian artery to the celiac artery
  - Zone II
    - Extends from the celiac artery to the most caudal renal artery
    - Approximately 3 cm long
    - REBOA balloon not recommended in this zone
  - Zone III
    - Extends from the most caudal renal artery to the aortic bifurcation

INDICATIONS FOR REBOA BALLOON IN UNSTABLE ABDOMINAL TRAUMA

- Blunt abdominal trauma
  - Zone I REBOA
    - Positive Focused Assessment with Sonography in Trauma (FAST) suggestive for intraabdominal hemorrhage
    - Negative FAST with negative pelvic x-ray for fractures
  - Zone III REBOA
    - Negative FAST with positive pelvic x-ray for fractures

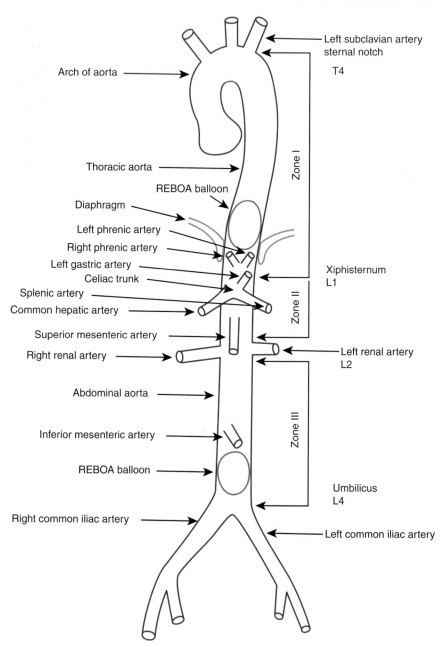

Illustration: Zones of aorta for REBOA placement

- Penetrating abdominal trauma
  - Zone I REBOA
    - Hemodynamically unstable patient
  - Zone III REBOA
    - Pelvic or groin injury with uncontrolled hemorrhage
    - Junctional vascular injury (iliac or common femoral vessels)

CONTRAINDICATIONS FOR REBOA

- High clinical/radiological suspicion of thoracic aortic injury

POST-REBOA PLACEMENT

- After Zone I REBOA placement, proceed for an emergent exploratory laparotomy, if possible, within 15 minutes.
- After Zone III REBOA placement, proceed for an emergent exploratory laparotomy, or preperitoneal packing, or an angioembolization.
- Compared to Zone I REBOA, Zone III REBOA is tolerated for a slightly longer period.
- Partial inflation of the balloon at either location may prolong the duration of REBOA to a maximum of 60 minutes.
- The balloon should be deflated as soon as possible.
- The catheter and sheath should be removed as soon as possible.

COMPLICATIONS OF REBOA

- Complication from femoral arterial access
  - Hematoma at the access site
  - Arterial disruption
  - Arterial dissection
  - Pseudoaneurysm
  - Thromboembolism
  - Extremity ischemia
- Aortoiliac injury
  - Intimal injury
  - Thrombosis
  - Dissection
  - Arterial rupture
  - Limb loss
- Rupture of the balloon due to overinflation
- Prolonged aortic occlusion
  - Spinal cord injury due to prolonged ischemia
  - Cardiac events
  - Renal complications

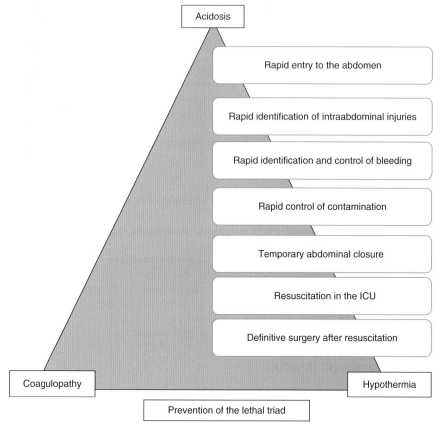

Illustration: Principles of damage control laparotomy

Must-Know Essentials: Principles of Damage-Control Laparotomy

- Damage-control laparotomy is an abbreviated and focused procedures to prevent the vicious cycle and the lethal triad
  - Rapid entry to the abdomen
  - Rapid identification of intraabdominal injuries
  - Rapid identification and control bleeding
  - Rapid control of contamination
  - Temporary abdominal closure
- Continued resuscitation in the ICU
- Definitive surgery after resuscitation

Must-Know Essentials: Damage-Control Laparotomy (also see Chapter 24)

RAPID ENTRY TO THE ABDOMEN

- Perform an exploratory laparotomy with midline incision.
- Enter the peritoneal cavity just proximal to the umbilicus because, in this area, the peritoneum is very thin with minimal preperitoneal fat.
- If possible, avoid entering the abdomen using the old abdominal surgical incision.
- Make a bilateral subcostal incision (rooftop incision) in patients with multiple previous abdominal incisions.

RAPID IDENTIFICATION OF INJURIES AND CONTROL OF BLEEDING

- Perform a rapid control of intraperitoneal bleeding.
    - Blunt trauma: Perform abdominal packing in each quadrant of the abdominal cavity.
    - Penetrating trauma: Perform direct control of the bleeding with sutures or clamps.
- Identify the source of bleeding.
    - Intraabdominal injuries may involve intraperitoneal and retroperitoneal structures.
    - Common sources of intraperitoneal bleeding in blunt trauma
        - Solid-organ injuries, such as liver and spleen
        - Mesenteric vascular injuries
        - Small bowel injuries
        - Retroperitoneal bleeding communicating to the peritoneal cavity
    - Common sources of intraperitoneal bleeding in penetrating trauma
        - Liver
        - Small bowel
        - Diaphragm
        - Colon
        - Intraperitoneal vascular injury
    - Retroperitoneal vascular injury in both blunt and penetrating trauma
    - Combination of intraperitoneal and retroperitoneal structures in penetrating trauma depending on the trajectory of injury.
- Damage-control or definitive control of specific bleeding based on injuries.

RAPID CONTROL OF CONTAMINATION

- In patients with bowel injuries
    - Resect the bowel using a stapler and perform a delayed anastomosis after resuscitation.
    - Ligate the bowel and perform resection and anastomosis after resuscitation.

TEMPORARY ABDOMINAL CLOSURE AFTER DAMAGE-CONTROL LAPAROTOMY

- Objectives in temporary abdominal closure
    - Closure of the abdomen without any risk of intraabdominal hypertension (IAH) or abdominal compartment syndrome (ACS)
    - Prevention of evisceration and contamination
    - Evacuation of abdominal fluid and reduction of bowel edema
    - Prevention of adhesions

- Prevention of bowel injury and fistula formation
- Prevention of injury to fascial edges and fascial retraction
- Prevention of skin injury
- Easy access to the abdominal cavity for planned reexploration of the abdomen for a second look and definitive procedures after resuscitation
- Definitive fascial closure as early as clinically feasible

COMPLICATIONS OF THE OPEN ABDOMEN

- Systemic effects
  - Fluid loss resulting in fluid and electrolyte imbalance
  - Sepsis
  - Systemic inflammatory response
- Local effects
  - Gastrointestinal fistula
  - Adhesions
  - Wound infection
  - Intraabdominal abscesses
  - Difficulty closing abdominal fascia can lead to:
    - closure of the abdomen with split-thickness skin graft after granulation of the abdominal wound.
    - ventral hernia

TECHNIQUES OF TEMPORARY ABDOMINAL CLOSURE

- No ideal techniques of temporary closure.
- Methods used
  - closure of the skin using multiple towel clips
  - Bogota bag closure
    - Suture or staple the sterile irrigation bag or sterile x-ray cassette cover to the skin or fascia.
    - Prevents evisceration, IAH, and ACS
    - Does not allow the effective removal of intraperitoneal fluid.
    - Does not prevent the loss of abdominal domain.
  - Wittmann Patch
    - Velcro-like device sutured to the fascia as a bridge for reapproximating the abdominal wall
    - Overlap of the patch is adjusted to accommodate the intraabdominal swelling.
    - May be used with or without a wound vac
    - Helps prevent the lateral retraction of the fascia and loss of abdominal domain
  - Negative pressuire therapy (NPT)
    - Abdominal wound V.A.C. Therapy System (3 M/KCI, St. Paul, MN, USA)
      - Fenestrated nonadherent protective layer over the bowel
      - Polyurethane foam over the protective covering
      - Suction tubing connected to collection canister and a continuous negative pressure suction pump
      - Prevents fascial retraction
      - Prevents adhesions between the bowel and anterior abdominal wall
      - Helps in abdominal reexploration and closure of the fascia
      - Actively removes intraperitoneal contamination

- ABTHERA (3 M/KCI, St. Paul, MN, USA)
  - Negative pressure system for temporary abdominal closure consists of a visceral protective layer, fenestrated foam, semiocclusive adhesive drape, tubing with interface pad, and a pump.
- High negative pressure in NPT may aggravate bleeding; may consider initial low negative pressure

Must-Know Essentials: Pelvic Packing (also see Chapter 33)

TYPES OF PELVIC PACKING

- Extraperitoneal
- Intraperitoneal

INDICATIONS FOR EXTRAPERITONEAL PELVIC PACKING

- Pelvic ring disruption with hemorrhagic shock
  - Post-REBOA placement
    - Failed angioembolization
    - Nonavailability of angioembolization
    - Persistent hypotension
  - Nonavailability of REBOA
  - Venous pelvic bleeding

INDICATIONS OF INTRAPERITONEAL PELVIC PACKING

- Combined pelvic and intraperitoneal abdominal injury

POST-PACKING MANAGEMENT

- Pelvic stabilization for unstable pelvic fracture
- Angiogram with angioembolization indicated for:
  - persistent bleeding based as suggested by base deficit, dropping hemoglobin, and hemodynamic instability.
  - persistent bleeding after resuscitation, correction of coagulopathy, and pelvic stabilization.
  - active arterial bleeding seen in CT scan with IV contrast.
  - Empiric embolization of the internal iliac arteries is not recommended due to concern for pelvic ischemia after embolization.
- After pelvic packing close the fascia for tamponade effect.
- Packing should be removed following resuscitation, correction of coagulopathy, and pelvic stabilization, usually after 24–48 hours.

Must-Know Essentials: Resuscitation in the Intensive Care Unit After a Damage-Control Laparotomy

GOALS

- No single hemodynamic value or lab result is helpful as an endpoint of resuscitation.
- Optimization of end-organ perfusion

- Optimization of tissue oxygen delivery
- Prevention of hypothermia
- Correction of coagulopathy
- Correction of acidosis
- Prevention of complications of overresuscitation

CLINICAL PARAMETERS OF RESUSCITATION

- Level of consciousness: an indicator of cerebral perfusion
- Urine output
  - Is the direct measurement of renal perfusion
  - Goal urine output: >0.5 mL/kg in adults
- Heart rate, respiratory rate, blood pressure, pulse pressure, and mean arterial pressure (MAP) do not predict the outcome in trauma patients.
- Hypotension predicts a bad outcome after head injury.

METABOLIC PARAMETERS OF RESUSCITATION

- Lactate level
  - Measures the extent of shock
  - Clearance of lactate level over time is more predictive of mortality than an isolated value.
    - 0%–10% mortality if cleared within 24 hours after injury
    - 25% mortality if cleared by 24–48 hours after injury
    - 80%–86% mortality if cleared >48 hours after injury
- Base deficit
  - Is a marker of reduced tissue perfusion
  - Severity of the base deficit
    - Mild: 2–5 mmol/L
    - Moderate: 6–14 mmol/L
    - Severe: >15 mmol/L
  - An absolute base deficit is a measurement of severity of shock, but a single value cannot be used as an endpoint.
  - The trend of base deficit over time is more useful to predict the outcome.
  - Persistently high or worsening base deficits may suggest:
    - ongoing hemorrhage.
    - abdominal compartment syndrome.
    - increased risk of multiple organ dysfunction.
    - diminished oxygen consumption.
    - predicts mortality in trauma patients.
  - Base deficit due to hyperchloremic acidosis is not associated with increased mortality.
  - Serum bicarbonate level correlates with base deficit, but it is affected by the ventilatory status of the patient.

OTHER PARAMETERS AND GOALS OF RESUSCITATION

- Central venous oxygen saturation ($ScvO_2$)
  - Low $ScvO_2$ reflects tissue hypoxia.
  - Normal $ScvO_2$ is >70%.
- Arterial blood gas (ABG): pH >7.36 has shown significant reduction of multisystem organ failure.

- Hemoglobin
  - 7 g/dL in normovolemic patients
  - 8–10 g/dL in severely injured patients
- Coagulation
  - International normalized ratio (INR) <1.5
  - Correction of thromboelastogram (TEG)-based parameters if available
- Hypocalcemia: Lower ionized calcium (<1.0 mmol/L) is associated with increased mortality.
- Temperature: Core temperature: >35°C

COMPLICATIONS OF OVERRESUSCITATION WITH CRYSTALLOID SOLUTIONS

- Compartment syndrome
- Coagulopathy
- Congestive heart failure in patients with cardiac disease

Must Know Essentials: Abdominal Compartment Syndrome

BACKGROUND

- Normal intraabdominal pressure (IAP): <5 mm Hg
- Intra-abdominal hypertension (IAH): IAP >12 mm Hg on separate occasions
- Abdominal perfusion pressure (APP): MAP – IAP
- Abdominal compartment syndrome (ACS): Sustained or repeated IAP >20 mm Hg or APP <60 mm Hg with evidence of new-onset organ failure
- ACS is an independent risk factor for mortality and morbidity.
- APP has been proven to be superior to both IAP and global resuscitation end points such as arterial pH, base deficit, and lactate level to predict outcome in patients with IAH and ACS.

ETIOLOGY

- Primary ACS
  - Hemorrhage from blunt/penetrating trauma
  - Abdominal packing
  - Pelvic packing
  - Bowel edema
  - Coagulopathy with intraabdominal bleeding
- Secondary ACS
  - Large-volume resuscitation

PATHOPHYSIOLOGY

- Splanchnic hypoperfusion
  - Bowel mucosal ischemia
    - Bacterial translocation
    - Bowel edema
    - Free radical release
    - Multisystem organ dysfunction

- Hepatic ischemia
  - Coagulopathy
- Cardiovascular dysfunction
  - Reduced venous return
  - Reduced cardiac output
  - Edema of the extremities
- Renal dysfunction
  - Oliguria due to:
    - reduced renal blood flow and glomerular filtration rate.
    - renal parenchymal pressure.
    - increased renal venous pressure.
- Pulmonary dysfunction
  - Increase in intrathoracic pressure with restriction in lung expansion
  - Increase in peak airway pressure
  - Increase in peak inspiratory pressure
  - Decrease in dynamic compliance of the lung, ventilation perfusion mismatch, and intra-pulmonary shunt
- Central nervous system
  - Increase in intracranial pressure (ICP), especially in patients with traumatic brain injury
- Musculoskeletal dysfunction
  - Increased incidence of abdominal wound complications due to reduced blood flow to abdominal wall

MANIFESTATIONS

- Hypotension due to reduced cardiac output
- Renal failure due to renal hypoperfusion
- Respiratory failure
- Increased ICP
- Splanchnic hypoperfusion
  - Hepatic dysfunction
  - Bowel edema

DIAGNOSIS

- High index of suspicion in patients with risk factors
- Bladder pressure measurement
- Evidence of organ dysfunction
- Metabolic acidosis
- Oliguria
- Elevated peak airway pressure
- Respiratory failure with hypercarbia and hypoxia
- Increase in ICP

TREATMENT

- Decompressive laparotomy with specific management of the etiology of ACS
- Temporary abdominal closure
- Supportive care
  - Fluid/electrolyte balance

- Ventilatory support
- Paralytic agents
- In patients where fascial closure is difficult
  - Closure using an absorbable mesh bridge closure followed by skin graft
  - Closure using synthetic or biological meshes with component separation

Must-Know Essentials: Reexploration and Definitive Abdominal Closure of the Abdomen After Resuscitation

TIMING OF REEXPLORATION AND DEFINITIVE ABDOMINAL CLOSURE

- Patient should be reexplored, and abdomen should be closed as soon as possible, usually within 24-48 hours.
- Requirements
  - Hemodynamically stable
  - No coagulopathy, no hypothermia, and no acidosis
  - Further evaluations of injuries
    - Angiograms: In patients with pelvic packing or after perihepatic packing
    - CT scans
    - Endoscopic retrograde cholangiopancreatography (ERCP) or magnetic resonance cholangiopancreatography (MRCP) in patients with pancreatic/pancreaticoduodenal injuries

PROCEDURES DURING REEXPLORATION

- Remove the abdominal packing.
- Perform definitive debridement or resection as indicated.
- Assess and manage the specific injuries.
- Perform abdominal closure.
  - Primary fascial closure
    - If no risk of tension or abdominal compartment syndrome
    - Repair under tension may result in fascial dehiscence or delayed incisional hernia.
  - Staged fascial closure
    - Progressive primary closure of the fascia using interrupted sutures in patients with persistent bowel edema or intraabdominal hypertension (IAH)

CHAPTER 23

Evaluation and Management of Hemodynamically Stable Abdominal Penetrating/Blunt Trauma

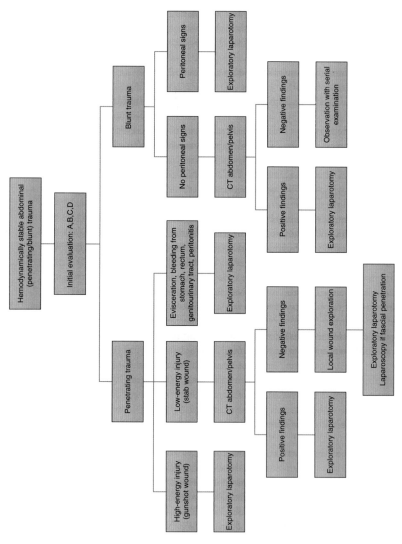

Algorithm: Evaluation & management of hemodynamically stable abdominal penetrating/blunt trauma

Must-Know Essentials: Anatomy of the Abdomen

SURFACE ANATOMY

- External abdomen extends from the diaphragm to the infragluteal fold.
- Divided into:
  - anterior abdomen
  - posterior abdomen
  - intrathoracic abdomen
  - flank.
- Anterior abdomen
  - Extension
    - Superior: Transverse line through bilateral fourth intercoastal space (nipple level)
    - Inferior: Bilateral inguinal ligament
    - Lateral: Bilateral posterior axillary line
  - Divided into:
    - upper abdomen:
      - Extends between nipple line to transpyloric line (imaginary horizontal line between the suprasternal notch and the superior border of pubic symphysis)
      - Further divided into:
        - right hypochondrium
        - epigastrium
        - left hypochondrium.
    - Mid abdomen:
      - Extends between transpyloric line to intertubercular line (line between iliac tubercles)
      - Further divided into:
        - right flank
        - umbilical region
        - left flank.
    - Lower abdomen:
      - Extends between the intertubercular line and the inguinal ligaments
      - Further divided into:
        - right groin
        - hypogastric (suprapubic) region
        - left groin.
- Posterior abdomen
  - Extension
    - Superior: Transverse line through the eighth intercostal space (angle of the scapula)
    - Inferior: Bilateral infragluteal fold
    - Lateral: Bilateral posterior axillary line
- Intrathoracic abdomen
  - Extension
    - Superior: Transverse line through bilateral fourth intercoastal space (nipple level)
    - Inferior: Bilateral costal margins
    - Lateral: Area between the anterior and posterior axillary lines extending from the sixth intercostal space superiorly and costal margins inferiorly
    - Posterior: Area between eighth intercostal space (angle of the scapula superiorly to costal margins inferiorly)
- Flank: Area between midclavicular line and posterior axillary line extending from the costal margin superiorly to the iliac crest inferiorly

INTRAABDOMINAL STRUCTURES

- Intraperitoneal
  - Supramesocolic (above the mesentery of the transverse colon) structures
    - Liver
    - Stomach
    - Spleen
  - Inframesocolic sutures
    - Small intestine and its mesentery
    - Transverse colon and mesocolon
    - Uterus
- Retroperitoneal (see illustration)
  - Supramesocolic (above the mesentery of the transverse colon) structures
    - Duodenum
    - Pancreas
    - Suprarenal midline vessels
  - Inframesocolic structures
    - Infrarenal midline vessels
    - Bilateral kidneys
    - Bilateral ureters
    - Urinary bladder
    - Ascending colon
    - Descending colon
    - Upper 2/3 of the rectum
    - Cervix

Must-Know Essentials: Mechanism of Injury and Organs Involved

- Blunt trauma
  - Most common cause of injury
  - Mechanism
    - Compression
    - Crushing
    - Shearing
    - Deceleration
- Penetrating trauma
  - Low energy
  - High energy

COMMON ORGANS INVOLVED

- Blunt trauma
  - Spleen: 40%–50%
  - Liver 35%–45%
  - Bowe: 5%–10%
- Penetrating trauma
  - Low energy
    - Liver 40%

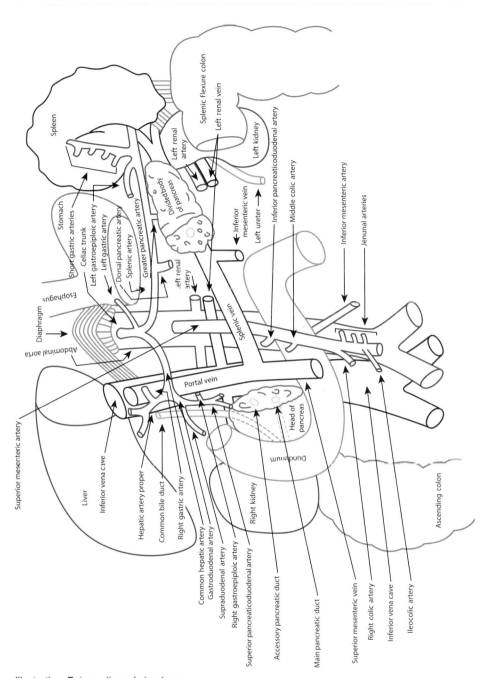

Illustration: Retroperitoneal structures

- Small bowel 30%
- Diaphragm 20%
- Colon 15%
- High energy
  - Small bowel 50%
  - Colon 40%
  - Liver 30%
  - Abdominal vascular 25%

Must-Know Essentials: Evaluation of Stable Abdominal Trauma

INITIAL EVALUATION AND MANAGEMENT

- Airway and protection of cervical spine
- Breathing
- Circulation
- Neurological deficit

PHYSICAL EXAMINATION OF THE ABDOMEN

- Clinical examination including:
  - inspection
  - auscultation
  - percussion
  - palpation.
- Limitations of clinical examination in patients with:
  - intoxication
  - head injury
  - spinal cord injury
  - spine fractures
  - ribs fractures
  - pelvic fractures.

FOCUSED ASSESSMENT WITH SONOGRAPHY FOR TRAUMA (FAST)

- Bedside procedure for a rapid assessment of the abdomen in blunt or penetrating trauma
- It can evaluate:
  - hemopericardium
  - hemoperitoneum
  - pneumothorax by extending the examination to bilateral hemithorax (Extended Focused Assessment with Sonography for Trauma [eFAST]).
- Sensitivity: 85%–96%
- Specificity: more than 98%
- Operator dependent
- Limitations
  - Distortion due to bowel gas and subcutaneous air

- Fails to diagnose:
  - bowel injury
  - diaphragm injury
  - pancreatic injuries.
- Techniques
  - Subxiphoid view
    - Evaluation of hemopericardium
      - Can detect as little as 20 mL of blood
      - Cardiac tamponade findings include:
        - right ventricular collapse during ventricular diastole
        - distended inferior vena cava (IVC).
  - Right upper quadrant (RUQ) view for blood in the:
    - hepatorenal recess (Morrison's pouch)
    - right paracolic gutter
    - hepatodiaphragmatic area.
  - Left upper quadrant (LUQ) view for blood in the:
    - splenorenal recess.
    - subphrenic space.
    - left paracolic gutter.
  - Suprapubic view for blood in the:
    - rectovesical pouch in men
    - rectouterine (pouch of Douglas) and vesicouterine pouches in women.

DIAGNOSTIC PERITONEAL LAVAGE

- Diagnostic peritoneal lavage (DPL) is a bedside invasive procedure for assessment of blunt or penetrating abdominal trauma.
- Sensitivity: 96%–99%
- Specificity: >98%
- Fails to diagnose retroperitoneal and diaphragmatic injuries
- Contraindications
  - Previous abdominal surgery
  - Morbid obesity
  - Coagulopathy
  - Pelvic fracture
- Complications
  - Injury to intraabdominal organs and/or vessels
  - Incision site bleeding or hematoma
- Techniques
  - Place a nasogastric tube.
  - Place a Foley catheter.
  - Prep and drape the abdomen.
  - Access the peritoneal cavity.
    - Closed percutaneous Seldinger technique
      - Insert an 18-gauge introducer needle 2 cm below the umbilicus in the midline angled at 45 degrees toward the pelvis in the peritoneal cavity.
  - Semiopen technique
    - Make a small vertical midline skin incision below the umbilicus.
    - Identify the fascia and insert the introducer needle directly through the fascia.
  - Aspirate the needle; if >10 mL of blood, gastrointestinal contents, or bile in the aspirated fluid, DPL is considered as positive.

- If no blood, GI content, or bile is aspirated, place a guidewire through the needle toward the pelvis.
- Remove the needle.
- Make a small skin incision at the guidewire entry site and advance the peritoneal dialysis catheter over the guidewire using the percutaneous Seldinger technique.
- Remove the guidewire.
- Connect the bag of warmed lavage solution to the catheter with IV tubing and allow the fluid to flow into the peritoneal cavity.
- Infuse 1 L warm lactated Ringer's (LR) solution into the peritoneal cavity.
- After infusion of LR in the peritoneal cavity, lower the empty bag below the level of the abdomen to return the fluid into the bag.
- Recover as much fluid as possible, but as little as 250 mL is adequate for the analysis.
- Send the fluid for analysis.
- Remove the catheter and place a dressing.
- DPL is considered positive if:
  - >10 mL of gross blood on aspiration
  - Gastrointestinal contents, or bile on aspiration
  - Gram stain positive for bacteria
  - WBC: >500 mm^3
  - RBC: >100,000 mm^3

CT ABDOMEN

- Gold standard for diagnosing intraabdominal injuries in blunt and penetrating trauma patients
- Can detect as little as 100 cc of intraperitoneal fluid
- Most specific for injuries
- Not recommended for unstable trauma patients

Must-Know Essentials: Management of Abdominal Trauma

INDICATIONS FOR EXPLORATORY LAPAROTOMY IN BLUNT ABDOMINAL TRAUMA

- Hypotension
- Peritonitis
- Positive FAST
- Positive DPL
- CT findings positive for injury
  - Pneumoperitoneum
  - Extravasation of contrast
  - Two of the following findings:
    - Free fluid in the absence of solid organ injury
    - Bowel wall thickening
    - Mesenteric fat streaking
    - Mesenteric hematoma

INDICATIONS OF LAPAROTOMY IN PENETRATING INJURY

- Hypotension
- Peritonitis
- Evisceration
- Bleeding from stomach, rectum, genitourinary tract
- High-energy abdominal injury such as gunshot wound (GSW)
- Low-energy injury such as stab wound with positive anterior fascial penetration after local wound exploration
- Positive FAST
- Positive DPL
- CT abdominal findings positive for injury in low-energy abdominal injury
- Impaled object

STEPS IN TRAUMA EXPLORATORY LAPAROTOMY (ALSO SEE CHAPTER 24)

- Use broad-spectrum preoperative antibiotics.
- Place a nasogastric tube.
- Place a Foley catheter.
- Prepare and drape the chest, abdomen, and both lower extremities up to the knees.
- Abdominal incision
  - Make a midline incision from the xiphoid process to the pubis.
  - Avoid entering the abdomen using the old abdominal surgical incision.
  - Make a bilateral subcostal incision (rooftop incision) in patients with multiple previous abdominal incisions.
- Enter the peritoneal cavity.
- Perform evisceration of bowel.
  - Small bowel loops up and to the patient's right in order to avoid traction injury on the mesentery
  - Transverse colon cranially
- Perform rapid temporary control of intraperitoneal bleeding.
  - Perform abdominal packing in each quadrant of the abdominal cavity in patients with blunt trauma.
  - Direct control of the bleeding with sutures or clamps in penetrating trauma.
  - May require cross-clamping of the aorta if indicated
- Identify the injuries.
  - Explore the peritoneal cavity.
  - Explore the retroperitoneum if indicated.
- Manage the specific injuries.
  - Definitive management in stable patients
  - Damage-control procedures for unstable patients with: Hypotension, hypothermia, acidosis, and coagulopathy
- Close the abdomen.
  - Definitive closure
  - Temporary abdominal closure
    - Indications
      - If significant bowel edema or ileus
      - Gross intraperitoneal contamination
      - After damage-control procedures

- Techniques of temporary abdominal closure
  - Closure of the skin using multiple Towel Clips.
  - Bogota bag closure
  - Wittmann Patch
  - Negative pressure therapy (NPT)
    - Abdominal wound V.A.C. system (3M/KCI, St. Paul, MN, USA).
    - ABTHERA (3M/KCI, St. Paul, MN, USA)
    - High negative pressure in NPT may aggravate bleeding; consider initial low negative pressure.

CHAPTER 24

Trauma Exploratory Laparotomy

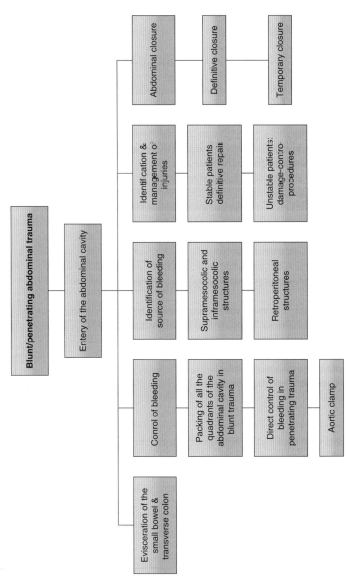

Algorithm: Trauma exploratory laparotomy

Must-Know Essentials: Principles of Trauma Exploratory Laparotomy

PREPARATION

- Use broad-spectrum preoperative antibiotics.
- Type and cross-match for blood.
- Place a nasogastric tube.
- Place a Foley catheter.
- Prepare and drape the chest, abdomen, and both lower extremities up to the knees.

ABDOMINAL INCISION AND ENTRY OF THE ABDOMINAL CAVITY

- Make a midline incision from the xiphoid process to the pubis.
- If possible, avoid entering the abdomen using the old abdominal surgical incision.
- Make a bilateral subcostal incision (rooftop incision) in patients with multiple previous abdominal incisions.
- Enter the peritoneal cavity just proximal to the umbilicus, because in this area the peritoneum is very thin with minimal preperitoneal fat.

EVISCERATION OF THE BOWEL

- Eviscerate small bowel loops up and to the patient's right in order to avoid traction injury on the mesentery.
- Eviscerate the transverse colon cranially.

TEMPORARY CONTROL OF INTRAPERITONEAL BLEEDING

- Blunt trauma
  - Perform abdominal packing in each quadrant of the abdominal cavity.
    - Above and below the right lobe of the liver
    - Right paracolic gutter
    - Superior and medial surface of the spleen
    - Superior surface of the left lobe of the liver
    - Left paracolic gutter
    - Pelvis
- Penetrating trauma
  - Perform direct control of the bleeding with sutures or clamps.
  - Aortic clamping if indicated (described below)

IDENTIFICATION OF THE SOURCE OF THE BLEEDING AND INJURIES

- Sources of bleeding in abdominal trauma
  - Intraperitoneal structures
  - Retroperitoneal structures
  - Combination of intraperitoneal and retroperitoneal structures.

- Intraperitoneal source of bleeding
  - Common sources in blunt trauma
    - Solid-organ injuries such as liver and spleen

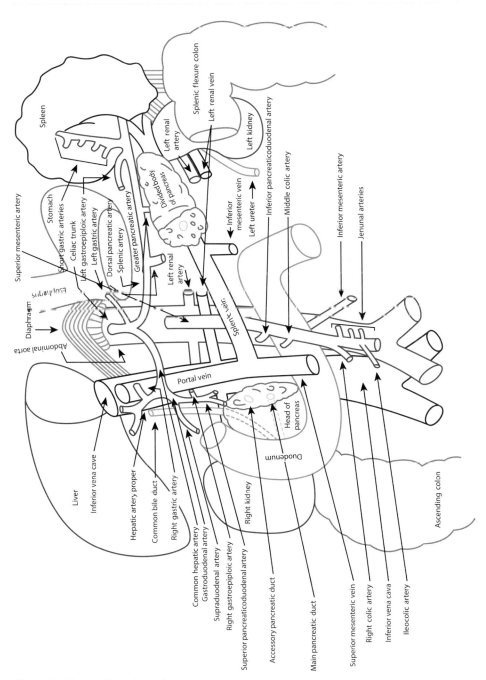

Illustration: Retroperitoneal structures

- Mesenteric vascular injuries
  - Distal superior mesenteric artery (SMA) and branches of the celiac trunk result in intraperitoneal bleeding.
  - Proximal SMA and celiac trunk are retroperitoneal structures.
- Small bowel injuries
- Retroperitoneal bleeding communicating to the peritoneal cavity
- Common sources in penetrating trauma
  - Liver
  - Small bowel
  - Diaphragm
  - Colon
  - Intraperitoneal or retroperitoneal vascular injury
  - Additional injury based on the trajectory of the weapon used
- Retroperitoneal source of bleeding
  - Blunt and penetrating trauma due to retroperitoneal vascular injuries
  - Exposure techniques (described below)

IDENTIFICATION AND MANAGEMENT OF INJURIES

- Intraperitoneal injuries
  - Supramesocolic (above the mesentery of the transverse colon) structures
    - Liver
    - Stomach
    - Spleen
  - Inframesocolic
    - Small intestine and its mesentery
    - Transverse colon and mesocolon
    - Uterus
- Retroperitoneal injuries
  - Supramesocolic (above the mesentery of the transverse colon) structures
    - Duodenum
    - Pancreas
    - Suprarenal midline vessels
  - Inframesocolic structures
    - Infrarenal midline vessels
    - Bilateral kidneys
    - Bilateral ureters
    - Urinary bladder
    - Ascending colon
    - Descending colon
    - Upper 2/3 of the rectum
    - Cervix
- Definitive or damage-control procedures of specific injuries

CLOSURE OF THE ABDOMEN

- Definitive closure
- Temporary abdominal closure
  - Indications
    - Risk of abdominal compartment syndrome

   Significant bowel edema or ileus
   Concern of ongoing intraperitoneal bleeding
   Gross intraperitoneal contamination
 After damage-control procedures
■ Techniques of temporary abdominal closure
 Closure of the skin using multiple towel clips
 Bogota bag closure
 Wittmann Patch
   Negative pressure therapy (NPT)
   Abdominal wound V.A.C. system (3 M/KCI, St. Paul, MN, USA)
   ABTHERA (3 M/KCI, St. Paul, MN, USA)
   High negative pressure in NPT may aggravate bleeding; may consider initial low
   negative pressure.

Must-Know Essentials: Aortic Clamping
INDICATIONS

■ Failure to control exsanguinating bleeding or hematoma with abdominal packing
■ Persistent hypotension due to exsanguination
■ Cardiac arrest in exsanguinating patients
■ Injury to the abdominal aorta and its branches, including the celiac trunk and superior
mesenteric artery

TECHNIQUES OF AORTIC CLAMP

■ Direct control of supraceliac aorta
 ■ Rapid temporary control of the supraceliac aorta
 ■ Requires minimal dissection
 ■ Steps
  ▨ Open the lesser sac and place a U-shaped handheld aortic compression device over the
    supraceliac aorta and apply constant anteroposterior pressure.
  ▨ May control proximal abdominal aorta at the hiatus of the diaphragm by digital com-
    pression or compression using a sponge stick.
■ Transabdominal subdiaphragmatic control of supraceliac aorta
 ■ A useful technique for more definitive control of the proximal aorta
 ■ Steps
  ▨ Mobilize the left lobe of the liver by dividing the round ligament, falciform ligament,
    and the left triangular ligament of the liver.
  ▨ Expose the esophageal hiatus by folding the left lobe of the liver medially.
  ▨ Expose the gastrohepatic ligament and the right crus of the diaphragm by retracting
    the stomach to the patient's left and downward.
  ▨ Dissect the esophagus circumferentially at the gastroesophageal junction and place a
    Penrose drain for traction.
  ▨ Make a vertical incision in the gastrohepatic ligament at least 1 cm to the right of
    the esophagus and extending along the upper margin of the lesser curvature of the
    stomach.
  ▨ Incise the posterior peritoneum over the right crus and bluntly dissect the aorta from
    the right crus. The aorta is located posteriorly to the right crus of the diaphragm.
  ▨ Divide the right crus of the diaphragm at the avascular 2 o'clock position.

- Free the medial and lateral wall of the aorta by blunt digital dissection.
- To avoid injury to posterior arterial branches, do not perform posterior dissection of the aorta..
- Place a curved vascular clamp (DeBakey or Cooley aortic aneurysm clamp) under finger guidance.
- Transthoracic control of the aorta with left anterolateral thoracotomy
  - Indicated in high supramesocolic hematoma where infradiaphragmatic exposure of the aorta is difficult.
  - Steps
    - Perform a left anterolateral thoracotomy (see Chapter 20 for detailed description).
    - Divide the inferior pulmonary ligament and retract the lung anteriorly and superiorly.
    - Open the pleura overlying the aorta with scissors.
    - Dissect the thoracic aorta anteriorly and posteriorly and place vascular clamp on the aorta.
  - Complications
    - Avulsion of intercostal arteries during dissection of the aorta resulting in with significant bleeding
    - Esophageal injury during anterior dissection of the aorta. Palpation of a previously placed nasogastric tube may help in rapid identification of the esophagus.
    - Injury to the inferior pulmonary vein leading to massive bleeding during mobilization of the lung by cutting the inferior pulmonary ligament.
- Control after exposure of the abdominal aorta with left medial visceral rotation (Mattox maneuver)
  - Advantages
    - Subdiaphragmatic proximal control of aorta.
    - Access to the abdominal aorta as well as most of its branches, including the celiac, superior mesenteric, left renal, and left iliac arteries

Must-Know Essentials: Exposure of Retroperitoneal Injuries

MANEUVERS FOR THE EXPOSURE OF THE RETROPERITONEUM

- Left medial visceral rotation (Mattox Maneuver)
- Right medial visceral rotations
  - Mobilization of duodenum (Kocher maneuver)
  - Mobilization of the ascending colon (Cattell maneuver).
  - Mobilization of the small bowel mesentery (Cattell-Braasch maneuver)
- Aird maneuver for the exposure of the body and tail of the pancreas

LEFT MEDIAL VISCERAL ROTATION (MATTOX MANEUVER)

- Indications
  - Subdiaphragmatic proximal control of aorta
  - Exposure of the abdominal aorta and its branches, including the celiac, superior mesenteric, left renal, and left iliac arteries
  - Inspection of the posterior surface of the pancreas

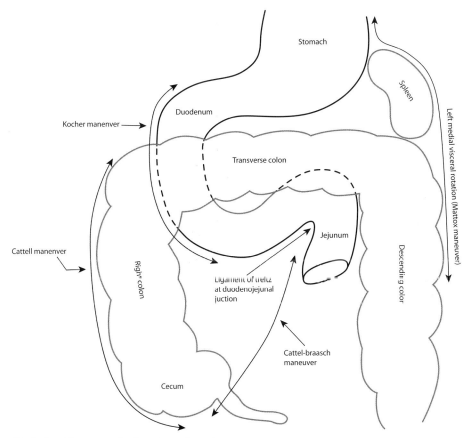

Illustration: Maneuvers for the retroperitoneal exposure

- Steps
  - Incise the left white line of Toldt to mobilize the descending colon, sigmoid colon, and splenic flexure toward the midline.
  - Extend the incision upward lateral to the spleen and divide the splenophrenic ligament.
  - Rotate the stomach, spleen, pancreas, and left kidney toward the midline from the posterior abdominal wall all the way up to the diaphragmatic hiatus.
  - Retract the gastroesophageal junction anteriorly to expose the anterolateral suprarenal abdominal aorta, celiac trunk, superior mesenteric artery, left renal artery, and left iliac arteries.
  - Modified left medial visceral rotation
    - Rotate the stomach, left colon, spleen, and tail of the pancreas medially and anterior to the left kidney.
    - It restricts the exposure of the anterolateral aspect of the aorta.
    - The left renal vein, left renal artery, and left ureter will be vulnerable to injury.
    - May consider for the exposure of the left kidney or the renal vessels.

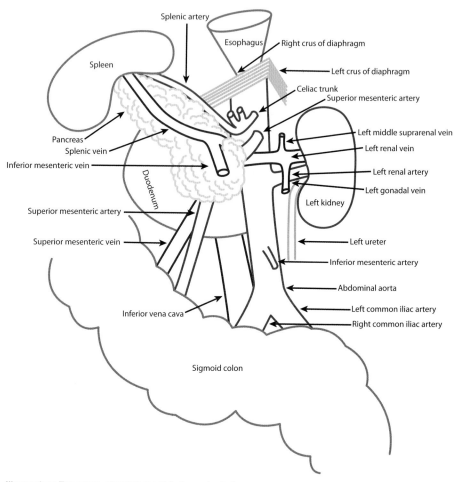

Illustration: Exposure after left medial visceral rotation

- Complications
  - Splenic injury
  - Avulsion of the left descending lumbar vein, which is a branch from the left renal vein that crosses over the lateral aspect of the aorta immediately below the left renal artery.

RIGHT MEDIAL VISCERAL ROTATION

- Complete right medial visceral rotation involves:
  - mobilization of the duodenum (Kocher maneuver)
  - mobilization of the ascending Colon (Cattell maneuver)
  - mobilization of the small bowel mesentery (Cattell-Braasch maneuver).
- Exposure after the complete right medial visceral rotation
  - Entire inframesocolic retroperitoneum with access to the infrarenal aorta and inferior vena cava (IVC)
  - Bilateral renal arteries, bilateral renal veins, and bilateral iliac vessels
  - Third and fourth parts of the duodenum

- Superior mesenteric vessels
- Head of the pancreas
- Intrapancreatic portion of the common bile duct

MOBILIZATION OF THE DUODENUM (KOCHER MANEUVER)

- Indications
  - Exposure of the posterior surface of the head of the pancreas, intrapancreatic portion of the common bile duct (CBD), inferior vena cava (IVC), and right renal hilum with renal vessels
  - Exposure of the posterior surface of the pancreas, third and fourth parts of the duodenum, the superior mesenteric vessels, and the portal vein with extended Kocher maneuver
- Steps
  - Make an incision in the posterior peritoneum immediately lateral to the duodenum.
  - Mobilize the duodenal loop en bloc using blunt dissection to expose the posterior aspect of the head of the pancreas and its uncinate process.

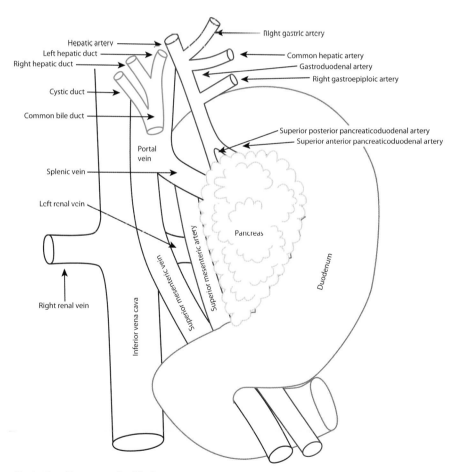

Illustration: Exposure after Kocher maneuver

- Watch for an accessory right hepatic artery, which comes from the superior mesenteric artery and situated posterior to the duodenum and the pancreas.
- Reflect the duodenal loop and head of the pancreas medially to expose the IVC, the right renal hilum, and the common bile duct.
- Avoid injury to the right gonadal vein as it enters the IVC at this level.
- Extended Kocher maneuver
  - Extend the peritoneal dissection along the duodenum to the ligament of Treitz along the superior leaf of the transverse mesocolon.
  - Continue mobilizing the duodenal loop from the common bile duct superiorly to the superior mesenteric vein (SMV) inferiorly.

MOBILIZATION OF THE RIGHT COLON (CATTELL MANEUVER)

- Indications
  - Exposure of the entire infrahepatic IVC
  - Exposure of the right kidney and the renal hilum with the right renal vessels
  - Exposure of the right iliac vessels
- Steps
  - Extend the lateral peritoneal Kocher incision in the posterior peritoneum along the white line of Toldt lateral to the hepatic flexure of the right colon and extend it caudally to the cecum.
  - Mobilize the right colon from the hepatic flexure to the cecum.
  - Protect and avoid injury to the duodenum as hepatic flexure overlies the lower part of the duodenal loop.

MOBILIZE THE SMALL BOWEL MESENTERY (CATTELL-BRAASCH MANEUVER)

- Indications
  - Exposure of the entire infrahepatic IVC, from the inferior border of the liver (suprarenal portion) to its bifurcation
  - Exposure of the right kidney
  - Exposure of the bilateral renal vessels
  - Exposure of the infrarenal abdominal aorta
  - Exposure of the superior mesenteric vessels
  - Exposure of the bilateral iliac vessels
  - Exposure of the third and fourth parts of the duodenum
- Steps
  - Perform mobilization of the duodenum (Kocher maneuver) and the right colon (Cattell maneuver), as previously described.
  - Retract the small bowel to the right and cranially to expose the small bowel mesentery, which is attached to the posterior abdominal wall in an oblique line extending from the cecum to the ligament of Treitz.
  - Make an incision in the posterior peritoneum along the line of the small bowel mesentery from the medial side of the cecum to the ligament of Treitz.
  - Retract the small bowel and the right colon upward to expose the retroperitoneal structures.
  - Divide the ligament of Treitz on the right side of the duodenojejunal junction. The SMA is located on the left side of the duodenojejunal junction.

- Complications
  - Injury to the SMV at the root of the mesentery
  - Avulsion of the right colic vein off the SMV

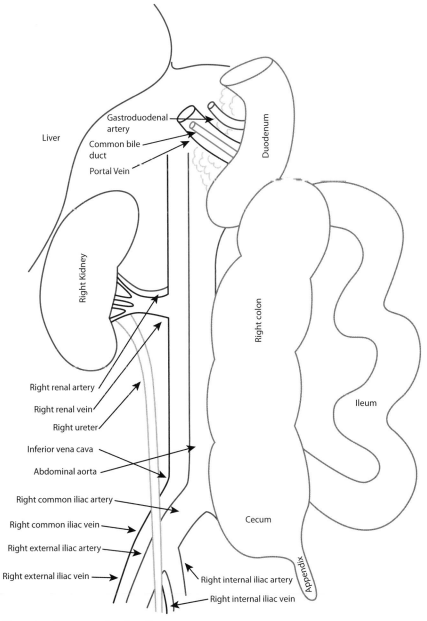

Illustration: Exposure after Cattell maneuver

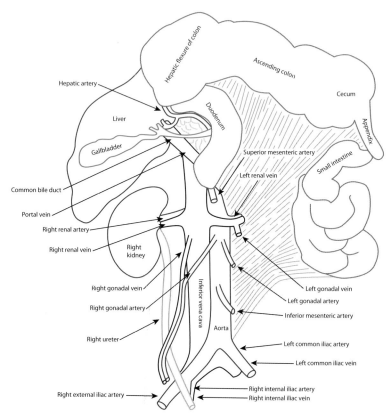

Illustration: Exposure after Cattell-Braasch maneuver

AIRD MANEUVER

- Indication
  - Exposure of the posterior aspect of the body and tail of the pancreas
- Steps
  - Divide the splenophrenic and splenorenal ligament.
  - Mobilize the spleen along with the tail of the pancreas from Gerota's fascia.
  - Rotate the spleen and the tail of the pancreas medially and anteriorly to expose the posterior aspect of the body and tail of the pancreas.

CHAPTER 25

Management of Liver Injuries

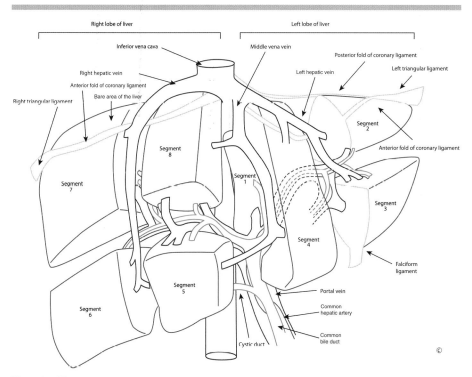

Illustration: Liver anatomy

Must-Know Essentials: Anatomy of the Liver (see illustration of liver anatomy)

LIGAMENTS OF THE LIVER

- Falciform ligament
  - Attaches the anterior surface of the liver to the anterior abdominal wall
  - Free edge of the Falciform ligament contains the remnant of umbilical vein and known as round ligament of the liver. It is also called the ligamentum of teres.
  - Round ligament divides the left lobe of the liver into a medial section (segment 4) and lateral sections (segments 2 and 3).
  - The left hepatic bile duct, left hepatic artery, and left portal vein enter the undersurface of the liver near the falciform ligament.
  - The portal venous supply to the medial segment of the left lobe can be injured during dissection of the falciform ligament.

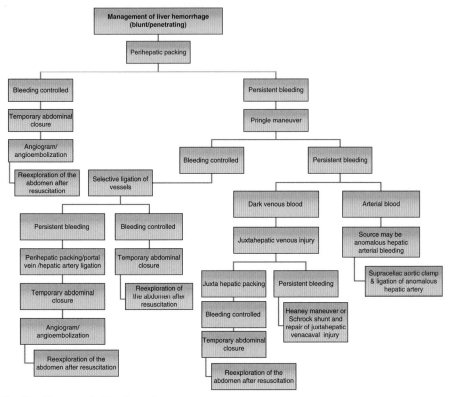

Algorithm: Management of liver hemorrhage

- Coronary ligament (anterior and posterior folds)
  - Attaches the superior surface of the liver to the inferior surface of the diaphragm
  - Demarcates the bare area of the liver
  - The anterior and posterior folds fuse to form the triangular ligaments on the right and left lobes of the liver.
- Triangular ligaments (left and right)
  - The left triangular ligament is formed by the union of the anterior and posterior layers of the coronary ligament and attaches the left lobe of the liver to the diaphragm.
  - The right triangular ligament is formed in a similar fashion adjacent to the bare area and attaches the right lobe of the liver to the diaphragm.
  - The right triangular ligament is divided for mobilization of the right lobe of the liver. The retrohepatic inferior vena cava (IVC) and the retrohepatic veins should be protected during mobilization of the right lobe of the liver.
  - The left triangular ligament is divided for mobilization of the left lobe of the liver. The phrenic vein should be protected during mobilization of the left lobe of the liver.
- Lesser omentum
  - Attaches the liver to the lesser curvature of the stomach and the first part of the duodenum
  - Consists of the hepatoduodenal ligament (extends from the duodenum to the liver) and the hepatogastric ligament (extends from the stomach to the liver)

- The hepatoduodenal ligament surrounds the portal triad (hepatic artery, common bile duct, and portal vein).

SEGMENTAL ANATOMY OF THE LIVER (COUINAUD CLASSIFICATION)

- Eight functionally independent segments of the liver
- Each segment has its own vascular inflow, outflow, and biliary drainage.

CANTLIE LINE

- An imaginary line from the left of the inferior vena cava, just left of the gallbladder fossa through the liver
- Separates the liver into right and left lobes
- The middle hepatic vein is situated within this line.
- Separates segment 4 from segments 5 and 8

PORTA HEPATIS

- Approximately 5-cm-long transverse deep fissure in the liver extending transversely beneath the left portion of the right lobe of the liver
- Separates the quadrate lobe (segment 4) from the caudate lobe (segment 1)

ROUVIERE'S SULCUS

- Fissure in the liver between the right lobe and the caudate process
- This sulcus should be identified during laparoscopic cholecystectomy before the dissection in Calot's triangle and considered as an important landmark for safe cholecystectomy.
- It is recommended that all dissection should be performed above or anterior to this sulcus to prevent injury to the common bile duct at the porta hepatis.

BLOOD SUPPLY OF THE LIVER

- Hepatic artery (proper hepatic artery)
  - Branch from common hepatic artery
  - Common hepatic artery is a branch from the celiac trunk.
  - The hepatic artery divides into right and left hepatic arteries.
  - The cystic artery is a branch from the right hepatic artery.
  - Variation in hepatic artery
    - Seen in 40%–60% of people
    - Accessory hepatic artery
      - Additional artery to the liver along with normal hepatic arteries
      - Accessory left hepatic artery: a branch from left gastric artery and the most common accessory hepatic artery
    - Replaced hepatic artery
      - Anomalous origin of hepatic arteries
      - The right hepatic artery arising from the superior mesenteric artery (SMA) and the replaced left hepatic artery arising from the left gastric artery are commonly replaced hepatic arteries.

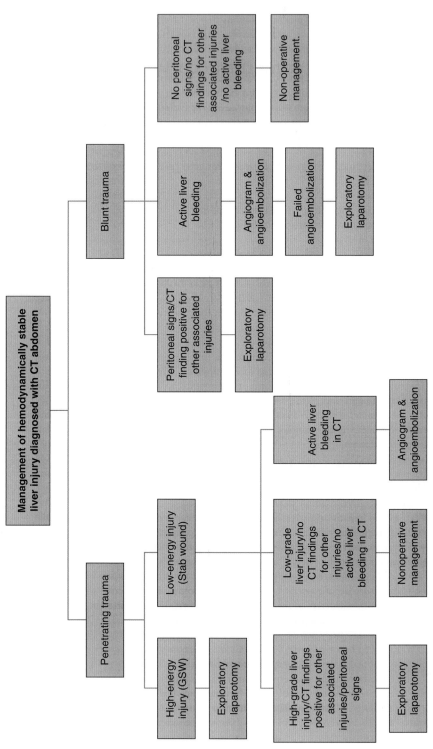

Algorithm: Management of hemodynamically stable liver injury

- Portal vein
  - Supplies approximately 75% of total blood to the liver
  - Formed by the superior mesenteric vein (SMV) and the splenic vein.
- Hepatic vein
  - Three hepatic veins (right, middle, and left) drain to the IVC.

Must-Know Essentials: The American Association for the Surgery of Trauma (AAST) Grading of Liver Injury

GRADES

- Grade I
  - Hematoma
    - Subcapsular <10% surface area
  - Laceration
    - Capsular tear or parenchymal laceration <1 cm deep
- Grade II
  - Hematoma
    - Subcapsular 10%–50 % of the surface area
  - Laceration
    - Intraparenchymal <10 cm diameter
    - Capsular tear or parenchymal laceration 1–3 cm deep, <10 cm in length.
- Grade III
  - Hematoma
    - Subcapsular >50% surface area
    - Ruptured subcapsular or parenchymal hematoma
    - Intraparenchymal hematoma >10 cm or expanding hematoma
  - Laceration
    - 3-cm-deep parenchymal laceration
- Grade IV
  - Laceration
    - Parenchymal disruption involving 25%–75% hepatic lobe or 1–3 Couinaud's segments
- Grade V
  - Laceration
    - Parenchymal disruption >75% hepatic lobe or >3 Couinaud's segments within a single lobe
  - Vascular
    - Juxtahepatic venous injury (retrohepatic vena cava/central major hepatic veins)
- Grade VI
  - Vascular
    - Hepatic avulsion. *Advance one grade for multiple injuries up to grade III.*

Must-Know Essentials: Management of Liver Injuries

INDICATIONS FOR EXPLORATORY LAPAROTOMY IN PATIENTS WITH LIVER INJURY

- Hemodynamically stable blunt trauma
  - Signs of peritonitis

- CT findings positive for injury
  - Pneumoperitoneum
  - Two of the following findings:
    - Free fluid in the absence of solid organ injury
    - Bowel wall thickening
    - Mesenteric fat streaking
    - Mesenteric hematoma
  - Persistent liver bleeding after angioembolization
- Hemodynamically stable penetrating trauma
  - All high-energy injuries such as gunshot wounds (GSWs)
  - Low-energy injuries such as stab wounds
    - Signs of peritonitis
    - Evisceration
    - Pneumoperitoneum
    - Free intraperitoneal fluid
    - Hemoperitoneum
    - High-grade liver injury
- Unstable
  - All blunt and penetrating trauma

INDICATIONS FOR ANGIOGRAM AND ANGIOEMBOLIZATION

- Stable blunt trauma with active liver bleeding without any other indications for an exploratory laparotomy
- Stable low-energy penetrating trauma with active liver bleeding without other indications for an exploratory laparotomy
- Unstable patient after hepatic packing before reexploration of the abdomen

Must-Know Essentials: Operative Procedures for Liver Injury

PERIHEPATIC PACKING

- The most important damage-control procedure
- Most liver bleeding can be controlled by liver packing, including retrohepatic vena cava bleeding.
- Mobilization of the liver should not be performed for perihepatic packing.
- Mobilization of the liver in retrohepatic hematoma and retrohepatic venous injury can make the situation worse due to loss of tamponade effect.
- Packing is more effective in right lobe injuries than in left lobe injuries because it is difficult to compress the left lobe against the chest wall and the diaphragm.
- Technique of packing
  - Place lap pads/gauze posterior and anterior to the liver, plus one or two in the hepatorenal space.
  - Anterior packing compresses the liver against the anterior abdominal wall and anterior chest wall.
  - Posterior packing compresses the liver against the posterior chest wall, diaphragm, and retroperitoneum.
  - Do not place packing in the retrohepatic space.

- May place an absorbable mesh such as Polyglactin or other hemostatic agents over the laceration site before placement of the lap pad/gauze.
- May use commercially available hemostatic packing gauze (e.g., QuikClot).
- Complications of hepatic packing
  - Compression of IVC may result in hypotension due to the drop in cardiac venous return.
  - Portal vein thrombosis
  - Hypoventilation due to increase in peak airway pressure

PRINGLE MANEUVER

- Inflow occlusion of hepatic artery and portal vein at the portal triad
- Technique
  - Make an opening in the avascular portion of the lesser omentum on the left side of the portal triad.
  - Perform a blunt dissection through the foramen of Winslow encircling the hepatoduodenal ligament.
    - The hepatoduodenal ligament contains the common bile duct, hepatic artery, and portal vein.
  - Place a noncrushing vascular clamp or an umbilical tape with a Rummel tourniquet around the hepatoduodenal ligament.
  - Portal triad occlusion for 30–45 minutes may be considered safe. Longer occlusion of the portal triad can cause splanchnic hypervolemia/systemic hypovolemia, liver ischemia, and gallbladder ischemia.
- Continued bleeding after this maneuver suggests the source of bleeding may be:
  - retrohepatic inferior vena cava (IVC) injury.
  - hepatic venous injuries.
  - replaced left hepatic artery injury.
  - The replaced left hepatic artery is a branch from the left gastric artery that cannot be controlled with the Pringle maneuver.
  - The replaced right hepatic artery is commonly a branch from the SMA that lies in the hepatoduodenal ligament and is included in the Pringle maneuver.

MOBILIZATION OF THE LIVER

- Indicated for the direct control of bleeding in complex liver laceration if bleeding continues after perihepatic packing
- Peripheral and anterior laceration can be repaired without mobilizing the liver.
- Technique
  - Exposure of the posterior lateral surface of the left lobe.
    - Mobilize the left lobe by dividing the:
      - falciform ligament.
      - anterior and posterior coronary ligaments on the left side.
      - left triangular ligament.
  - Exposure of the posterior lateral surface of the right lobe.
    - Mobilize the right lobe by dividing the:
      - falciform ligament.
      - right anterior coronary ligament.
      - right triangular ligament.
  - Complications during mobilization of the liver
    - Injury to the left portal vein during division of the falciform ligament

- Injury to the retrohepatic IVC and hepatic veins during division of the right triangular ligament to mobilize the right lobe
- Injury to the phrenic vein during division of the left triangular ligament to mobilize the left lobe
- Avoid mobilization of the right lobe if there is any concern for retrohepatic venous injury.

HEPATOTOMY USING FINGER FRACTURE TECHNIQUE AND SELECTIVE LIGATION OF BLEEDERS

- Extend the liver laceration using the finger fracture technique.
- Identify the bleeding vessels and control with:
  - suture ligation.
  - clips.
  - electrocautery.
  - argon beam coagulator.
- After control of bleeding
  - Repair the deep liver lacerations with figure-of-eight, tension-free sutures using 0-chromic catgut on a large blunt-tip liver needle.
  - If repair is not possible
    - Pack the cavity with hemostatic agents (Fibrin glue, Floseal) and gauze or Combat Gauze.
    - The pedicle of the greater omentum may also be used to pack the cavity.
- Complications
  - Significant bleeding
  - Iatrogenic injury to a major hepatic duct or hilar vessel

NONANATOMICAL RESECTION/DEBRIDEMENT OF THE LIVER

- Indications
  - Significant destruction of the hepatic lobe with profuse bleeding
  - Laceration of the edges of the liver with bleeding
- Techniques
  - Resection using electrocautery: Resect the liver immediately outside the injured area in healthy hepatic tissue.
  - Finger fracture technique
    - After finger fracture, perform selective ligation of vessels and ducts.
    - Perform resection of the liver using electrocautery.
  - Resection of the liver using a vascular-load linear cutting stapler.
  - Using large clamps, resect the liver by underrunning the clamp with 0- chromic catgut sutures to close the raw surface of the liver.

REPAIR OF LACERATION (HEPATORRHAPHY)

- Perform repair of the linear laceration with intact capsule with 0-chromic catgut on a blunt-tip, large, curved needle using horizontal mattress/figure-of-eight/simple-through-and-through suture technique.
- Adjuncts of repair
  - Omental flap to reinforce the repair
  - Hemostatic agents (fibrin glue, Floseal, etc.)
  - Packing using hemostatic-agent-coated gauze, such as QuikClot) or regular gauze.

HEPATIC ARTERY AND PORTAL VEIN LIGATION FOR PERSISTENT LIVER BLEEDING

- Persistent bleeding after hepatotomy or liver packing but controlled with Pringle maneuver may require ligation of the portal vein or the hepatic artery as a damage-control procedure.
- Hepatic artery ligation
  - Perform if bleeding appears arterial in nature.
  - Ligate the artery at the porta hepatis.
  - Perform cholecystectomy once the patient is stable.
- Portal vein ligation
  - Perform if bleeding appears venous in nature.
  - Ligate the portal vein at the porta hepatis.
  - It is tolerated well in patients with patent hepatic artery.
  - Complications
    - May result in mesenteric venous congestion and reduced systemic venous return, causing shock and possible cardiac arrest, a condition known as splanchnic hypervolemia/systemic hypovolemia syndrome
    - Bowel ischemia
    - Portal hypertension

INTRAHEPATIC BALLOON TAMPONADE FOR BLEEDING CONTROL

- An effective method of bleeding control in centrally located penetrating through-and-through liver injury
- Techniques
  - Wider tract (>2 cm in diameter)
    - Insert a Sengstaken-Blackmore tube into the tract so that the gastric balloon comes out of the exit wound of the liver
    - Inflate the gastric balloon with air outside the exit wound of the liver.
    - After inflation of the gastric balloon, gently inflate the esophageal balloon in the tract until bleeding stops.
  - Narrow tract or short for a Sengstaken-Blakemore tube
    - Create a balloon from a red rubber catheter and a Penrose drain.
    - Tie off one end of the Penrose drain with two heavy silk ties.
    - Place the open end of the Penrose drain over a red rubber catheter and tie it around the catheter to create a sausage-shaped balloon.
    - Check the balloon for leaks by injecting saline through the red rubber catheter and clamping it.
    - Insert the balloon into the tract and inflate the balloon until bleeding stops, then clamp the catheter.

TRACTOTOMY WITH BLEEDING CONTROL

- It is a most effective method of bleeding control in peripherally located penetrating injuries.
- It is not recommended for centrally located penetrating injuries due to the risk of significant bleeding.
- Techniques
  - Use a linear stapler to open the tract and obtain hemostasis.
  - Use finger fracture technique and obtain hemostasis by ligation of the vessels.

PROCEDURES FOR RETROHEPATIC VENOUS INJURY

- Diagnosed when dark venous bleeding is seen behind the liver that cannot be controlled by manual compression or the Pringle maneuver.
- Exploration is usually not recommended. It can result in worsening of bleeding due to loss of the tamponade effect.
- It is usually treated with liver packing without mobilizing the liver.
- Packing should be placed between the liver and anterior abdominal wall and under the inferior surface of the liver to compress the liver against the IVC and create a tamponade.
- Packing should not be placed in the retrohepatic space.
- Repair of injury is recommended in persistent bleeding after liver packing.
- Repair requires complex procedures such as:
  - total hepatic isolation (Heaney maneuver) (see Chapter 31 for details).
  - atriocaval shunt placement (see Chapter 31 for details).
- Associated with high mortality, including cardiac arrest

INJURY TO PORTAL TRIAD

- Structures of the portal triad include:
  - the extrahepatic portal vein.
  - the extra hepatic artery
  - the extrahepatic bile duct.
- Injury to the extrahepatic portal vein and extrahepatic hepatic artery is also called Zone 4 injury.
- Portal vein injury
  - Exposure
    - Perform Pringle maneuver before exploring the hematoma.
    - Explore the injury through the hematoma and place vascular clamp for proximal and distal control.
    - Consider extended Kocher maneuver for better exposure of the portal vein.
    - In penetrating injury, consider division of the neck of the pancreas with a TA stapler. It provides good exposure of the portal vein. Place the stapler in the avascular plane at the neck of the pancreas anterior to the superior mesenteric vessels and the portal vein.
  - Treatment
    - Hemodynamically stable patients
      - Smaller injury: Repair with 4-0/5-0 polypropylene suture
      - Larger injury: Reconstruction with autologous saphenous vein graft
    - Damage control in hemodynamically unstable patients
      - Ligation of portal vein
        - Well tolerated in patients with patent hepatic artery
        - May result in mesenteric venous congestion and reduced systemic venous return, causing shock and possible cardiac arrest, a condition known as splanchnic hypervolemia/systemic hypovolemia syndrome
        - Syndrome of splanchnic hypervolemia/systemic hypovolemia also seen after superior mesenteric vein ligation but is more common after portal vein ligation
        - May result in bowel ischemia, portal hypertension, and abdominal compartment syndrome
- Hepatic artery injury
  - Ligate the hepatic artery if the portal vein is intact.
  - Perform a cholecystectomy after ligation of the hepatic artery once the patient is stable.

REEXPLORATION AFTER DAMAGE-CONTROL LAPAROTOMY IN LIVER INJURY

- Reexploration of the abdomen is performed after:
  - adequate resuscitation.
  - correction of hypothermia, acidosis, and coagulopathy.
  - angiography with selective angiographic embolization if indicated:
    - No definite recommendation about the benefit from hepatic angiography after packing in stable patient
    - Complications of angioembolization
      - Liver necrosis
      - Bile leak
      - Liver abscess
- Procedures
  - Remove the hepatic packing.
  - Reevaluate the liver injury for bleeding and bile leak.
  - Evaluate for any associated nonhepatic injuries.
  - Perform local resection of nonviable liver parenchyma.
  - Perform abdominal closure.

Must-Know Essentials: Management of Extrahepatic Biliary Injuries

THE AMERICAN ASSOCIATION FOR THE SURGERY OF TRAUMA (AAST) GRADING OF BILIARY INJURIES

- Grade I
  - Gallbladder contusion/hematoma
  - Contusion of portal triad
- Grade II
  - Partial gallbladder avulsion from the liver bed with intact cystic duct
  - Laceration or perforation of gallbladder
- Grade III
  - Complete gallbladder avulsion from the liver bed
  - Cystic duct laceration
- Grade IV
  - Partial or complete right hepatic duct laceration
  - Partial or complete left hepatic duct laceration
  - Partial common hepatic duct laceration (<50%)
  - Partial common bile duct laceration (<50%)
- Grade V
  - >50% laceration of common hepatic duct
  - >50% laceration of common bile duct
  - Combined right and left hepatic duct injuries
  - Intraduodenal or intrapancreatic bile duct injuries *Advance one grade up for multiple injuries up to Grade III.*

EVALUATION FOR BILIARY INJURY

- Indications for evaluation
  - Concern of biliary injury during exploratory laparotomy for liver injury

- Bilious drainage in intraoperatively placed drains
- Elevated bilirubin or liver enzymes after abdominal trauma
- High-grade liver injuries, both blunt and penetrating
- Methods of evaluation
  - Intraoperative cholangiogram
  - Hepatobiliary iminodiacetic acid (HIDA) scan
  - Magnetic resonance cholangiopancreatography (MRCP)
  - Endoscopic retrograde cholangiopancreatography (ERCP)

TREATMENT OF GALLBLADDER INJURY

- Indications of cholecystectomy
  - Severe gallbladder contusion
  - Laceration or perforation of the gallbladder
  - Partial or complete avulsion of the gallbladder from the liver bed
  - Injury to the cystic duct
  - Injury to the cystic artery
- Damage-control in unstable patient
  - Do not perform cholecystectomy in an unstable coagulopathic patient due to the risk of bleeding from the liver bed. Options include:
    - Repair the laceration with a single layer of absorbable suture.
    - Drain the gallbladder with a cholecystostomy tube inserted through the injured fundus and secure it with a purse-string suture.
- Cholecystectomy after patient becomes stable

TREATMENT OF BILE DUCT INJURY

- Damage-control options for common bile duct injury
  - External biliary drainage
  - Ligating or clipping the common duct
  - Placement of a T-tube in the common bile duct
- Definitive repair of extrahepatic biliary injuries
  - Performed during reexploration of the abdomen once patient becomes stable
  - Simple laceration with involvement of <50% of the circumference: Repair with an absorbable 5-0 PDS interrupted suture with placement of an external drain.
  - Laceration with involvement of >50 % of the circumference: Debridement and end-to-end anastomosis with a T-tube placement
  - Complex laceration with tissue loss: Biliary (hepatic duct or common bile duct) enteric Roux-en-Y reconstruction
- Endoscopic treatment with stent
  - Bile leak after biliary surgery
  - Small biliary injury detected on evaluation in patients being treated nonoperatively.

CHAPTER 26

Evaluation and Management of Pancreatic Injuries

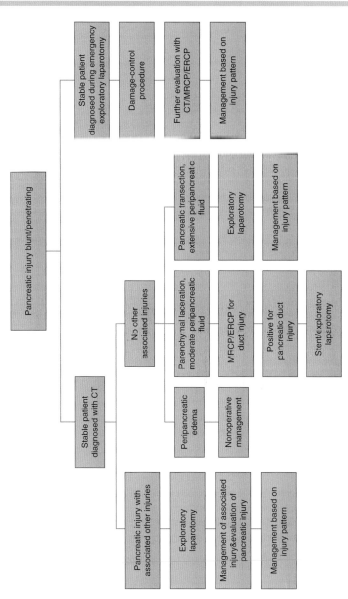

Algorithm: Evaluation of pancreas injury

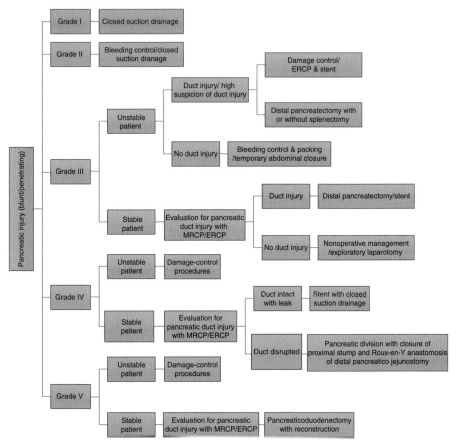

Algorithm: Management of pancreatic injury

Must-Know Essentials: Anatomy of the Pancreas

LOCATION

- Retroperitoneum
- Extends obliquely at the level of L1 and L2 vertebra

DIVISION OF THE PANCREAS

- Head of the Pancreas
  - Located in the C-loop of the duodenum
  - On the right side of the superior mesenteric vessels
  - Important structures posterior to the head:
    - Inferior vena cava (IVC)
    - Hilum of the right kidney
    - Right renal vein
    - Common bile duct (CBD)
  - Medial side of the head is in close contact with the duodenum.

- Uncinate process of the pancreas
  - Extension of the head of the pancreas
  - Situated posterior to the superior mesenteric vessels
- Neck of the pancreas
  - Situated anterior to the superior mesenteric vessels
  - Important posterior structures
    - Superior mesenteric artery
    - Superior mesenteric vein
    - Proximal portal vein
- Body and tail of the pancreas
  - Situated on the left side of the mesenteric vessels
  - Important structures posterior to the body
    - Suprarenal aorta
    - Left renal vessels
    - Splenic vein
    - Inferior mesenteric vein, which joins the splenic vein
  - Splenic artery runs along the superior border of the pancreas.
  - Tail of the pancreas is in close contact with the hilum of the spleen.

PANCREATIC DUCTS

- Main pancreatic duct (Wirsung duct)
  - Runs in the entire length of the pancreas
  - Joins the CBD to drain into the ampulla of Vater
  - Ampulla of Vater drains into the medial wall of the second part of the duodenum (D2) through the major papilla.
  - Both the CBD and the pancreatic duct enter the duodenum through a separate ampulla in 10% of the population.
- Accessary pancreatic duct (duct of Santorini)
  - Present in approximately 30% of the patient population
  - Drains into the second part of the duodenum, usually proximal and dorsal to the main pancreatic duct through the minor papilla (70%), or may drain directly (30%) into the main pancreatic duct
  - In pancreas divisum (failure of the fusion of the ventral and dorsal pancreatic ductal systems), the majority of the pancreas is drained through the accessory duct into the minor papilla.

ARTERIAL SUPPLY

- Head of the pancreas
  - Superior pancreaticoduodenal artery
    - Branch from gastroduodenal artery
    - Divides to form anterior and posterior pancreaticoduodenal arcades
  - Inferior pancreaticoduodenal artery
    - Branch from superior mesenteric artery.
    - Divides to form anterior and posterior pancreaticoduodenal arcades.
- Body and tail of the pancreas
  - Branches from the splenic artery including the:
    - greater pancreatic artery.
    - dorsal pancreatic artery.

VENOUS DRAINAGE

- Follows the arteries to provide tributaries to the splenic vein and superior mesenteric vein
- Superior mesenteric vein joins the splenic vein and forms the portal vein posterior to the neck of the pancreas.

Must-Know Essentials: American Association for the Surgery of Trauma (AAST) Grading of Pancreatic Injuries

GRADES

- Grade I
  - Hematoma: Minor contusion without duct injury
  - Laceration: Superficial laceration without duct injury
- Grade II
  - Hematoma: Major contusion without duct injury or tissue loss
  - Laceration: Major laceration without duct injury or tissue loss
- Grade III
  - Laceration: Distal transection (left of the superior mesenteric vessels)
  - Laceration: Distal parenchymal injury with duct injury (left of the mesenteric vessels)
- Grade IV
  - Laceration: Proximal transection (right of superior mesenteric vein) or parenchymal injury involving ampulla
- Grade V
  - Laceration: Massive disruption of the pancreatic head *Advance one grade up for multiple injuries up to Grade III.*

Must-Know Essentials: Evaluation of Pancreatic Injuries

UNSTABLE PATIENT

- Emergency exploratory laparotomy and intraoperative evaluation of pancreatic injury

STABLE PATIENT

- CT abdomen with IV contrast is an initial modality of choice.
  - Finding(s) suggestive of pancreatic injury
    - Pancreatic hematoma/contusion
    - Peripancreatic stranding
    - Pancreatic laceration
    - Transection of pancreas
    - Fluid collection or hematoma in the lesser sac
  - Indirect findings suggestive for pancreatic injury
    - Inflammation of anterior renal fascia
    - Inflammation of peripancreatic fat
    - Extraperitoneal or intraperitoneal fluid
    - Fluid in lesser sac
    - Associated splenic, duodenal, or hepatobiliary injury

- Evaluation of pancreatic duct injury
  - CT scan has low sensitivity (79%) and specificity (62%) for the diagnosis of main pancreatic duct injury.
  - Indications
    - CT findings concerning of pancreatic duct injury in stable patients
    - Intraoperative findings suspicious of ductal injury
    - Damage-control laparotomy after patients become hemodynamically stable
  - Methods of evaluation
    - Magnetic resonance cholangiopancreatography (MRCP)
      - High sensitivity and specificity for the detection of pancreatic ductal injury
    - Endoscopic retrograde cholangiopancreatography (ERCP)
      - Most accurate diagnostic test for ductal evaluation
      - Can also be used to for the treatment of pancreatic duct injury with stent

Must-Know Essentials: Management of Pancreatic Injuries

EXPOSURE OF PANCREATIC INJURY DURING EMERGENCY EXPLORATORY LAPAROTOMY

- Intraoperative findings suggestive for pancreatic injuries
  - Peripancreatic hematoma
  - Peripancreatic edema
  - Presence of retroperitoneal bile
  - Hematoma at the base of the transverse mesocolon
  - Central retroperitoneal hematoma
- Intraoperative findings suggestive of major ductal injury
  - Direct visualization of the ductal injury
  - Complete transection of the pancreas
  - Transverse laceration involving >50% of the gland
  - Central laceration of the pancreas

EXPLORATORY LAPAROTOMY AND EXPOSURE FOR PANCREATIC INJURY-BASED CT ABDOMEN IN STABLE PATIENTS

- CT abdomen findings with:
  - pancreatic injury with other associated injuries.
  - pancreatic transection.
  - large peripancreatic hematoma.
  - large laceration with bleeding.
  - large peripancreatic fluid.
- Pancreatic duct injury diagnosed with MRCP/ERCP
  - May be treated with stent
  - Exploratory laparotomy if stent not possible

TECHNIQUES OF EXPOSURE OF THE PANCREAS

- Exposure of the anterior surface of the pancreas
  - Best exposed through the lesser sac
  - Steps

- Divide the gastrocolic ligament just below the arcades of right and left gastroepiploic vessels using a LigaSure, or suture ligation of the vessels starting from the splenic flexure of the colon to the duodenum.
- Divide the membranous attachment between the posterior surface of the stomach and anterior surface of the pancreas after entering the lesser sac.
- Identify the splenic artery along the posterior surface of the upper border.
- Exposure of the posterior surface of the pancreas
  - Limited exposure of the posterior surface is obtained by mobilizing the inferior border.
  - Steps
    - Divide the superior leaf of the transverse mesocolon to expose the inferior border of the pancreas.
    - Apply gentle upward traction at the inferior border to expose the posterior surface of the pancreas.
    - This also exposes the middle colic vessels, superior mesenteric vein, and inferior mesenteric vein.
  - Full exposure of posterior surface of the pancreas
    - Perform extended Kocher maneuver for exposure of the posterior surface of the pancreas (see Chapter 24 for details).
    - Perform left medial visceral rotation anterior to the left kidney for the exposure of the posterior surface of the body and tail of the pancreas (see Chapter 24 for details).
- Exposure of the superior mesenteric vessels and portal vein in penetrating pancreatic injury
  - Perform the extended Kocher maneuver for exposure of the superior mesenteric vein and portal vein, which can also be exposed by dividing the neck of the pancreas.
  - Steps
    - Dissect the avascular plane between posterior surface of the neck of the pancreas and vessels (portal vein and the superior mesenteric vessels) to create a space.
    - Divide the neck of the pancreas with a TA stapler.
    - It provides exposure of the portal vein and the superior mesenteric vessels.

TREATMENT OF PANCREATIC INJURIES BASED ON GRADING

- Grades I and II
  - Intraoperative diagnosis
    - Surgical hemostasis
    - Topical hemostatic agents
    - Close suction drain placement
  - Diagnosed with CT scan of the abdomen
    - Nonoperative management
- Grade III
  - Intraoperative diagnosis
    - No pancreatic duct injury
      - Debridement of nonviable tissue and bleeding control
        - Surgical hemostasis
        - Topical hemostatic agents
      - Close suction drain placement
      - Damage control for continued bleeding with hemodynamic instability
        - Packing with hemostatic gauze such as QuikClot
        - Temporary abdominal closure
        - Reexploration and abdominal closure after hemodynamic stability

- Pancreatic duct injury
  - Distal pancreatectomy with or without splenectomy
  - In stable patient may consider:
    - bleeding control.
    - closed suction drain placement.
    - postoperative ERCP and stent placement.
- Diagnosed with CT scan of the abdomen
  - Evaluation for pancreatic duct injury with MRCP/ERCP
  - Treatment options if there is no pancreatic duct injury
    - Exploratory laparotomy
    - Hemostasis
    - Closed suction drain placement
    - Nonoperative management; may need drain placement by interventional radiology
  - Treatment options if there is pancreatic duct injury
    - ERCP and pancreatic duct stent
    - Exploratory and distal pancreatectomy with or without splenectomy
- Grade IV and V injuries
  - Usually associated with:
    - duodenal injury.
    - injury to ampulla of Vater.
    - intrapancreatic CBD injury.
  - Damage-control procedures
    - Control of bleeding
      - Surgical hemostats
      - Local hemostatic agents
      - Packing with hemostatic agent gauze
    - Closed suction drainage
    - Temporary abdominal closure
    - Pancreaticoduodenectomy for damage-control in severe pancreatic injury with associated duodenal injury should be avoided due to high morbidity and mortality.
  - Reexploration of the abdomen and definitive treatment
    - After hemodynamic stability and resolution of coagulopathy, hypothermia, and acidosis
    - After evaluation of ducts with ERCP or MRCP
    - Treatment based on injuries
      - Stent for the pancreatic duct/CBD leak in ERCP without disruption of the duct
      - Injury to the head of the pancreas without duodenal injury (Grade IV)
        - Pancreatic resection at the neck with oversewing of the proximal pancreatic stump
        - Reconstruction with distal Roux-en-Y end–end pancreaticojejunostomy
        - Consider a feeding jejunostomy.
      - Injury to the head of the pancreas with duodenal injury (Grade V)
        - Pancreaticoduodenectomy with reconstruction including Pancreaticojejunostomy, choledochojejunostomy, and gastroenterostomy
        - Consider a feeding jejunostomy.

STEPS OF DISTAL PANCREATECTOMY WITH SPLENECTOMY

- Mobilize the body or tail of the pancreas starting at the point of the injury.
- Incise the peritoneum at the inferior border of the pancreas.
- Develop a plane behind the pancreas using blunt dissection with finger or a clamp.

- Resect the pancreas just proximal to the site of injury using a gastrointestinal anastomosis (GIA)/TA stapler.
- Identify the pancreatic duct, splenic artery, and splenic vein and individually perform suture ligation with nonabsorbable sutures.
- Also identify, ligate, and divide small vascular branches to the pancreatic parenchyma.
- Mobilize the resected distal pancreas toward the splenic hilum.
- Complete the splenectomy by dividing the:
  - gastrosplenic ligament.
  - splenocolic ligament.
  - splenorenal ligament.
  - splenophrenic ligaments.
- Alternatively, mobilize the spleen first by dividing the above-mentioned ligaments, followed by resection of the pancreas just proximal to the injury site using a GIA/TA stapler.

COMPLICATIONS OF PANCREATIC INJURIES

- Traumatic pancreatitis
- Pancreatic fistula
- Pseudocyst
- Pancreatic ascites
- Abscess
- Erosion of surrounding vessels with bleeding
- Stricture of main pancreatic duct
- Sepsis
- Multiple organ failure

CHAPTER 27

Evaluation and Management of Spleen Injuries

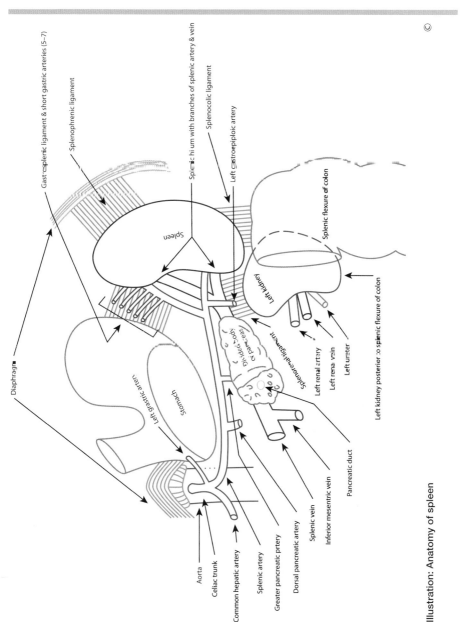

Gast roplenic ligament & short gastric arteries (5–7)

Splenophrenic ligament

Splenic hi um with branches of splenic artery & vein

Splenocolic ligament

Left gastroepiploic artery

Splenic flexure of colon

Spleen

Left kidney

Diaphragm

Left gastric artery

Stomach

Di idec body of pancreas

Splenorenal ligament

Left renal artery

Left rena vein

Left ureter

Left kidney posterior to splenic flexure of colon

Aorta

Celiac trunk

Common hepatic artery

Splenic artery

Greater pancreatic prtery

Dorsal pancreatic artery

Splenic vein

Inferior mesentric vein

Pancreatic duct

Illustration: Anatomy of spleen

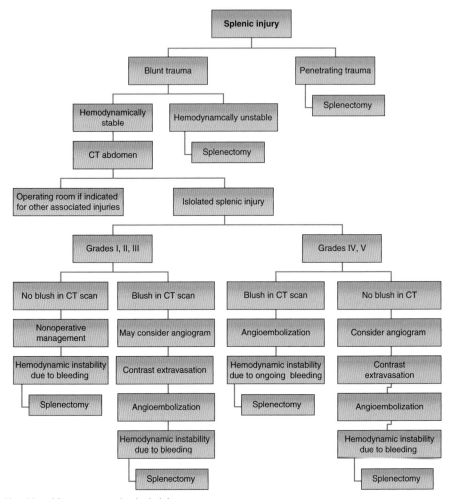

Algorithm: Management of splenic injury

Must-Know Essentials: Evaluation and Management of Splenic Injury

ANATOMY OF THE SPLEEN

- Location
  - Situated under the left diaphragm at the level of ribs 9–11
  - Important relations
    - Lateral to the stomach
    - Anterosuperior to the left kidney
    - Tail of the pancreas is in proximity to the hilum.
- Ligaments
  - Four ligaments attach to the spleen.
    - Splenophrenic ligament

- Connects posterolateral surface of the spleen to the diaphragm
  - Splenorenal ligament
    - Connects posterolateral surface of the spleen to the Gerota fascia of the left kidney
    - Also attached to the splenic hilum, splenic vessels, and tail of the pancreas
  - Gastrosplenic ligament
    - Connects medial surface of the spleen to the greater curvature of the stomach
    - Is the only vascular ligament
    - Contains 5–7 short gastric vessels
  - Splenocolic ligament
- Connects the inferior pole of the spleen to the splenic flexure of the colon
- Structures at the hilum
  - Splenic artery
    - Branch of the celiac trunk
    - Runs along the superior surface of the pancreas toward the splenic hilum
    - Divides into upper and lower pole branches at the hilum
    - Branches of the splenic artery
      - Short gastric arteries (5–7)
      - Left gastroepiploic artery
      - Dorsal pancreatic artery
      - Greater pancreatic artery
  - Splenic vein
    - Upper and lower pole veins form the splenic at the hilum.
    - It runs posterior and inferior to the splenic artery.
    - The inferior mesenteric vein drains into the splenic vein.
    - The superior mesenteric vein joins the splenic vein and forms the portal vein posterior to the neck of the pancreas.
  - The tail of the pancreas is closely related to the hilum.

AMERICAN ASSOCIATION FOR THE SURGERY OF TRAUMA (AAST) GRADING

- Grade I
  - Hematoma
    - Subcapsular <10% surface area
  - Laceration
    - Capsular tear
    - <1 cm parenchymal depth
- Grade II
  - Hematoma
    - Subcapsular 10%–50% surface area
    - Intraparenchymal <5 cm diameter
  - Laceration
    - 1–3 cm parenchymal depth, not involving a parenchymal vessel
- Grade III
  - Hematoma
    - Subcapsular >50% surface area or expanding
    - Ruptured subcapsular or parenchymal hematoma
    - Intraparenchymal hematoma >5 cm diameter
  - Laceration
    - >3 cm parenchymal depth
    - Involving trabecular vessels

- Grade: IV
  - Laceration
    - Segmental or hilar vessels producing major devascularization (>25% of spleen)
- Grade V
  - Laceration
    - Completely shattered spleen
    - Hilar vascular injury with devascularized spleen

INDICATIONS FOR SPLENECTOMY IN TRAUMA PATIENTS

- Hemodynamically unstable blunt trauma patient with splenic laceration
- Penetrating trauma with splenic laceration
- Initially stable patient who becomes hemodynamically unstable due to persistent bleeding
- Failed angioembolization
- Postembolization splenic abscess

TECHNIQUES OF SPLENECTOMY

- Patients without exsanguinating splenic hemorrhage
  - Steps
    - Divide the avascular splenophrenic and splenorenal ligaments after applying medial and inferior traction on the spleen.
    - Divide the vascular gastrosplenic ligament containing short gastric arteries (5–7) using LigaSure or sutures after applying gentle medial retraction of the stomach.
    - Stay closer to the spleen during division of the gastrosplenic ligament in order to prevent injury to the greater curvature of the stomach.
    - Divide the splenocolic ligament with gentle traction on the splenic flexure of the colon.
    - Ligate the splenic artery and vein separately, if possible, to prevent a rare complication of arteriovenous fistula.
    - Ligate the vessels close to the hilum to prevent injury to the tail of the pancreas.
    - Divide the hilum to complete the splenectomy.
    - If the tail of the pancreas is very close to the hilum, divide the splenic vessels with the tail of the pancreas using a gastrointestinal anastomosis (GIA) or TA stapler.
- Patients with exsanguinating splenic hemorrhage
  - Steps
    - Pack the splenic bed with several laparotomy pads.
    - Control the bleeding using one of the following techniques:
      - Direct digital compression of the splenic parenchyma
      - Digital compression at the hilum between the fingers of the left hand
      - Placing a vascular clamp across the hilum
    - Ligate the artery and the vein together and divide it, which rarely can result in an arteriovenous fistula.
    - If the tail of the pancreas is very close to the splenic hilum, divide the hilum, including the hilar vessels, with a GIA or TA stapler.
    - Once bleeding is controlled, divide the ligaments to complete the splenectomy.
- Place a closed suction drain in the pancreatic bed if there is a concern of:
  - incomplete hemostasis.
  - injury of the pancreatic tail.

COMPLICATIONS OF SPLENECTOMY

- Bleeding
  - Intraoperative bleeding
    - Injury to the splenic capsule from excessive traction of the gastrosplenic ligaments
    - Bleeding from short gastric vessels
    - Injury to the splenic capsule at the inferior pole from excessive traction of the splenocolic ligament
  - Immediate postoperative bleeding from the following sources:
    - Superior pancreatic artery injury near the tail of the pancreas
    - Short gastric vessels at the greater curvature of the stomach
    - Treatment
      - Hemodynamically stable: Angioembolization
      - Hemodynamically unstable: Reexploration of the abdomen to control the bleeding
- Ischemia of the greater curvature of the stomach
- Overwhelming postsplenectomy infection (OPSI)
  - The spleen provides immunity against infection with encapsulated organisms (*Streptococcus pneumoniae*, *Neisseria meningitidis*, and *Haemophilus influenzae*).
  - May be seen in 7% of the population after splenectomy
  - Common during the first year after splenectomy but may occur later
  - More common in pediatric population
  - Characterized by fulminant infection from encapsulated organisms leading to bacteremia, pneumonia, and meningitis
  - Associated with very high mortality
  - Immunization against encapsulated organisms can prevent OPSI.
  - *Streptococcus pneumoniae* vaccination should be repeated every 3–5 years.
- Increased incidence of deep vein thrombosis (DVT) due to hypercoagulable state 36–48 hours after splenectomy
- Pancreatic fistula due to injury of the pancreatic tail
  - Treatment
    - ERCP and pancreatic stent
    - Drain placement for controlled drainage of the leak
- Subphrenic abscess
  - Treatment
    - IR-guided drain placement

ANGIOEMBOLIZATION AND SPLENIC SALVAGE FOR SPLENIC INJURY

- Indication of angiogram with angioembolization
  - Hemodynamically stable patients with Grades I, II, and III injury with contrast extravasation in CT scan
    - May consider angiogram with angioembolization for active bleeding
  - Hemodynamically stable Grades IV and V injury without contrast extravasation in CT scan
    - Consider angiogram with angioembolization for active bleeding
  - Hemodynamically stable Grades IV and V injury with contrast extravasation in CT scan
    - Consider angiogram with angioembolization for active bleeding
  - CT with findings suggestive for pseudoaneurysm or arteriovenous fistula

- Types of splenic artery embolization
  - Proximal
    - Performed for active bleeding in the splenic artery
    - Helps to control bleeding by decreasing the perfusion pressure of the splenic parenchyma without causing splenic infarction
    - The splenic artery is occluded just distal to its main pancreatic artery branches with a coil pack or absorbable gelatin.
    - Preserves the pancreatic collaterals for splenic perfusion
  - Distal
    - Performed for specific focal extravasation from the spleen
  - Proximal and distal combined
    - In patients with continued bleeding with proximal or distal embolization
- Preservation of immunologic function of the spleen after proximal or distal embolization is controversial.
  - Studies suggest sufficient immunity against *Haemophilus influenzae* after splenic embolization.
- Complications of angioembolization
  - Splenic abscess
    - Seen in both proximal and distal embolization
  - Infraction of the spleen
    - Proximal splenic artery embolization is associated with less frequent and smaller volumes of splenic infarct than distal embolization.
  - Rebleeding
    - No difference in rebleeding rate in proximal versus distal embolization
    - Treated with splenectomy
  - Postembolization syndrome
    - Features include:
      - fever.
      - nausea.
      - left upper quadrant abdominal pain.

CHAPTER 28

Evaluation and Management of Stomach and Duodenal Injuries

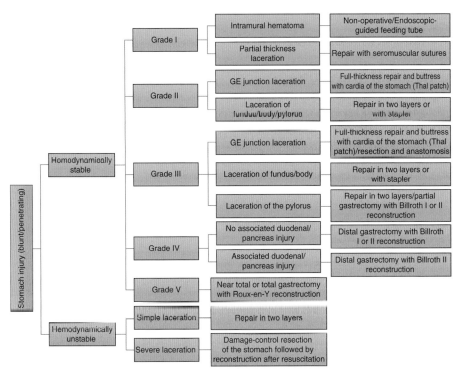

Algorithm: Management of stomach injury

Must-Know Essentials: Anatomy of the Stomach

PARTS OF THE STOMACH

- Cardia
  - Superior part of the stomach that contains the cardiac sphincter
  - Situated at T11 vertebra level
- Fundus
  - Part of the stomach superior and left of the cardia
- Body
  - Largest part of the stomach
- Antrum
  - Below the body of the stomach

- Pylorus
  - Inferior part of the stomach that connects to the duodenum.
  - Divided into the antrum, pyloric canal, and pyloric sphincter

POSTERIOR RELATION OF THE STOMACH

- Pancreas
- Lesser sac
- Left kidney
- Left adrenal
- Spleen
- Splenic artery
- Left portion of the transverse colon

ARTERIES OF THE STOMACH

- Lesser curvature
  - Left gastric artery: branch from the celiac trunk
  - Right gastric artery: branch from the proper hepatic artery
- Greater curvature
  - Right gastroepiploic artery: branch from the gastroduodenal artery
  - Left gastroepiploic artery: branch from the splenic artery
- Fundus
  - Short gastric arteries from the splenic artery

VENOUS DRAINAGE

- Veins run parallel to the arteries.
- Right and left gastric veins drain into the portal vein.
- Short left gastric veins and right gastroepiploic veins drain into the superior mesenteric vein.

Must-Know Essentials: American Association for the Surgery of Trauma (AAST) Grading of Stomach Injuries

GRADES

- Grade I
  - Contusion/intramural hematoma
  - Partial-thickness laceration
- Grade II
  - Laceration <2 cm in gastroesophageal (GE) junction or pylorus
  - Laceration <5 cm in proximal 1/3 stomach
  - Laceration <10 cm in distal 2/3 stomach
- Grade III
  - Laceration >2 cm in GE junction or pylorus
  - Laceration >5 cm in proximal 1/3 stomach
  - Laceration >10 cm in distal 2/3 stomach
- Grade IV
  - Tissue loss or devascularization <2/3 stomach

- Grade V
  - Tissue loss or devascularization >2/3 stomach

  Advance one grade for multiple lesions up to Grade III.

Must-Know Essentials: Management of Stomach Injuries

EXPOSURE OF STOMACH INJURIES

- Midline incision extending up to epigastric area left to xiphoid process
- May require excision of xiphoid for better exposure
- Exposure of the posterior surface of the stomach
  - Divide the gastrocolic ligament to enter the lesser sac to expose the posterior surface of the stomach.
- Exposure of the GE junction
  - Expose the lateral side of the GE junction by dividing the falciform and left triangular ligaments of the liver.
  - Expose the medial side of the GE junction by dividing the gastrohepatic ligament (lesser omentum).
  - May divide the short gastric arteries along the greater curvature, and the left crus of the diaphragm for better exposure of the distal esophagus.

TREATMENT OF STOMACH INJURIES

- Grade I
  - Intramural hematoma without gastric outlet obstruction
    - No specific treatment
    - Normal feeding
  - Intramural hematoma with gastric outlet obstruction
    - Endoscope-guided feeding tube placement distal to obstruction and tube feeding
  - Partial-thickness laceration
    - Repair with seromuscular sutures using absorbable 3-0 Polyglactin or nonabsorbable 3-0 Silk suture
- Grade II
  - Laceration repair in two layers
    - First layer: Running absorbable 3-0 Polydioxanone suture
    - Second layer: Seromuscular interrupted absorbable 3-0 Polyglactin or nonabsorbable 3-0 Silk suture
    - May use a stapler to repair the laceration.
  - Laceration at GE junction: Full-thickness closure using interrupted absorbable 3-0 Polydioxanone suture and buttress of the repair with cardia of the stomach (Thal patch)
- Grade III
  - Laceration near pylorus
    - Repair in two layers as described for grade II laceration if possible
    - Resection of the stomach with Billroth I or Billroth II reconstruction if repair is not possible:
  - Laceration at GE junction
    - Repair possible: Full-thickness closure using interrupted absorbable 3-0 Polydioxanone suture and buttress of the repair with the cardia of the stomach (Thal patch)
    - Repair not possible: Resection and anastomosis using stapling device or hand sewing

- Grade IV
  - No associated injuries to the duodenum or pancreas
    - Distal gastrectomy with Billroth I (gastroduodenostomy) or Billroth II (gastrojeju-nostomy) reconstruction
  - Associated with injuries to the duodenum or pancreas
    - Distal gastrectomy with Billroth II reconstruction
- Grade V
  - Near total or total gastrectomy with Roux-en-Y reconstruction

DAMAGE-CONTROL PROCEDURES FOR STOMACH INJURIES

- Simple injury
  - Repair of laceration in two layers or using a stapler
- Severe injury
  - Resection of the stomach using a clamp or stapler
  - Reconstruction after resuscitation

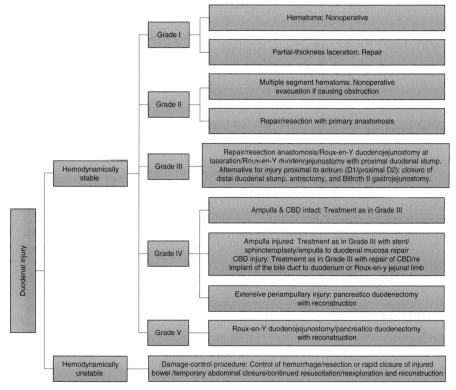

Algorithm: Management of duodenal injury

Must-Know Essentials: AAST Grading of Duodenal Injuries

GRADES

- Grade I
  - Hematoma
    - Involving single portion of the duodenum
  - Laceration
    - Partial thickness, no perforation
- Grade II
  - Hematoma
    - Involving more than one portion of the duodenum
  - Laceration
    - Disruption <50% of the circumference of the duodenum
- Grade III
  - Laceration
    - Disruption of 50%–75% of the circumference of the D2 segment of the duodenum
    - Disruption of 50%–100% of the circumference of the D1, D3, and D4 segments of the duodenum
- Grade IV
  - Laceration
    - Disruption >75% of the circumference of the D2 segment of the duodenum
    - Involving ampulla or intrapancreatic portion (distal) common bile duct
- Grade V
  - Laceration
    - Massive disruption of duodenopancreatic complex
  - Vascular
    - Devascularization of the duodenum
    Advance one grade for multiple injuries up to Grade III.

Must-Know Essentials: Anatomy of the Duodenum

LOCATION

- Majority of the duodenum is a retroperitoneal except for the first 2–3 cm of D1 and the most distal part D4, which is intraperitoneal.
- Situated at the L1–L3 vertebra level

SEGMENTS OF THE DUODENUM

- Starts at the pylorus and ends at the ligament of Treitz
- Approximately 20–30 cm long and consists of four segments
- First part (segment D1)
  - Starts at pylorus and ends at the level of the mmon bile duct superiorly and gastroduodenal artery inferiorly

- Approximately 5 cm long
- Attached to hepatoduodenal ligament
- Important relations
  - Anterior: liver and gallbladder
  - Posterior: common bile duct, inferior vena cava, portal vein
  - Superior: epiploic foramen
  - Inferior: pancreatic head
- Second part (segment D2)
  - The descending part, which starts at the superior duodenal flexure
  - Situated anterior and right to inferior vena cava and lateral to pancreatic head
  - The ampulla of Vater (major duodenal papilla) opens in middle part of D2 on its medial wall.
  - The ampulla of Vater is surrounded by the sphincter of Oddi, which controls the flow of bile and pancreatic juice into the duodenum; it also prevents the reflux of duodenal contents, bile, and pancreatic juice into the bile and pancreatic ducts.
  - Accessory pancreatic duct (minor duodenal papilla) opens proximal and dorsal to the ampulla of Vater on the medial wall.
  - Important relations
    - Anterior: transverse colon
    - Posterior: right kidney, right ureter, right adrenal gland, right renal vessels
    - Superior: liver, gallbladder
    - Inferior: loops of the jejunum
    - Lateral: ascending colon, hepatic flexure
    - Medial: pancreatic head
- Third part (segment D3):
  - A horizontal part of the duodenum, traverses from right to left
  - Situated inferior to the uncinate process of the pancreas
  - Important relations
    - Anterior: superior mesenteric artery, superior mesenteric vein
    - Posterior: right psoas major muscle, inferior vena cava, left psoas major muscle
    - Superior: pancreas
- Fourth part (segment D4)
  - Ascends to the left side of the aorta and continues as jejunum at the duodenojejunal flexure, where it is attached to the ligament of Treitz
  - The ligament of Treitz is a continuation of the left crus at the left border of L2 vertebra.
  - Important relations
    - Superior: stomach
    - Inferior: jejunal loops
    - Posterior: left psoas (major muscle), abdominal aorta

ARTERIAL SUPPLY

- Superior pancreaticoduodenal artery
  - Branch from gastroduodenal artery
  - Divides into anterior and posterior branches
- Inferior pancreaticoduodenal
  - Branch from the superior mesenteric artery
  - Divides into anterior and posterior branches

- The anterior and posterior branches of the superior and inferior pancreaticoduodenal arteries form the anterior and posterior pancreaticoduodenal arcade, which supply the D2 segment of the duodenum and head of the pancreas.

VENOUS DRAINAGE

- Follows the arteries
- The superior pancreaticoduodenal drains into the portal vein.
- The inferior pancreaticoduodenal vein drains into the superior mesenteric vein.

Must-Know Essentials: Management of Duodenal Injuries

EXPOSURE OF DUODENAL INJURIES

- Divide the hepatoduodenal ligament to expose the superior aspect of the D1 segment.
- Exposure of the posterior wall of the D1, D2, and D3 segments and the posterior surface of the head and neck of the pancreas.
  - Mobilize the hepatic flexure of the colon.
  - Perform Kocher's maneuver (see Chapter 24 for details).
- Exposure of the posterior surface of the D1 segment, the medial aspect of the D2 segment, and the anterior surface of the pancreas
  - Divide the gastrocolic ligament and enter the lesser sac.
  - Divide the retroperitoneum inferior to the pancreas to inspect the posterior pancreas after mobilizing and lifting the inferior edge of the pancreas.
- Exposure of the D3 and D4 segments
  - Perform the Cattell-Braasch maneuver (see Chapter 24 for details).
- Exposure of the D4 segment
  - Incise the ligament of Treitz after retracting the transverse colon superiorly and the small bowel inferiorly and to the right.
  - Identify and protect the superior mesenteric vessels, which are located on the right side of the ligament of Treitz.
- Full-thickness duodenal injury in the region of the ampulla requires full evaluation of the ampulla, bile ducts, and pancreatic ducts using cholangiopancreatography.

TREATMENT OF DUODENAL INJURIES

- Grade I injury
  - Duodenal hematoma
    - No duodenal obstruction
      - Nonoperative treatment
    - Duodenal obstruction
      - Gastrointestinal decompression
      - Parenteral nutritional support
      - Repeat imaging after 5–7 days to evaluate the patency of the duodenum.
      - Evacuation of hematoma: Persistent hematoma after 10–14 days
    - Intraoperative finding of duodenal hematoma in penetrating/blunt injury:
      - Explore the hematoma to identify any perforation.
  - Partial-thickness injury without perforation
    - Repair with interrupted seromuscular sutures using a nonabsorbable 3-0 Silk suture.

- Grade II injury
  - Hematoma
    - No duodenal obstruction
      - Nonoperative treatment
    - Duodenal obstruction
      - Gastrointestinal decompression
      - Parenteral nutritional support
      - Evacuation of hematoma
    - Intraoperative finding of duodenal hematoma in penetrating/blunt injury:
      - Explore the hematoma to identify any perforation.
  - Laceration
    - Transverse primary closure in two layers
      - Inner layer: running absorbable 3-0 Polydioxanone or Polyglactin suture
      - Outer layer: interrupted seromuscular closure using 3-0 nonabsorbable Silk or absorbable 3-0 Polyglactin sutures
    - Concern of significant stenosis after repair
      - Gastrojejunostomy
    - Extensive (>5 cm) injury
      - Resection with primary end-to-end anastomosis in two layers, inner layer with running absorbable 3-0 Polydioxanone or Polyglactin and outer seromuscular layer using interrupted layer with 3-0 nonabsorbable Silk or absorbable 3-0 Polyglactin suture.
    - Laceration on the medial aspect of the D2 segment
      - Repair of laceration from inside after a lateral duodenotomy
      - Mobilization of the pancreas for repair from the outside can cause duodenal ischemia.
- Grade III injury
  - Laceration involving 50%–75 % circumference of the D2 segment
    - Transverse primary repair in two layers if possible as described earlier for grade II laceration
    - Segmental resection and end-to-end to anastomosis in two layers as described earlier for grade II laceration if repair is not possible
      - Mobilization during resection is limited due to the ampulla of Vater and the common blood supply of the duodenum and the head of the pancreas.
    - If repair or resection anastomosis is not possible
      - Roux-en-Y duodenojejunostomy at the laceration site
      - Closure of distal duodenal stump and proximal Roux-en-Y duodenojejunostomy
      - Alternative treatment for injury proximal to ampulla of Vater (D1 and proximal D2 segments): Antrectomy and Billroth II gastrojejunostomy
- Grade IV injury
  - Laceration with intact ampulla and common bile duct (CBD)
    - Management as in Grade III injury with primary repair/resection and anastomosis/ Roux-en-Y duodenojejunostomy
  - Laceration with injured ampulla with intact CBD
    - Management as in Grade III injury with primary repair/resection and anastomosis/ Roux-en-Y duodenojejunostomy
    - Management of injured ampulla
      - Stent placement

   Sphincteroplasty

   Ampulla to D2 mucosa repair.

- Laceration with injured CBD:
  - Management as in Grade III injury with primary repair/resection & anastomosis/ Roux-en- Y duodenojejunostomy
  - Injured CBD may require:
    - Repair of CBD with interrupted 4-0 Polydioxanone absorbable suture.
    - Reimplantation of CBD in the duodenum (choledochoduodenostomy)
    - Reimplantation of CBD in the Roux-en-Y jejunal limb (choledochojejunostomy)
- Extensive periampullary injury
  - Pancreaticoduodenectomy with reconstruction
- Grade V injury
  - Roux-en-Y duodenojejunostomy if possible
  - Usually requires pancreaticoduodenectomy with reconstruction

DAMAGE CONTROL IN DUODENAL INJURIES

- Recommended in unstable patients with complex injuries (Grade IV or V)
- Procedures include:
  - Control of bleeding:
    - Surgical hemostasis
    - Local hemostatic agents
    - May require packing with hemostatic-agent-coated gauze
  - Resection/debridement of devitalized tissues without anastomosis
  - Ends of the resected bowel may be closed temporarily with suture or umbilical tape.
  - Temporary abdominal closure
- Reexploration with pancreaticoduodenectomy and reconstruction

ADJUNCTIVE PROCEDURES AFTER REPAIR OF DUODENAL INJURIES

- Adjunctive procedures may be considered after:
  - high-grade duodenal injury repair.
  - tenuous repair.
- Pyloric exclusion with gastrojejunostomy
  - Closure of pylorus with purse-string suture through an anterior gastrotomy along the greater curvature using a size-0 Polydioxanone suture with a loop gastrojejunostomy
  - Stapling of the postpyloric duodenum with TA stapler and a loop gastrojejunostomy is an alternative method of pyloric exclusion.
  - Pylorus reopens spontaneously in 3–6 weeks.
- Gastrostomy for duodenal decompression

CHAPTER 29

Management of Small Bowel, Colon, and Rectal Injuries

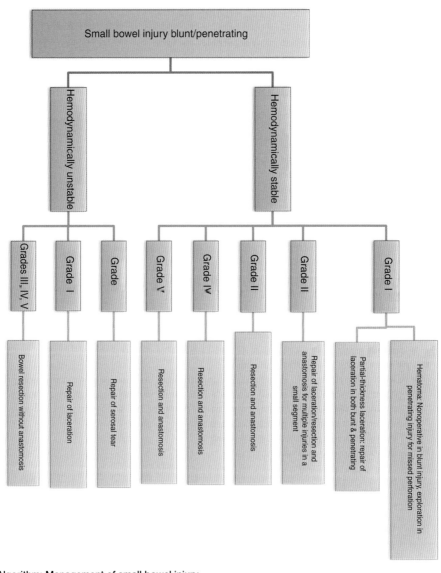

Algorithm: Management of small bowel injury

Must-Know Essentials: Management of Small Bowel Injuries

ANATOMY OF SMALL BOWEL

- Divisions of the small bowel
  - The small bowel is 4–6 meters long and divided into the duodenum, jejunum, and ileum.
  - Duodenum (see Chapter 28 for details)
  - Jejunum
    - Continuation of the fourth part of the duodenum at duodenojejunal flexure situated on the left side of L2 vertebra
    - It is fixed to the retroperitoneum by the ligament of Treitz.
    - The aorta and the superior mesenteric vessels are located on the right, and the inferior mesenteric vein is located on the left side of the ligament of Treitz.
    - It constitutes about two-fifths of the proximal small intestine.
    - Features to identify jejunum
      - Situated in the left upper and central abdomen
      - Thicker wall and a wider lumen than the ileum
      - Less mesenteric fat compared to mesentery of the ileum, mesenteric vessels more visible
  - Ileum
    - Continuation of jejunum; terminates at the ileocecal junction
    - Constitutes the distal three-fifths of the small bowel
    - Features to identify ileum
      - Thinner wall and a smaller lumen
      - Situated in the central and right lower abdomen and pelvis
      - Abundant mesenteric fat; mesenteric vessels are not well visualized
- Mesentery of the small bowel
  - Double-folded peritoneum attached to the posterior abdominal wall
  - The root of the mesentery extends obliquely from the left L2 vertebra level to the right sacroiliac joint.
  - The mesentery crosses the third part of the duodenum, aorta, inferior vena cava (IVC), and right ureter.
  - The mesenteric vessels and lymph nodes are situated between the two leaves of the mesentery.
- Blood supply of small bowel
  - Arterial supply
    - Jejunal and ileal branches of the superior mesenteric artery (SMA) arise from the left side of the SMA
    - Jejunal and ileal arterial branches form 2–3 arterial arcades in the jejunum, and 4-5 in the ileum to supply the small bowel.
    - Right colic artery, middle colic artery, and ileocolic artery arises form the right side of the SMA.
  - Venous drainage
    - Veins from the jejunum and ileum drain into the superior mesenteric vein (SMV).
    - Veins run parallel to the arteries.
    - The SMV lies slightly anterior and to the right of the SMA anterior to the uncinate process and third part of the duodenum.
    - The SMV and splenic vein join to form the portal vein posterior to the neck of the pancreas.

PATTERN OF INJURIES BASED ON MECHANISM

- Blunt injury
  - Shearing force: Perforation of the small bowel, usually at the antimesenteric border
  - Traction injury: Injury at the point of fixation, such as at the ligament of Treitz or ileocecal junction
  - Deceleration injury: Bucket handle tear of the mesentery causing small bowel ischemia

AMERICAN ASSOCIATION FOR THE SURGERY OF TRAUMA (AAST) GRADING OF SMALL BOWEL INJURIES

- Grade I injury
  - Minor hematoma
  - Partial-thickness laceration
- Grade II injury
  - Full-thickness laceration involving <50% of the circumference
- Grade III injury
  - Full-thickness laceration involving >50% of the circumference without complete transection
- Grade IV injury
  - Complete transection without devascularization
- Grade V injury
  - Mesenteric disruption causing devascularized bowel
  - Transection with segmental tissue loss
  - *Advance one grade for multiple injuries up to Grade III.*

DAMAGE CONTROL IN SMALL BOWEL INJURIES

- Indications
  - Hemodynamically unstable patients
  - Bowel injury with:
    - significant edema.
    - significant bowel distention (ileus).
    - gross intraperitoneal contamination.
  - Mesenteric injury with concern of bowel ischemia
- Damage-control options in small bowel injury
  - Grade I injury
    - Minor hematoma: Nonoperative treatment
    - Partial thickness laceration: Repair with interrupted seromuscular sutures using non-absorbable 3-0 Silk or absorbable 3-0 Polydioxanone/Polyglactin sutures
  - Grade II injury
    - Laceration: Repair (enterorrhaphy) transversely in two layers, inner layer with full thickness running absorbable 3-0 Polydioxanone/Polyglactin sutures, and outer layer with interrupted seromuscular absorbable 3-0 Polydioxanone/Polyglactin or nonabsorbable 3-0 Silk sutures.
  - Grade III/IV/V injuries
    - Bowel resection using stapler or ligation of injured bowel without anastomosis
    - Temporary abdominal closure
    - Reexploration after hemodynamic stability, and resolution of coagulopathy, acidosis, and hypothermia
      - Bowel resection/anastomosis
      - Definitive abdominal closure if possible

DEFINITIVE TREATMENT OF SMALL BOWEL INJURIES

- Grade I injury
  - Minor hematoma
    - Blunt injury: Nonoperative treatment
    - Penetrating injury
      Hematoma should be explored to examine for perforation.
      Missed bowel perforation is common at the mesenteric border hematoma.
  - Partial-thickness laceration: Repair with interrupted seromuscular sutures using 3-0 nonabsorbable or absorbable sutures.
- Grade II injury
  - Laceration: Repair (enterorrhaphy) transversely in two layers: inner layer with full thickness running absorbable 3-0 Polydioxanone/Polyglactin sutures, and outer layer with interrupted seromuscular absorbable 3-0 Polydioxanone/Polyglactin or nonabsorbable 3-0 Silk sutures.
- Grades III/IV/V
  - Bowel resection with stapled anastomosis or hand-sewn anastomosis in two layers: inner full thickness with running absorbable 3-0 Polydioxanone/Polyglactin sutures, and outer interrupted seromuscular layer using absorbable 3-0 Polydioxanone/Polyglactin or nonabsorbable 3-0 Silk sutures.
  - Hand-sewn anastomosis should be considered in patients with significant bowel edema.
  - In multiple lacerations, multiple anastomosis should be avoided.
  - Bowel resection may result in short bowel syndrome.
    - Approximately 100 cm of small bowel without ileocecal valve or 60 cm of small bowel with ileocecal valve is essential to prevent short bowel syndrome.
    - Resection of up to 70% of the small bowel is usually tolerated well if the terminal ileum and ileocecal valve are preserved.
    - Proximal bowel resection is tolerated better than distal resection because the ileum can adapt and increase its absorptive capacity more efficiently than the jejunum.

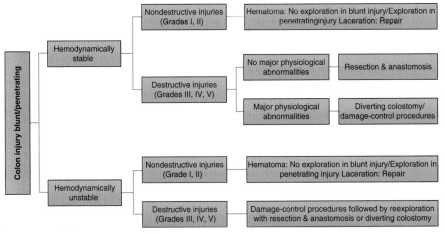

Algorithm: Management of colon injury

Must-Know Essentials: Management of Colon Injuries

ANATOMY OF THE COLON

- Division of the colon
  - Colon begins at the cecum and ends at the rectum.
  - Approximately 1.5 meters long
  - Divided into four parts
    - Cecum
      - First part of colon
      - Intraperitoneal structure
      - Contains ileocecal valve
      - Connected to the appendix
    - Ascending colon
      - Retroperitoneal
    - Transverse colon
      - Intraperitoneal
      - Extends between the hepatic flexure and the splenic flexure
      - Attached to the mesocolon
    - Descending colon
      - Retroperitoneal
    - Sigmoid colon
      - Intraperitoneal
      - Attached to sigmoid mesocolon
      - Attached to the rectum
- Characteristics of the colon
  - Haustra: Sacculation
  - Semilunar folds
  - Taeniae coli: Three longitudinal muscle folds
  - Epiploic appendices. Adipose-tissue-filled serosa
- Arteries of the colon (Please see illustration: blood supply of the colon)
  - Branches from the SMA
    - Ileocolic artery: Supply to the appendix and cecum
    - Right colic artery: Supply to the right colon
    - Middle colic artery: Supply to the transverse colon
  - Branches from the inferior mesenteric artery (IMA)
    - Left colic artery: Supply to descending colon
    - Sigmoid arteries: Supply to sigmoid colon
- Marginal artery of Drummond (MAD)
  - Blood supply to the colon from SMA branches ends at the distal portion of the transverse colon.
  - Blood supply to the colon from the IMA starts at the splenic flexure of the colon.
  - The MAD is a vascular arcade along the mesenteric border of the entire length of the colon and its branches provide collateral circulation to the colon.
  - Communication between SMA and IMA
  - Very important collateral circulation of the colon

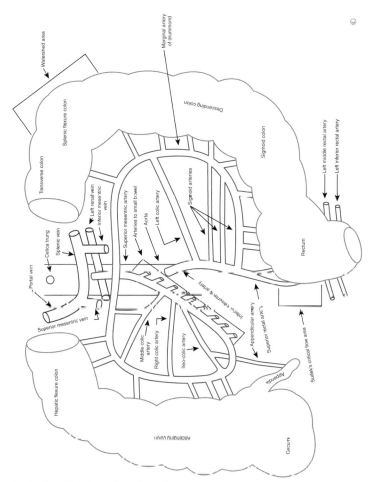

Illustration: Blood supply of the colon

- ■ Variations of the MAD
  - ▫ May be absent at the splenic flexure (Griffiths point), a major watershed area prone to ischemia
  - ▫ Inconsistent between right colic and ileocolic arteries
  - ▫ Absent in the sigmoid colon
- ■ Arc of Riolan
  - ■ Inconsistent artery that connects proximal SMA or one of its primary branches to the inferior mesenteric artery branches
  - ■ Commonly, the connection is between the middle colic artery branch of the SMA with the left colic branch of the IMA.
  - ■ Important collateral circulation of the colon
- ■ Veins of the colon
  - ■ Veins run parallel to the arteries.
  - ■ SMV connects to the splenic vein and forms the portal vein.
  - ■ Inferior mesenteric vein (IMV) drains into the splenic vein.

MECHANISM OF COLON INJURIES

- Penetrating trauma:
  - Most common cause of colon injury
  - Gunshot wounds (GSWs) frequently involve the ascending colon and transverse colon.
  - Stab wounds frequently involve the descending colon and sigmoid colon.
- Blunt trauma:
  - Less common cause of colon injury
  - Commonly due to motor vehicle collision (MVC)
  - Usually involve transverse colon and sigmoid colon
  - May result in:
    - serosal tears
    - contusions
    - devascularizations

AAST GRADING OF THE COLON INJURY

- Grade I injury
  - Hematoma: Contusion or hematoma without devascularization
  - Laceration: Partial thickness, no perforation
- Grade II injury
  - Laceration: <50 % of circumference
- Grade III injury
  - Laceration: >50% of circumference without transection
- Grade IV injury
  - Laceration: Transection of the colon
- Grade V injury
  - Laceration: Transection of the colon with segmental tissue loss
  - Vascular: Devascularized segment
  - *Advance one grade for multiple injuries up to Grade III.*

NONDESTRUCTIVE INJURIES

- AAST Grades I and II injuries

DESTRUCTIVE COLON INJURIES

- AAST colon injury Grades III, IV, or V
- >50% circumference involvement
- Transection of the colon
- Tissue loss
- Vascular injury

TREATMENT OF COLON INJURIES IN HEMODYNAMICALLY STABLE PATIENTS

- Nondestructive injuries
  - Grade I injury
    - Hematoma in blunt injury
      - Nonoperative treatment

 Hematoma in penetrating injury
      Exploration of the hematoma to rule out perforation
      Seromuscular closure with interrupted absorbable 3-0 Polydioxanone/Polyglactin
      or nonabsorbable 3-0 Silk sutures
 Partial-thickness laceration
      Repair with interrupted absorbable 3-0 Polydioxanone/Polyglactin or nonabsorb-
      able 3-0 Silk sutures
- Grade II injury
   - Laceration repair transversely in two layers: inner layer with full-thickness running or
     interrupted using absorbable 3-0 Polydioxanone/Polyglactin sutures, and outer layer
     with interrupted seromuscular absorbable 3-0 Polydioxanone/Polyglactin absorbable
     or nonabsorbable 3-0 Silk sutures
- Destructive (Grades III, IV, and V) injuries
   - If no physiological abnormalities
      Resection and stapled or hand-sewn anastomosis
   - If physiological abnormalities
      Diverting colostomy or damage-control procedures followed by delayed resection
      anastomosis versus diverting colostomy

DAMAGE-CONTROL PROCEDURE IN TREATMENT OF COLON INJURIES IN HEMODYNAMICALLY UNSTABLE PATIENTS

- Damage-control procedures are indicated in patients with:
- Hemodynamically instability.
- Lethal triad (hypothermia, coagulopathy, acidosis)
- May be considered in hemodynamically stable high-grade destructive injuries with major
  physiological abnormalities.
   - Blood transfusion requirement >6 units
   - Prolonged hypotension
   - Severe fecal contamination
   - Associated medical comorbidities
- Damage control procedures
- Nondestructive (Grades I, II) injuries
   - Grade I injury
      Hematoma in blunt injury: Nonoperative treatment
      Hematoma in penetrating injury: Exploration to rule out perforation
      Partial-thickness laceration: Repair with interrupted absorbable 3-0 Polydioxanone/
      Polyglactin or nonabsorbable 3-0 Silk sutures
   - Grade II injury
      Laceration repair transversely in two layers: inner layer with full-thickness run-
      ning or interrupted absorbable 3-0 Polydioxanone/Polyglactin sutures, and outer
      layer with interrupted seromuscular absorbable 3-0 Polydioxanone/Polyglactin or
      nonabsorbable 3-0 Silk sutures
- Destructive (Grades III/IV/V) injuries
   - Control of hemorrhage.
   - Resection using a GIA stapler or closure of the ends with ties to control contamination.
   - No anastomosis
   - No colostomy
   - Temporary abdominal closure

REEXPLORATION AFTER DAMAGE-CONTROL PROCEDURE

- Perform after hemodynamic stability and correction of lethal triad.
- Resection and stapled or hand-sewn anastomosis in patients with:
  - no major physiological abnormalities.
  - no other major associated injuries.
  - reexploration within 2–3 days.
    - High risk of bowel edema and anastomotic leak after 3 days of open abdomen with bowel in discontinuity
- Diverting colostomy in patients with:
  - major physiological abnormalities.
  - reexploration after 48–72 hours.
- Abdominal fascial closure
- Delayed or negative pressure wound therapy (NPWT) assisted skin closure

Must-Know Essentials: Management of Rectal Injuries

ANATOMY OF RECTUM

- Part of the large intestine that connects to the sigmoid colon and anal canal
- Approximately 12–15 cm in length
- Starts at S2–S3 vertebra level
- Divisions
  - Upper third: Intraperitoneal
  - Middle third: Retroperitoneal
  - Lower third: Extraperitoneal
- Upper two-thirds is considered intraperitoneal for the surgical management in trauma patients.
- Differentiated from the colon due to lack of taeniae, haustra, appendices epiploicae, and semilunar folds.
- Arterial supply
  - Superior rectal artery: Branch from the inferior mesenteric artery
  - Middle rectal artery: Branch from the internal iliac artery
  - Inferior rectal artery: Branch from the internal pudendal artery, which is a branch from the internal iliac artery
- Venous drainage
  - Superior rectal veins
    - Drain the upper part of the rectum into the IMV
    - IMV drains into the splenic vein of the portal venous system.
- Middle rectal veins
  - Drain the middle part of the rectum into the internal iliac vein of the systemic venous system
- Inferior rectal veins
  - Drain the lower part of the rectum into the internal pudendal vein
  - Internal pudendal vein drains into the internal iliac vein of the systemic venous system.

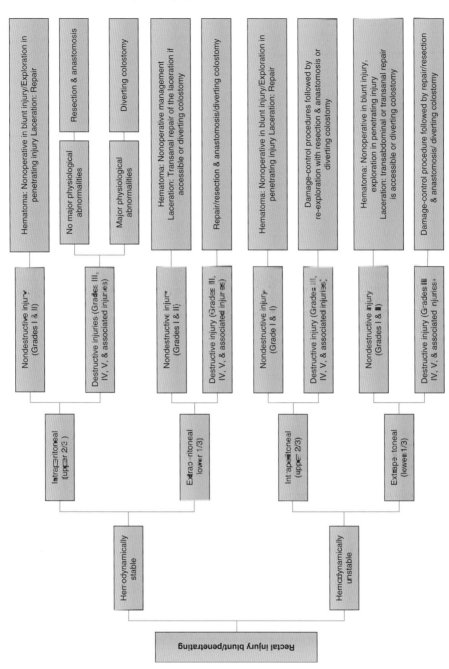

Algorithm: Management of rectal injury

EVALUATION

- Common mechanism of injury
  - Penetrating trauma
    - Most common cause of rectal injury
    - Majority from transpelvic GSW
    - Other causes
      - Stab wound
      - Foreign body
  - Blunt trauma
    - Bony fragments from pelvic fractures
    - Open book pelvic fracture dislocation
- Diagnosis
  - High index of suspicion in patients with:
    - penetrating trauma with injuries of lower anterior abdominal wall, buttock, pelvis, or perineum.
    - blunt trauma with pelvic fractures.
- Rectal examination
  - Blood on examination
  - Laceration in the rectal wall
  - Bone fragments through the rectal wall
- Rectal examination under anesthesia with proctoscopy if clinical examination suggestive of rectal injury
- CT abdomen and pelvis with IV and +/– rectal contrast
  - Evaluation for other associated injuries
  - Identification of missile trajectory in GSWs
- Evaluation for associated injuries
  - Pelvic blood vessel injuries
    - CT angiogram
  - Bladder and ureter injuries
    - CT cystogram

AAST GRADING OF RECTAL INJURY

- Grade I injury
  - Hematoma: Contusion or hematoma without devascularization
  - Laceration: Partial thickness
- Grade II injury
  - Laceration: <50 % of circumference
- Grade III injury
  - Laceration: >50% of circumference
- Grade IV injury
  - Laceration: Full-thickness laceration with extension into the perineum
- Grade V injury
  - Vascular: Devascularized segment
  - *Advance one grade for multiple injuries up to Grade III.*

NONDESTRUCTIVE INJURIES

- AAST injuries Grades I & II

DESTRUCTIVE RECTAL INJURIES

- AAST injuries Grades III, IV, or V
  - >50% circumference involvement
  - Full-thickness laceration
  - Laceration with extension into perineum
  - Devascularized segment
  - Associated pelvic fractures
  - Concomitant vascular injuries that can compromise the blood supply to the rectum

MAJOR PHYSIOLOGICALF ABNORMALITIES

- Blood transfusion requirement >6 units
- Prolonged hypotension
- Severe fecal contamination
- Associated medical comorbidities

TREATMENT OF HEMODYNAMICALLY STABLE RECTAL INJURIES

- Intraperitoneal nondestructive injuries
  - Grade I injury
    - Hematoma in blunt injury
      Nonoperative treatment
    - Hematoma in penetrating injury
      Exploration of the hematoma to rule out perforation
      Seromuscular closure with interrupted absorbable 3-0 Polydioxanone/Polyglactin or nonabsorbable 3-0 Silk sutures
    - Partial-thickness laceration
      Repair with interrupted absorbable 3-0 Polydioxanone/Polyglactin or nonabsorbable 3-0 Silk sutures.
  - Grade II injury
    - Laceration repair transversely in two layers: inner layer with full thickness running or interrupted using absorbable 3-0 Polydioxanone/Polyglactin sutures, and outer layer with interrupted seromuscular absorbable 3-0 Polydioxanone/Polyglactin or nonabsorbable 3-0 Silk sutures.
- Intraperitoneal destructive (Grades III, IV, V) and other associated injuries
  - If no physiological abnormalities
    - Resection and anastomosis
  - If physiological abnormalities
    - Diverting colostomy
- Extraperitoneal nondestructive injuries
  - Access to extraperitoneal injury
    - Transabdominal: May be possible in proximal extraperitoneal injury
    - Transanal: May be possible in distal extraperitoneal injury
  - Grade I injury
    - Hematoma in blunt injury: Nonoperative management
    - Hematoma in penetrating injury: exploration to exclude penetrating injuries
    - Partial-thickness laceration: Transanal repair is easily accessible or nonoperative.

- Grade II injury
  - Transabdominal/transanal repair if accessible
  - Diverting colostomy if repair is not possible
  - No role of rectal washout
- Extraperitoneal destructive injuries
- Resection and anastomosis if possible
  - May consider a protective diverting loop colostomy for a low anastomosis.
- Repair of the laceration if possible (transabdominal or transanal access)
- Diverting colostomy
- No role of rectal washout
- Presacral drainage
  - Current literature does not support
  - May be considered in:
    severely contaminated injuries.
    high-energy blunt trauma with pelvic fractures.

TREATMENT OF HEMODYNAMICALLY UNSTABLE RECTAL INJURIES

- Intraperitoneal nondestructive injuries:
  - Grade I injury
    - Hematoma in blunt injury
      Nonoperative treatment
    - Hematoma in penetrating injury
      Exploration of the hematoma to rule out perforation
      Seromuscular closure with interrupted absorbable 3-0 Polydioxanone/Polyglactin
      or nonabsorbable 3-0 Silk sutures
    - Partial-thickness laceration
      Repair with interrupted absorbable 3-0 Polydioxanone/Polyglactin or nonabsorbable 3-0 Silk sutures
  - Grade II
    - Laceration repair transversely in two layers: inner layer with full-thickness running or interrupted absorbable 3-0 Polydioxanone/Polyglactin sutures, and outer layer with interrupted seromuscular absorbable 3-0 Polydioxanone/Polyglactin or nonabsorbable 3-0 Silk sutures
- Intraperitoneal destructive (Grades III, IV, V) and other associated injuries
  - Damage-control procedures
    - Control of hemorrhage.
    - Resection using a GIA stapler or closure of the ends with ties to control contamination.
    - No anastomosis
    - No colostomy
    - Temporary abdominal closure
  - Reexploration after damage-control procedure
    - Performed after hemodynamic stability and correction of the lethal triad
    - Resection and anastomosis in patients with:
      no major physiological abnormalities.
      no other major associated injuries.
      reexploration within 2–3 days.
      High risk of bowel edema and anastomotic leak after 3 days of open abdomen with bowel in discontinuity

- Diverting colostomy in patients with:
  - major physiological abnormalities.
  - delayed reexploration after 48–72 hours.
  - associated pelvic fractures.
  - associated vascular injuries.
- Abdominal fascial closure
- Delayed or negative pressure wound therapy (NPWT) assisted skin closure
- Extraperitoneal nondestructive injuries
  - Grade I injury
    - Hematoma in blunt injury: Nonoperative management
    - Hematoma in penetrating injury: Exploration to exclude penetrating injuries
    - Partial-thickness laceration: Transanal repair is easily accessible or nonoperative.
  - Grade II injury
    - Repair of laceration (transabdominal or transanal access) if possible
    - Diverting colostomy if repair is not possible
    - No role of rectal washout
  - Extraperitoneal destructive injuries
    - Damage-control procedure
      - Control hemorrhage.
      - Resection using a GIA stapler or closure of the ends with ties to control contamination.
      - No colostomy
  - No role of rectal washout
  - No role of presacral drainage
  - Reexploration after hemodynamic stability and correction of the lethal triad
    - Repair if possible
    - Resection and low anastomosis if possible
      - May consider protective diverting loop ostomy.
    - Diverting colostomy if repair or resection and anastomosis are not possible

CHAPTER 30

Evaluation and Management of Urological Injuries

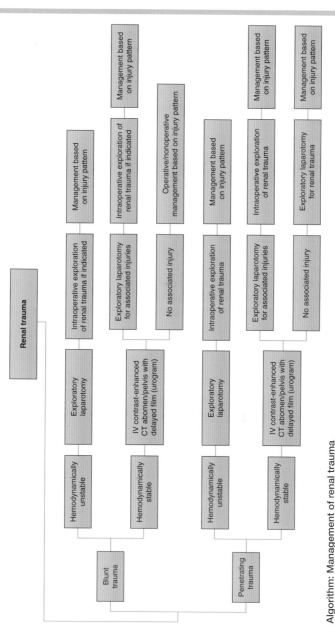

Algorithm: Management of renal trauma

Must-Know Essentials: Management of Renal Trauma

ANATOMY OF THE KIDNEYS

- Location
  - Paired retroperitoneal structures at the level of T12-L3 vertebra
  - Right kidney slightly inferior to the left due to liver
- Covered with superficial to the deep with:
  - pararenal fat.
  - renal fascia (Gerota's fascia or perirenal fascia): It encloses the kidneys and the suprarenal glands.
  - Perirenal fat.
  - Renal capsule.
- Renal hilum
  - Deep fissure on the medial margin of each kidney
  - Structures at the hilum from anterior to posterior
    - Renal vein
    - Renal artery
    - Ureter
- Anatomical relations
  - Left kidney
    - Superior
      - Left suprarenal gland
    - Anterior
      - Spleen
      - Pancreas
      - Stomach
      - Splenic flexure of the colon
    - Posterior
      - Diaphragm
      - 11th and 12th ribs
      - Psoas major, quadratus lumborum, and transversus abdominis muscles
      - Subcostal, iliohypogastric, and ilioinguinal nerves
  - Right kidney
    - Superior
      - Right suprarenal gland
    - Anterior
      - Liver
      - Duodenum
      - Right colic (hepatic) flexure
    - Posterior
      - Diaphragm
      - 12th rib
      - Psoas major, quadratus lumborum, and transversus abdominis muscles
      - Subcostal, iliohypogastric, and ilioinguinal nerves
- Arterial supply
  - Renal arteries
    - One for each kidney
    - Direct branch from the abdominal aorta, just distal to the origin of the superior mesenteric artery (SMA) at the level of L2 vertebra

Right renal artery is longer and lies posterior to the inferior vena cava (IVC).

Renal arteries enter the kidney at the renal hilum.

Renal artery divides into an anterior and a posterior division at the hilum.

Each division of the renal arteries further divides into five segmental arteries.

- Venous drainage
  - Renal veins

    Right and left renal veins drain directly into the IVC.

    Located anterior to the renal arteries at the renal hilum

    Left renal vein is longer and travels anteriorly to the abdominal aorta below the origin of the SMA.
  - Left renal vein receives:

    left adrenal vein.

    lumbar vein.

    left gonadal vein.

MECHANISM OF RENAL TRAUMA

- Blunt trauma
  - Most common mechanism of injury
  - Frequently due to high-velocity deceleration mechanism
- Penetrating trauma
  - Less common mechanism of injury
  - May be due to low-energy stab wound or high-energy gunshot wound (GSW)
  - Renal vascular injuries are more frequent after penetrating trauma.
  - Usually associated with other injuries

EVALUATION

- Focused Assessment with Sonography for Trauma (FAST)
  - Low sensitivity and specificity for renal trauma evaluation
- IV contrast-enhanced CT of the abdomen and pelvis with delayed urographic phase
  - Preferred test in hemodynamic stable blunt or penetrating injuries
- Intravenous urography
  - May be used to identify renal injuries intraoperatively in hemodynamically unstable patients where CT was not performed

AMERICAN ASSOCIATION FOR THE SURGERY OF TRAUMA (AAST) GRADING OF KIDNEY INJURY

- Grade I
  - Subcapsular hematoma and/or parenchymal contusion without laceration
- Grade II
  - Perirenal hematoma confined to Gerota's fascia
  - Renal parenchymal laceration <1 cm depth without urinary extravasation
- Grade III
  - Renal parenchymal laceration >1 cm depth without collecting system rupture or urinary extravasation
  - Any injury in the presence of a kidney vascular injury or active bleeding contained within Gerota's fascia
- Grade IV
  - Parenchymal laceration extending into urinary collecting system with urinary extravasation

- Renal pelvis laceration and/or complete ureteropelvic disruption
- Segmental renal vein or artery injury
- Active bleeding beyond Gerota's fascia into the retroperitoneum or peritoneum
- Segmental or complete kidney infarction(s) due to vessel thrombosis without active bleeding
- Grade V
  - Main renal artery or vein laceration or avulsion of hilum
  - Devascularized kidney with active bleeding
  - Shattered kidney with loss of identifiable parenchymal renal anatomy. *More than one grade of kidney injury may be present and should be classified by the higher grade injury. Advance one grade for multiple injuries up to Grade III.*

TREATMENT OF HEMODYNAMICALLY STABLE BLUNT KIDNEY TRAUMA

- Grades I, II, and III
  - Nonoperative management
    - If no other associated injuries that require abdominal exploration
    - Evaluation with angiogram for possible angioembolization indicated if CT positive for blush
- Grades IV and V
  - Nonoperative management
    - If no other associated injuries that require exploratory laparotomy
    - Evaluation with angiogram and possible angioembolization are possible if CT abdomen is suggestive for:
      arterial contrast extravasation.
      Extended perirenal hematoma
      Pseudoaneurysm
      Arteriovenous fistula
    - Non-self-limiting gross hematuria may need evaluation with angiogram and angioembolization.
    - Renal artery injury in CT should be evaluated for stent or stent graft.
    - Endoscopic evaluation for renal pelvic injury
      - May require ureteric stent or surgical management
  - Operative management
    - Indications
      Evidence of associated intraabdominal injuries in CT abdomen
      Severe renal arterial injury with persistent bleeding and failed embolization
      Main renal venous injury
      Peritonitis
      Expanding or pulsatile hematoma
      Pyeloureteral injury not amenable to endoscopic/percutaneous techniques/stent
    - Operative procedures may include:
      exploration of hematoma and bleeding control.
      Active bleeding
      Expanding hematoma
      Pulsatile bleeding
      Nephrectomy
      Shattered kidney
      Severe arterial injury
      Severe right renal venous injury requiring ligation. Ligation of the left renal vein does not require nephrectomy.

Partial nephrectomy for upper or lower pole renal injury
Repair of laceration
Repair of pyeloureteric injury
Repair of renal artery
Ligation of renal vein
Right renal vein ligation requires nephrectomy because lack of venous collaterals results in renal infarct.
Left renal vein ligation does not require nephrectomy because of its collaterals from suprarenal vein, lumbar vein, and left gonadal vein.
Renal salvage procedures for solitary or bilateral injuries
Segmental angioembolization
Percutaneous revascularization with stent or stent graft may be considered in patients with limited warm ischemia time (<240 min). Warm ischemia time >60 min results in significant losses in kidney function.
Repair of renal pelvis with nephrostomy tube and stent placement

TREATMENT OF HEMODYNAMICALLY STABLE PENETRATING KIDNEY TRAUMA

- Grades I, II, and III
  - Nonoperative management
    - If isolated low-energy injuries without any other associated injury
    - Evaluation with angiogram for possible angioembolization is indicated if CT is positive for blush.
  - Operative management
    - High-energy penetrating injury
    - Renal injury associated with other intraabdominal injuries
- Grades IV and V
  - Operative management including:
    - nephrectomy if nonsalvageable injury.
      - Shattered kidney
      - Severe arterial injury
      - Severe right venous injury requiring ligation. Ligation of left renal vein does not require nephrectomy.
    - Partial nephrectomy
    - Repair of laceration
    - Repair of pyeloureteric injury
    - Attempt for renal salvage for solitary or bilateral injuries as discussed in blunt injury

TREATMENT OF HEMODYNAMICALLY UNSTABLE BLUNT KIDNEY TRAUMA

- Exploratory laparotomy
  - Procedures depend on the grade of injury.
  - Grades I, II, and III
    - Retroperitoneal hematoma is explored if:
      - expanding.
      - ruptured.
      - pulsatile.
    - Control of bleeding
      - Surgical bleeding control

Packing with hemostatic agents
- Postoperative evaluation after resuscitation
  IV contrast-enhanced CT with urogram after resuscitation
  Postoperative evaluation with angiogram for angioembolization
- Grades IV and V
  - Nephrectomy
    Uncontrollable life-threatening hemorrhage with avulsion of the renal pedicle
    Pulsating and/or expanding retroperitoneal hematoma or renal vein lesion without self-limiting hemorrhage
    Shattered kidney
    Severe arterial injury
    Severe right renal venous injury. Ligation of left renal vein does not require nephrectomy.
  - Partial nephrectomy if injury is at the upper or lower pole.
  - Exploration of hematoma with control of bleeding/repair of laceration. Indications of exploration include:
    Active bleeding with hematoma
    Expanding hematoma
    Pulsatile bleeding
  - Repair of laceration
  - Ligation of vein
    Right renal vein ligation requires nephrectomy.
    Left renal vein ligation does not require nephrectomy.
  - Repair of pyeloureteric injury
    Endoscopic treatment or surgical treatment after resuscitation
  - Attempt for renal salvage for solitary or bilateral injuries as discussed in blunt injury
    IV contrast-enhanced CT abdomen with urogram after resuscitation
    Angiogram and evaluation for angioembolization
    Endoscopic evaluation after resuscitation for ureteric repair or stent
    Percutaneous revascularization with stent or stent graft may be considered in patients with limited warm ischemia time (<240 min). Warm ischemia time >60 min results in significant losses in kidney function.
    Repair of renal pelvis with nephrostomy tube and stent placement

TREATMENT OF HEMODYNAMICALLY UNSTABLE PENETRATING KIDNEY TRAUMA

- Exploratory laparotomy
- Procedures depending on the grade of injury
  - Grades I, II, and III
    - Retroperitoneal hematoma is explored to control bleeding/repair of laceration.
    - Postoperative evaluation after resuscitation
      IV contrast-enhanced CT with urogram after resuscitation
      Evaluation with angiogram if bleeding noted in CT
  - Grades IV and V
    - Nephrectomy
      Uncontrollable life-threatening hemorrhage renal pedicle injury
      Pulsating and/or expanding retroperitoneal hematoma or renal vein lesion without self-limiting hemorrhage
      Severe renal laceration

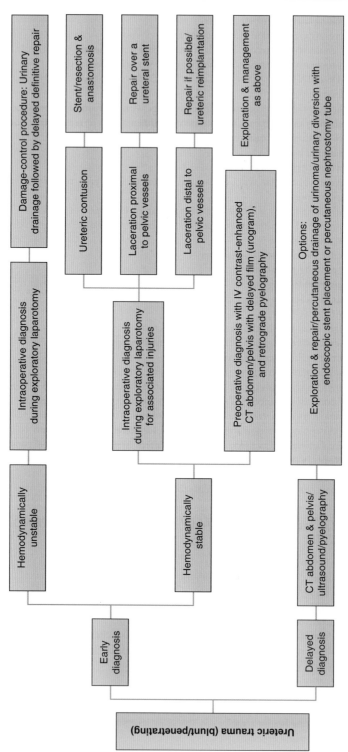

Algorithm: Management of ureteric trauma

Severe arterial injury

Severe right renal venous injury. Ligation of left renal vein does not require nephrectomy.

- Partial nephrectomy if injury at the upper or lower pole
- Exploration of hematoma with control of bleeding/repair of laceration
- Repair of laceration
- Ligation of vein

Right renal vein ligation requires nephrectomy.

Left renal vein ligation does not require nephrectomy.

- Repair of pyeloureteric injury

Endoscopic treatment or surgical treatment after resuscitation

- Attempt for renal salvage for solitary or bilateral injuries

Damage-control procedure to control bleeding

Postoperative evaluation after resuscitation and reexploration

IV contrast-enhanced CT abdomen with urogram after resuscitation

Angiogram and evaluation for angioembolization

Endoscopic evaluation after resuscitation for ureteric repair or stent

Percutaneous revascularization with stent or stent graft may be considered in patients with limited warm ischemia time (<240 min). Warm ischemia time >60 min results in significant losses in kidney function.

Repair of renal pelvis with nephrostomy tube and stent placement

COMPLICATIONS AFTER NONOPERATIVE MANAGEMENT FOR HIGH-GRADE RENAL TRAUMA

- Enlarging urinoma; can be treated with:
  - percutaneous drainage of urinoma.
  - percutaneous nephrostomy.
  - ureteral stent.
- Fistula
- Infection
- Ileus

Must-Know Essentials: Management of Ureteric Trauma

ANATOMY OF THE URETER

- 20 to 30 cm long
- Divided into three parts
  - Proximal third
    - Extends from the ureteropelvic junction to the area where it crosses the sacroiliac joint above the bifurcation of the iliac vessels
  - Middle third
    - Part that courses over the bony pelvis anterior to the bifurcation of the common iliac artery
  - Distal third
    - Extends below the internal iliac artery and connects to the urinary bladder
    - Intramural ureters are approximately 1.5 cm long
    - Terminal portion of the ureter may be subdivided into three sections.

- Juxtavesical
- Intramural
- Submucosal
- Relations
  - Courses along the anterior border of the psoas major muscle
  - Gonadal vessels cross the ureter anteriorly.
  - Crosses anterior to the bifurcation of the common iliac artery
- Arterial supply
  - Upper third, supplied by ureteric branches from the:
    - aorta.
    - renal artery.
  - Middle and lower third, supplied by branches from the:
    - iliac artery.
    - lumbar arteries.
    - vesicular artery.

MECHANISM OF INJURY

- Traumatic ureteral injury is rare.
- Most common after penetrating trauma
- Injury to the upper third of the ureter is more common than to the middle and lower thirds.
- Frequently associated with other injuries
- Penetrating trauma
  - GSWs are the most common cause of penetrating ureteral injury.
  - Injury in GSWs may be due to direct injury or blast effect.
- Blunt trauma
  - May cause approximately 25% of ureteric injuries
  - Injury at the ureteropelvic junction is common after high-energy deceleration injuries.

EVALUATION

- Evaluation for ureteral injuries should be performed in patients with a high index of suspicion based on the mechanism and location of the injury.
- Ureteral injury is suspected in patients with:
  - gross hematuria.
  - flank injury—flank pain and ecchymosis.
- IV contrast-enhanced CT with delayed film (urogram)
  - Investigation of choice hemodynamically stable patients
- Retrograde pyelography
  - Combination with CT is useful for an accurate diagnosis of ureteral injuries.
- Unstable patients
  - Intraoperative direct inspection during laparotomy
  - Single-shot intraoperative intravenous pyelogram

AAST GRADING OF URETERIC INJURY

- Grade I
  - Hematoma: Contusion or hematoma without devascularization
- Grade II
  - Laceration: >50% transection

- Grade III
  - Laceration: ≥50% transection
- Grade IV
  - Laceration: Complete transection with <2 cm of devascularization
- Grade V
  - Laceration: Avulsion with >2 cm of devascularization
  Advance one grade for bilateral injury up to Grade III.

TREATMENT OF URETERIC TRAUMA (BLUNT/PENETRATING) IN HEMODYNAMICALLY UNSTABLE PATIENT

- Exploratory laparotomy with evaluation of the ureter
- Ureteral injury may be visualized using intravenous or renal pelvic indigo carmine or methylene blue injection.
- Damage-control procedures
  - Urinary drainage
    - Percutaneous ureterostomy using a ureteric stent or an 8 F Foley catheter in the proximal ureter
    - Ligation of the proximal and distal ends of the injured ureter and a percutaneous nephrostomy tube placement intraoperatively or postoperatively by interventional radiologist
  - Foley catheter
  - Definitive ureteric repair after resuscitation and hemodynamic stability

TREATMENT OF URETERIC TRAUMA (BLUNT/PENETRATING) IN HEMODYNAMICALLY STABLE PATIENT

- Grade I
  - Diagnosed preoperatively with CT and pyelogram
    - Blunt trauma
      - No associated injury requiring an exploratory laparotomy
        - Nonoperative treatment with ureteric stent
        - Surgical repair if leaks
      - Exploratory laparotomy for other associated injury
        - Viable ureter: Ureteric stent
        - Nonviable ureter: Resection and ureteroureterostomy over a stent
    - Penetrating trauma
      - Exploratory laparotomy
        - Viable ureter: Ureteric stent
        - Nonviable ureter: Resection and ureteroureterostomy over a stent
- Grade II
  - Diagnosed preoperatively with CT and pyelogram
    - Blunt trauma
      - No associated injury requiring an exploratory laparotomy
        - Nonoperative management with ureteric stents
        - Surgical repair if leaks
      - Exploratory laparotomy for other associated injuries
        - Primary repair over a stent
    - Penetrating trauma
      - Exploratory laparotomy and primary repair over a stent

- Grades III, IV, and V
  - Surgical exploration is indicated in blunt and penetrating ureteric trauma.
  - Treatment depends on the location and extent of the injury.
  - Surgical principles for ureteric injury repair
    - Debridement of devitalized tissue
    - Careful mobilization of the ureter to prevent vascular compromise
    - Primary ureteroureterostomy is usually possible in injuries proximal to the pelvic vessels.
    - Injuries distal to the pelvic vessels usually require more complex procedures for reconstruction.
    - Isolation of the ureteric repair from other associated injuries
    - Adequate drainage of the retroperitoneum
  - Upper-third injury
    - Ureteroureterostomy
      - Tension-free spatulated end-to-end anastomosis over a stent using interrupted mucosa-to-mucosa 5-0 absorbable suture
    - Ureteropyelostomy
      - If ureteroureterostomy is not possible
      - Ureter is anastomosed to the renal pelvis over a stent using interrupted mucosa-to-mucosa 5-0 absorbable suture.
  - Middle-third injury
    - Ureteroureterostomy
      - Tension-free spatulated end-to-end anastomosis over a stent using interrupted mucosa-to-mucosa 5-0 absorbable suture if possible
    - Transureteroureterostomy
      - If ureteroureterostomy is not possible
      - End-to-end anastomosis of the injured ureter to the contralateral ureter over a stent using inturrupted mucosa-to-mucosa 5-0 absorbable suture
      - Injured ureter is brought through a window in the transverse mesocolon cephalad to the inferior mesenteric artery.
    - Anterior wall bladder flap (Boari flap)
      - Flap of anterior bladder wall is rotated cephalad to create a tube and the ureter is reimplanted into the tube.
      - May be considered as an alternative to transureteroureterostomy in distal middle-third injury
  - Lower third
    - Ureteroureterostomy
      - Tension-free spatulated end-to-end anastomosis over a stent using interrupted mucosa-to-mucosa 5-0 absorbable suture if possible
    - Direct ureteric reimplantation (ureteroneocystostomy)
      - A tunnel is created in the detrusor muscle on the posterolateral surface of the dome of the bladder.
      - An opening is made in the bladder mucosa and anastomosed to the ureteric mucosa over a stent using interrupted 5-0 absorbable sutures.
      - The detrusor muscle flap is sutured over the ureter with 4-0 absorbable sutures.
    - Ureteroneocystostomy (psoas hitch)
      - The bladder dome is pulled cephalad and sutured to the ipsilateral psoas tendon if tension-free reimplantation of the ureter into the bladder is not possible.
      - The ureter is then reimplanted into the dome of the bladder (as previously described).

- Complete disruption of the ureter may be treated with:
    - ureteric reconstruction using ileal segment interposition.
    - ureteric reconstruction using appendix as a conduit.
    - autotransplantation.

TREATMENT OF URETERIC TRAUMA (BLUNT/PENETRATING) WITH DELAYED DIAGNOSIS

- Missed or delayed diagnosis may result in:
    - retroperitoneal abscess.
    - urinoma.
    - stricture.
    - fistula.
- Incomplete disruption of ureter
    - Percutaneous drainage of urinoma
    - Urinary diversion
        - Percutaneous nephrostomy
        - Ureteric stent placement
- Complete disruption of ureter
    - Open repair (as previously described earlier in the treatment of hemodynamically ureteric injury)
- Surgery for complications such as stricture or fistula

Must-Know Essentials: Management of Bladder Trauma

ANATOMY OF THE BLADDER

- Situated in the pelvis behind the pubic symphysis
- Separated from the pubic symphysis by an anterior prevesical space (space of Retzius), which contains fibroadipose tissue, and prevesical fascia
- Dome and posterior surface of the bladder are covered by peritoneum.
- Bladder neck is fixed to neighboring structures by reflections of the pelvic fascia and by true ligaments of the pelvis.
- Inferior support of the bladder is provided by the pelvic diaphragm in women and the prostate in men.
- Lateral support of the bladder is provided by the obturator internus and levator ani muscles.
- Bladder neck
    - It serves as the internal sphincter in women.
    - It is contiguous with the prostate, and both structures function as the internal urethral sphincter in men.
- Trigone
    - Triangular portion of the bladder floor bordered by the internal urethral opening or bladder neck and the orifices of the right ureter and left ureter
    - The intravesical ureteral orifices are roughly 2–3 cm apart.
- Arterial supply
    - Internal iliac (hypogastric) arteries
        - Main source of blood supply
        - Branches that supply bladder
            - Umbilical artery
                - Gives rise to several superior vesicle branches

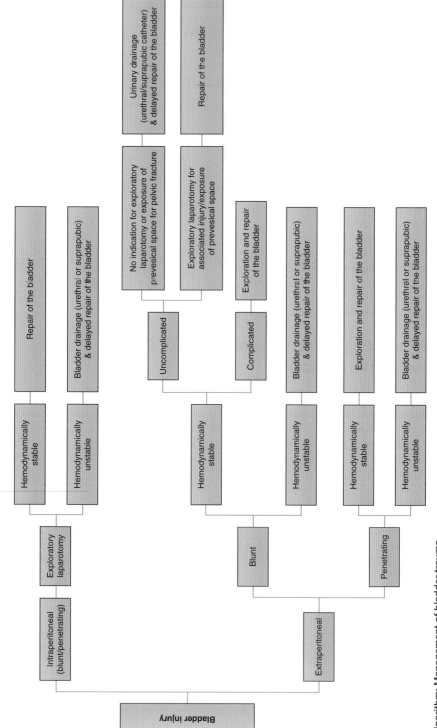

Algorithm: Management of bladder trauma

Inferior vesical arteries
  Direct branch in men
  From vaginal artery in women
  Obturator artery
  Inferior gluteal artery
- Venous drainage
  - Internal iliac vein

MECHANISM OF INJURY

- More common after blunt compared to penetrating trauma
- Penetrating trauma in the abdomen and buttock

EVALUATION

- Bladder injury should be suspected in patients with:
  - pelvic fractures.
  - gross hematuria.
- Retrograde cystography
  - Conventional radiography or using a CT scan
  - Investigation of choice for bladder injury
- IV contrast-enhanced CT with delayed phase (CT cystogram)
  - Less sensitive and less specific than retrograde cystography
- Cystoscopy
  - Evaluation of the bladder and the urethra
- Direct inspection of the intraperitoneal bladder during an emergency laparotomy
  - Intravenous injection of methylene blue or indigo carmine helps identify the injury.

AAST GRADING OF BLADDER INJURY

- Grade I
  - Hematoma: Contusion, intramural hematoma
  - Laceration: Partial thickness
- Grade II
  - Laceration: Extraperitoneal bladder wall laceration <2 cm long
- Grade III
  - Laceration: Extraperitoneal (>2 cm long) or intraperitoneal (<2 cm long) bladder wall laceration
- Grade IV
  - Laceration: Intraperitoneal bladder wall laceration >2 cm long
- Grade V
  - Laceration: Intraperitoneal or extraperitoneal bladder wall laceration extending into the trigone (bladder neck or ureteral orifice).
  Advance one grade for multiple lesions up to Grade III.

TYPES OF BLADDER INJURIES BASED ON LOCATION

- Intraperitoneal
- Extraperitoneal
  - Most common

- Frequently associated with pelvic fractures
- Urinary extravasation
  - May be limited to the pelvic region
  - May extend to the anterior abdominal wall, the scrotum, and the perineum
- Combined intraperitoneal and extraperitoneal

TREATMENT OF BLADDER INJURY

- Contusion
  - No specific treatment
- Intraperitoneal bladder injury (blunt/penetrating)
  - Exploratory laparotomy and primary repair of the bladder
- Blunt extraperitoneal bladder injury
  - Uncomplicated
    - Urinary drainage via urethral or percutaneous suprapubic catheter if no other indication for exploratory laparotomy
    - Surgical repair of the bladder
      During exploratory laparotomy for other indications
      During surgical exploration of the prevesical space for orthopedic fixations
      Persistent urine extravasation 4 weeks after nonsurgical management
  - Complicated
    - Including:
      Bladder neck injuries
      Associated pelvic ring fracture
      Vaginal injuries
      Rectal injuries
    - Exploration and surgical repair of the bladder during the management of associated injuries such as:
      internal fixation of pelvic fractures.
      management of vaginal injury.
      management of rectal injury.
- Penetrating extraperitoneal bladder injury
  - Both complicated and uncomplicated injuries are treated with surgical exploration and repair of the bladder.
- Damage control
  - Intraperitoneal bladder injury
    - Urinary diversion with a bladder catheter and perivesical drainage during exploratory laparotomy
    - Repair of bladder injury after resuscitation and hemodynamic stability
  - Extraperitoneal bladder injury
    - Urethral or suprapubic catheter
    - Suprapubic catheter recommended for associated perineal injuries
    - Repair of the bladder injury after resuscitation and hemodynamic stability
- Principles of bladder injury repair
  - Debridement of devitalized tissue
  - Inspection for additional bladder injury through the laceration or by extending the laceration
  - Extraperitoneal laceration may be repaired through the bladder with 3-0 absorbable sutures in a single layer.
  - Intraperitoneal bladder repair may be done with 3-0 absorbable sutures in two layers.

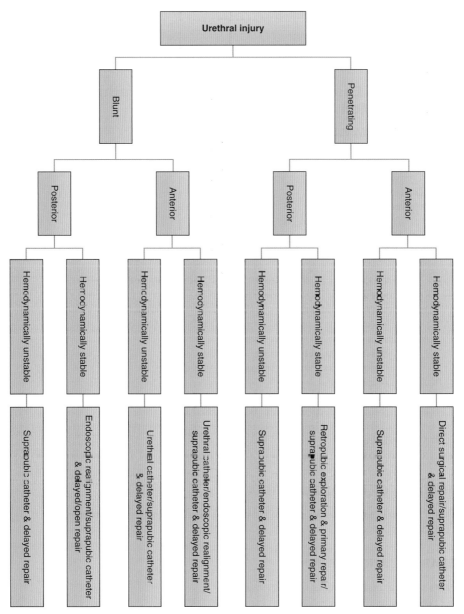

Algorithm: Management of urethral trauma in menv

- ■ Placement of perivesical drainage
- ■ Placement of urethral catheter without a suprapubic catheter is mandatory after surgical repair.

Must-Know Essentials: Management of Urethral Trauma in Men

ANATOMY OF MALE URETHRA

- ■ Extends from the bladder neck to the urethral meatus
- ■ Approximately 15–25 cm long in the adult
- ■ Divided into:
  - ■ prostatic urethra.
    - ▪ Approximately 2–3 cm long
    - ▪ Passes through the prostate gland
  - ■ Membranous urethra
    - ▪ Extends from the apex of the prostate to the bulb of the penis
    - ▪ Is the shortest part of the urethra, approximately 1 cm long
    - ▪ Susceptible to injury in pelvic fracture
  - ■ Penile (spongy) urethra
    - ▪ Divided into the pendulous urethra and the bulbous (or bulbar) urethra
  - ■ Urethra is also divided into two sections.
    - ▪ Anterior urethra: Penile urethra
    - ▪ Posterior urethra: Prostatic and membranous urethra
- ■ Arterial supply
  - ■ Prostatic urethra: Inferior vesical artery
  - ■ Membranous and bulbar urethra: Bulbourethral artery
  - ■ Pendulous urethra: Deep penile artery branch of the internal pudendal artery
- ■ Venous drainage
  - ■ Follows the arterial supply

ANATOMY OF FEMALE URETHRA

- ■ Extends from the bladder neck to the urethral meatus in the vaginal vestibule
- ■ Approximately 4 cm long

CLASSIFICATION OF INJURY

- ■ Types of urethral injuries based on location
  - ■ Anterior
    - ▪ Involves penile urethra
    - ▪ More common after blunt trauma
    - ▪ Rarely caused by penetrating trauma
  - ■ Posterior
    - ▪ Involves prostatic urethra and membranous urethra
    - ▪ Usually caused by blunt trauma such as anterior pelvic fractures and diastasis of the pubic symphysis

- Risk of urethral injury increases by 10% for every 1-mm increase in diastasis of the pubic symphysis.
- Extremely rare after penetrating trauma
■ Classification based on injury pattern
- Contusion
- Partial urethral injury
- Complete urethral injury

EVALUATION

■ Clinical manifestations
- Blood at the urethral meatus in patients with pelvic fracture is suggestive of a urethral injury.
- Hematuria
- High-riding prostate in men
- May be associated with the following:
  - Bladder injury
  - Rectal injury
  - Vaginal injury
■ Retrograde urethrography
- First test of choice
■ Selective urethroscopy
- Preferred over retrograde urethrography in patients with penile injuries
■ Combined bladder/urethral injury
- CT cystogram
- Cystourethrogram
- Cystoscopy

AAST GRADING OF URETHRAL INJURY

■ Grade I
- Contusion: Blood at urethral meatus; urethrography normal
■ Grade II
- Stretch injury: Elongation of urethra without extravasation on urethrography
■ Grade III
- Partial disruption: Extravasation of urethrography contrast at injury site with visualization in the bladder
■ Grade IV
- Complete disruption: Extravasation of urethrography contrast at injury site without visualization in the bladder; <2 cm of urethra separation
■ Grade V
- Complete disruption: Complete transaction with >2 cm urethral separation, or extension into the prostate or vagina

TREATMENT OF URETHRAL INJURY

■ Penetrating anterior urethral trauma
- Hemodynamically stable patient
  - Direct surgical repair if possible
  - If anastomotic urethroplasty is not feasible due to a large anatomic defect in bulbar or penile urethra

- Suprapubic urinary catheter followed by delayed anatomic reconstruction with graft or flap
- Hemodynamically unstable patient
  - Suprapubic urinary catheter and delayed reconstruction
  - Selected cases of incomplete penetrating trauma may be managed with transurethral catheter.
- Penetrating posterior urethral trauma
  - Hemodynamically stable patients without associated severe injuries
    - Retropubic exploration and primary repair of the injury if possible
    - If primary repair is not possible, suprapubic catheter and delayed urethroplasty
  - Hemodynamically unstable patient with associated severe injuries
    - Suprapubic catheter placement and delayed urethroplasty, preferably within 14 days from the injury
- Blunt anterior urethral blunt trauma
  - Hemodynamically stable patient
    - Urethral catheter placement if possible and delayed surgical treatment
    - If ureteral catheter placement unsuccessful
      - Endoscopic treatment with realignment
    - Failed urethral catheter or endoscopic realignment
      - Suprapubic catheter placement and delayed surgical urethroplasty
      - Patients with associated pelvic fractures, definitive surgery should be performed after the healing of pelvic ring fractures.
  - Hemodynamically unstable patient
    - Urethral catheter placement if possible and delayed surgical treatment
    - If urethral catheter placement is unsuccessful
      - Suprapubic catheter followed by delayed surgical urethroplasty
- Blunt posterior urethral trauma
  - Hemodynamically stable
    - Partial injury
      - Urinary drainage: Urethral catheter
      - Endoscopic realignment if failed urethral catheter
      - Suprapubic catheter if failed endoscopic realignment followed by delayed definitive surgical management after 14 days if no other indications for laparotomy
      - Open repair if there are other indications for an exploratory laparotomy
    - Complete injury
      - Immediate endoscopic realignment
        - Preferred over immediate urethroplasty
        - Associated with improved outcomes
      - Failed realignment
        - Suprapubic cystostomy
        - Delayed definitive surgical management
      - Open repair if other indications for laparotomy
        - Primary open realignment and primary open anastomosis are associated with high rates of stricture, urinary incontinence, and impotence.
    - Associated with complex pelvic fracture
      - Suprapubic catheter followed by delayed definitive surgical treatment with urethroplasty after the healing of pelvic ring injury
  - Hemodynamically unstable
    - Suprapubic catheter followed by delayed definitive surgical treatment

COMPLICATIONS OF URETHRAL INJURY

- Urethral stricture
- Erectile dysfunction
- Urinary incontinence

Vascular Trauma

CHAPTER 31

Evaluation and Management of Retroperitoneal Vascular Injuries

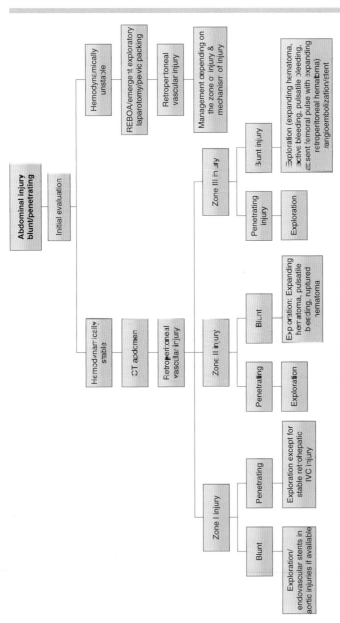

Algorithm: Evaluation and management of retroperitoneal vascular injuries

Must-Know Essentials: Anatomy of Retroperitoneal Vessels

ABDOMINAL AORTA

- The abdominal aorta originates at the T12-L1 vertebra level as a continuation of the thoracic aorta.
- It enters the abdomen through the aortic hiatus between the two crura of the diaphragm.
- It bifurcates into the left and right common iliac arteries at the L4-L5 vertebra level.
- The umbilicus is the external landmark for the bifurcation of the aorta.
- Branches
  - Inferior phrenic arteries
    - Paired first branches of the abdominal aorta
    - Originates from the anterolateral surface of the abdominal aorta
  - Celiac trunk
    - Originates immediately below the phrenic arteries at the T12 vertebra level and is 1–2 cm in length
    - Located along the upper border of the pancreas
    - Branches
      Common hepatic artery
      Left gastric artery
      Splenic artery
  - Superior mesenteric artery (SMA)
    - Located 1–2 cm below the celiac trunk posterior to the pancreas at the L1 vertebra level
    - Lies over the uncinate process of the pancreas and the third part of the duodenum and enters the root of the mesentery
    - Branches
      Inferior pancreaticoduodenal artery
      Middle colic artery
      Arterial arcade with 12–18 intestinal branches
      Right colic artery
      Ileocolic artery
  - Renal arteries
    - Originate 1–1.5 cm below the SMA at the L2 vertebra level
    - Right renal artery
      Located at a slightly higher level
      Courses posterior to the inferior vena cava (IVC)
  - Inferior mesenteric artery (IMA)
    - Located 2–5 cm above the aortic bifurcation at the L3 vertebra level
    - Branches
      Left colic artery
      Sigmoid artery
      Superior rectal artery
    - Communicates with the SMA through the marginal artery of Drummond
  - Subcostal arteries
    - Bilateral small arteries that originate from the posterior surface of the distal descending thoracic aorta
    - Courses beneath the 12th rib, it supplies to abdominal wall and also supply to the spinal cord

- Middle suprarenal arteries
  - Middle suprarenal arteries originate from the posterior surface of the abdominal aorta at the level of the SMA.
  - Superior suprarenal arteries originate from the inferior phrenic arteries.
  - Inferior suprarenal arteries originate from the renal arteries.
- Lumbar arteries
  - Four pairs of bilateral arteries on each side, originating from the posterior surface of the abdominal aorta
  - Located at the level of the corresponding upper four lumbar vertebrae
  - Supply to the muscles of the abdominal wall, skin, lumbar vertebrae, and spinal cord
- Median sacral artery
  - Unpaired artery originates from the posterior aspect of the abdominal aorta just superior to the bifurcation
  - Supplies the fourth and fifth lumbar vertebrae, sacrum, coccyx, and super posterior rectum

COMMON ILIAC ARTERIES

- Each common artery divides into the external and internal (hypogastric) iliac arteries.
- The ureter crosses over the bifurcation of the common iliac arteries.

EXTERNAL ILIAC ARTERIES

- Continue as femoral arteries under the inguinal ligament
- Branches
  - Inferior epigastric artery
  - Deep circumflex iliac artery

INTERNAL ILIAC (HYPOGASTRIC) ARTERIES

- Divides into anterior and posterior branches at the level of the greater sciatic foramen
- Branches from posterior division
  - Superior gluteal artery
    - Most common source of arterial bleeding in pelvic fractures
    - Gives rise to iliolumbar and lateral sacral arteries
- Branches from anterior division
  - Superior vesical artery
  - Obturator artery
  - Inferior vesical artery
  - Middle rectal artery
  - Internal pudendal artery
  - Inferior gluteal artery

INFERIOR VENA CAVA

- The IVC is formed at the level of L5 vertebra by the union of the common iliac veins posterior to the right common iliac artery.
- The IVC enters the chest at the T8 verebra level through an opening in the diaphragm and drains in the right atrium.
- Courses along the right side of the lumbar and thoracic vertebral bodies
- The right crus of the diaphragm separates the IVC from the aorta.

- Divided into:
  - infrarenal IVC—below the renal veins
  - retrohepatic IVC—usually 8–10 cm long
  - suprahepatic IVC—between the liver and the diaphragm and approximately 1 cm long
  - Intrathoracic (intrapericardial)
- Branches
  - Lumbar veins
    - Usually five pairs
    - First pair of lumbar veins usually drain in the ascending lumbar veins on each side
    - Left lumbar veins pass behind the abdominal aorta.
    - Second, third, and fourth lumbar veins may drain directly to the IVC or the ascending lumbar veins on each side.
    - Fifth lumbar veins drain in the right common iliac vein on the right side and iliolumbar vein on the left side.
    - Ascending lumbar veins are connected to the IVC through lumbar veins.
  - Right gonadal vein
  - Left gonadal vein drains in the left renal vein.
  - Right adrenal (suprarenal) vein
  - Left adrenal (suprarenal) vein drains in the left renal vein.
  - Renal veins
    - Left renal vein is situated anterior to the aorta.
    - Renal veins lie anterior to the renal arteries.
  - Hepatic veins
    - Major veins: right, middle, and left hepatic veins
    - Many accessary veins: from the caudate and right lobes
  - Phrenic veins

ASCENDING LUMBAR VEINS

- Paired veins on each side of the lumbar vertebral body
- Start from the common iliac veins
- First pair of lumbar veins usually drain in the ascending lumbar veins on each side.
- Second, third, and fourth lumbar veins may drain directly to the IVC or to the ascending lumbar veins on each side.

HEMIAZYGOS VEIN

- Arises as a continuation of the left ascending lumbar vein
- Enters the left chest through the diaphragm
- Connects to the azygos vein in the right chest at the level of T8 vertebra
- Branches
  - Left 9th–11th intercostal veins
  - Left 12th intercostal (subcostal) vein
- May connect to the left renal vein

AZYGOS VEIN

- Arises as a continuation of right ascending lumbar vein at the level of the right renal vein
- Passes through the diaphragm and enters the right chest and drains in the superior vena cava (SVC)

- Branches
  - Right 4th–9th intercostal veins
  - Right 12th intercostal (subcostal) vein
  - Hemiazygos vein
  - Accessory hemiazygos vein: Situated in the left posterior chest and drains left 4–8 intercostal veins
  - May have many anastomoses with IVC and vertebral venous plexuses
- An important connection between the IVC and SVC for an alternate drainage in patients with IVC obstruction

COMMON ILIAC VEINS

- Located posterior and to the right of the right common iliac artery
- Branches
  - External iliac vein: Continuation of femoral vein
  - Internal iliac veins
  - Median sacral vein (or middle sacral vein): A branch of the left common iliac vein or sometimes arises from the angle of junction of the two iliac veins

INTERNAL ILIAC (HYPOGASTRIC) VEINS

- Divides into anterior and posterior branches
- Branches of posterior division
  - Superior gluteal vein
  - Iliolumbar and lateral sacral veins are the branches from the superior gluteal vein
- Branches of anterior division
  - Obturator vein
  - Inferior gluteal vein
  - Internal pudendal vein
  - Vesical plexus
  - Rectal plexus

Must-Know Essentials: Evaluation and Management

COMMON RETROPERITONEAL VASCULAR INJURIES

- Blunt trauma in descending order
  - IVC
  - Aorta
  - Iliac arteries
  - Iliac vein
  - SMA
- Penetrating trauma in descending order
  - Aorta
  - Iliac arteries
  - SMA
  - Renal arteries
  - Splenic artery
  - Celiac trunk
  - Hepatic artery
  - IMA

INITIAL EVALUATION AND MANAGEMENT

- May present with retroperitoneal hematoma or free rupture into the peritoneal cavity
- Patients with contained retroperitoneal hematoma are usually stable.
- Patients with ruptured hematoma are unstable and present with:
  - hemorrhagic shock characterized by persistent hypotension (systolic blood pressure <90 mm Hg).
  - transient response to fluid resuscitation.
- Initial evaluation
  - Assessment of the airway
  - Definitive airway should be secured in unstable patients.
  - Protection of cervical spine
  - Assessment of breathing and management as indicated
  - Assessment of the circulation
  - Obtainment of venous access
  - Start resuscitation with crystalloid fluid.
  - In unstable patients consider:
    - central venous access.
    - femoral arterial line.
    - initiation of massive transfusion protocol.
    - evaluation for Resuscitative Endovascular Balloon Occlusion of Aorta (REBOA) if available
  - Assessment for neurological deficit

FURTHER EVALUATION AND MANAGEMENT

- Hemodynamically stable patients
  - Physical examination
    - Unstable pelvic fracture may be associated with retroperitoneal vascular injury.
    - Penetrating trauma to the back or flank may be associated with renal or great vessel injury.
    - Evaluation for any concomitant injuries; retroperitoneal injuries are often associated with intraabdominal injuries.
  - IV contrast-enhanced CT abdomen
    - Most useful for the diagnosis and location of the zone of retroperitoneal vascular injuries
    - Information about active bleeding if there is contrast extravasation
    - Information about concomitant intraabdominal injuries
  - Focused Assessment with Sonography in Trauma (FAST) exam is unreliable in the diagnosis of retroperitoneal vascular injuries.
  - Management of the specific injuries
- Hemodynamically unstable patients
  - REBOA
  - Exploratory laparotomy
  - Pelvic packing
  - Angioembolization

Must-Know Essentials: Anatomical Zones (Selivanov et al.) of Retroperitoneal Vascular Injuries

ZONE 1

- Extends from the aortic hiatus to the sacral promontory containing midline vessels
- Divided into the supramesocolic and inframesocolic regions
- Supramesocolic region contains:
  - suprarenal aorta.
  - celiac trunk.
  - proximal SMA.
  - superior mesenteric vein (SMV).
  - portal vein.
  - proximal renal arteries.
  - supra mesocolic IVC and its branches.
- Inframesocolic region contains:
  - infrarenal aorta.
  - IMA.
  - gonadal arteries.
  - right gonadal vein.
  - origins of renal arteries.
  - renal veins.
  - infrahepatic IVC.

ZONE 2

- Located in the paracolic gutters bilaterally and extends from the lateral diaphragm to the iliac crest
- It contains:
  - bilateral renal arteries.
  - bilateral renal veins.

ZONE 3

- Begins at the sacral promontory
- It contains:
  - bilateral common iliac arteries and its branches.
  - bilateral common iliac veins and its branches.
  - median sacral artery.
  - median sacral vein.

Must-Know Essentials: Treatment of Zone 1 Vascular Injuries

IMMEDIATE CONTROL OF BLEEDING IN UNSTABLE PATIENTS

- Immediate control of bleeding with one of the following:
  - REBOA if available (see Chapter 9 for details) in the emergency room or in the operating room
  - Emergent exploratory laparotomy and control of bleeding (see Chapter 24 for details)

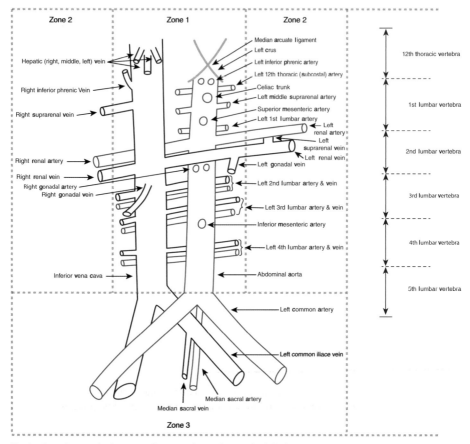

Illustration: Anatomical zones of retroperitoneal vascular injuries

- ▪ Abdominal packing with laparotomy pads
- ▪ Proximal control of abdominal aorta with one of the following techniques:
  - ▫ Direct control of supraceliac aorta through the lesser sac
  - ▫ Transabdominal subdiaphragmatic control of supraceliac aorta with mobilization of the left lobe of the liver
  - ▫ Left medial visceral rotation and control of proximal aorta
- ▪ Transthoracic cross-clamping of the distal thoracic aorta through the left anterolateral thoracotomy (see Chapter 20 for details) may be an alternative option for the proximal control of the aorta.

INDICATIONS FOR EXPLORATION IN ZONE I INJURIES DURING AN EMERGENT EXPLORATORY LAPAROTOMY

- ▪ Aortic injuries
  - ▪ All patients (stable or unstable) with penetrating aortic injuries
  - ▪ Unstable patients with blunt aortic injuries with contained hematoma
  - ▪ Stable patients with blunt aortic injuries with contained hematoma may be treated with an exploration or endovascular stent if available.

- Celiac trunk injuries
  - All penetrating celiac trunk injuries
  - Unstable blunt celiac trunk injuries with hematoma
  - Stable blunt celiac trunk injuries with contained hematoma may be treated with an exploration or endovascular stent if available.
- Proximal SMA injury
  - All penetrating proximal SMA injuries
  - Unstable blunt proximal SMA injuries with hematoma
  - Stable blunt proximal SMA injuries with contained hematoma may be treated with exploration or endovascular stent if available.
- IMA injury
  - All penetrating injuries
  - Unstable blunt injuries
  - Stable blunt injuries with contained hematoma may be treated with an exploration or endovascular stent.
- IVC injury
  - All blunt or penetrating infrahepatic IVC injury
  - Unstable blunt or penetrating retrohepatic IVC injury
    - Exploration is not recommended in stable patients with nonexpanding hematoma.
  - Unstable blunt or penetrating suprahepatic intraabdominal IVC injury
    - Exploration is not recommended in stable patients with nonexpanding hematoma.
  - All blunt or penetrating suprahepatic intrathoracic injuries

TECHNIQUES OF EXPOSURE OF RETROPERITONEAL INJURIES DURING EXPLORATORY LAPAROTOMY

- Supramesocolic diaphragmatic aorta may be exposed with one of the following:
  - Left medial visceral rotation with division of the left crus in the 2:00 position
  - Through the lesser sac by dividing the gastrohepatic and left triangular ligaments
  - Left anterolateral thoracotomy
- Supramesocolic suprarenal aorta
  - Left medial visceral rotation with division of the left crus in the 2:00 position
- Inframesocolic (infrarenal) aorta
  - Exposure at the base of the transverse mesocolon
    - Eviscerate the small bowel to the patient's right.
    - Lift the transverse mesocolon cephalad.
    - Open the retroperitoneum in the midline, beginning at the ligament of Treitz at the duodenojejunal junction to expose the infrarenal aorta.
    - Dissect until the left renal vein is exposed.
  - Left medial visceral rotation
- Celiac trunk
  - Left medial visceral rotation
  - Exposure through the lesser sac by dividing the gastrohepatic and left triangular ligaments
- SMA with one of the following techniques:
  - Left medial visceral rotation
  - Exposure through the lesser sac with or without the transection of the neck of the pancreas for direct exposure
  - Exposure through the base of the transverse mesocolon
- Proximal IMA
  - Through the base of the transverse mesocolon

- IVC
  - Infrahepatic IVC including both infrarenal, juxtarenal, and supra renal
    - Requires complete right medial visceral rotation by mobilizing the duodenum (Kocher maneuver), right colon (Cattell maneuver) and small bowel mesentery (Cattell-Braasch maneuver).
    - Superior retraction of the edge of the right lobe of the liver for further exposure of the suprarenal IVC for distal control of the IVC above the renal veins may be required.
    - Injury to lumbar veins can occur during posterior dissection of the infrarenal IVC.
    - There are no lumbar veins posterior to the suprarenal IVC.
  - Retrohepatic IVC
    - Usually requires additional subcostal incision or right thoracotomy incision through 6th or 7th intercostal space for the exposure of retrohepatic IVC
    - The liver is mobilized after division of the falciform, right triangular, and right coronary ligaments.
    - Division of the central tendon of the diaphragm is also required for exposure of the retrohepatic IVC.
    - A partial hepatectomy or enlargement of the liver laceration site may be needed in patients with associated liver laceration to control bleeding and exposure of retrohepatic IVC.
  - Suprahepatic IVC
    - Intraabdominal
      - As in retrohepatic IVC
    - Intrathoracic
      - Stable: Midline abdominal incision with extension to median sternotomy/right thoracotomy
      - Unstable: Midline abdominal incision with left anterolateral thoracotomy with clamshell extension
- SMV and portal vein
  - Pringle maneuver for bleeding control
  - Exploration of the injury through the hematoma and placement of a vascular clamp for proximal and distal control
  - An extended Kocher maneuver provides exposure of the superior mesenteric vein and portal vein.
  - In a penetrating injury, division of the neck of the pancreas with a TA stapler provides good exposure. The stapler is placed in the avascular plane at the neck of the pancreas anterior to the superior mesenteric vessels and the portal vein.

Exposure of Zone 1 vascular injuries

Zone I Vessel Injuries	Exposure Techniques
Supramesocolic diaphragmatic abdominal aorta	Midline laparotomy with left medial visceral rotation/exposure through the lesser sac/exposure through the left anterolateral thoracotomy
Supramesocolic suprarenal abdominal aorta	Midline laparotomy with left medial visceral rotation
Inframesocolic abdominal aorta	Midline laparotomy with exposure through the base of the transverse mesocolon/left medial visceral rotation
Celiac trunk and proximal branches	Midline laparotomy with left medial visceral rotation/exposure through the lesser sac
Proximal superior mesenteric artery	Midline laparotomy with left medial visceral rotation/exposure through the base of the transverse mesocolon/exposure through the lesser sac with or without transection of the neck of the pancreas

Exposure of Zone 1 vascular injuries

Zone I Vessel Injuries	Exposure Techniques
IMA	Midline laparotomy with exposure through the base of the transverse mesocolon
Infrahepatic inferior vena cava	Midline laparotomy with complete right medial visceral rotation
Retrohepatic inferior vena cava and suprahepatic intraabdominal inferior vena cava	Midline laparotomy with additional subcostal incision or right thoracotomy through 6th or 7th intercostal space, mobilization of the right lobe of the liver and division of the central tendon of the diaphragm
Suprahepatic intrathoracic inferior vena cava	Stable patient: Midline laparotomy with median sternotomy or right thoracotomyUnstable patient: Midline laparotomy with left anterolateral thoracotomy and clamshell extension
Superior mesenteric vein and portal vein	Pringle maneuver/extended Kocher maneuver/division of the neck of the pancreas with a stapler

TREATMENT OF ABDOMINAL AORTIC INJURIES

- Types of aortic injury
  - Supramesocolic
    - Diaphragmatic aortic injury
    - Suprarenal aortic injury
  - Inframesocolic (infrarenal) aortic injury
- Proximal and distal control of the aorta
  - Diaphragmatic aortic injury
    - Proximal aortic clamp with one of the following:
      - Cross-clamp the distal thoracic aorta through the left anterolateral thoracotomy
      - Left medial visceral rotation to control the proximal aorta
    - Distal control
      - Cross-clamping of the aorta proximal to the bifurcation
  - Suprarenal aortic injury
    - Proximal aortic control with one of the following:
      - Direct control of supraceliac aorta through the lesser sac
      - Transabdominal subdiaphragmatic control of supraceliac aorta with mobilization of the left lobe of the liver
      - Left medial visceral rotation and control of the proximal aorta
      - Cross-clamp the distal thoracic aorta through the left anterolateral thoracotomy
    - Distal control
      - Cross-clamping of the aorta proximal to the bifurcation.
  - Inframesocolic (infrarenal) aortic injury
    - Proximal aortic control with one of the following:
      - Direct control of supraceliac aorta through the lesser sac
      - Transabdominal subdiaphragmatic control of the supraceliac aorta with mobilization of the left lobe of the liver
      - Cross-clamp of the distal thoracic aorta through the left anterolateral thoracotomy
      - Left medial visceral rotation and control of the proximal aorta
      - Below the left renal vein after direct exposure of the aorta at the base of the transverse mesocolon

- Distal control
  - Cross-clamping of the aorta proximal to the bifurcation
- Repair of the injuries
  - Supramesocolic injuries
    - Hemodynamically stable patients
      - Small injury
        - Repair of the injury with 3-0 or 4-0 running polypropylene sutures.
      - Large injuries
        - Larger defect or risk of narrowing with aortorrhaphy: Patch angioplasty repair with autogenous vein (saphenous vein) or with polytetrafluoroethylene (PTFE) graft.
        - Interposition graft with a 12–18 mm PTFE or Dacron graft for defects > 2 cm.
        - Primary end-to-end anastomosis is not possible due to limited mobility of the aorta.
    - Damage-control procedures for hemodynamically unstable patients
      - Ligation of aorta is not an option.
      - Temporary intravascular shunt (TIVS)
        - Limited success
        - Use a chest tube or Javid or Argyle shunt.
        - Shunt is secured with silk ties, vessel loops, or umbilical tape.
        - Shunt tube should be flushed with heparinized saline.
        - Systemic heparinization is not required.
  - Infrarenal aortic injury
    - Hemodynamically stable patients
      - Small injury: Repair of the injury with 3-0 or 4-0 running polypropylene sutures.
      - Large injuries
        - Larger defect or risk of narrowing with aortorrhaphy: Patch angioplasty repair with autogenous vein (saphenous vein) or with PTFE.
        - Interposition graft with a 12–18 mm PTFE or Dacron graft for defects >2 cm.
        - Primary end-to-end anastomosis is not possible due to limited mobility of the aorta.
      - Extensive infrarenal aortic injury with gross contamination: Options include:
        - Aortic ligation with bilateral axillofemoral grafts
        - Unilateral axillofemoral graft with femorofemoral graft
        - Unilateral axillofemoral with end-to-end iliac anastomosis
    - Damage-control procedures for hemodynamically unstable patients
      - TIVS
        - Limited success
        - Use a chest tube or Javid or Argyle shunt.
        - Shunt is secured with silk ties, vessel loops, or umbilical tape.
        - Shunt tube should be flushed with heparinized saline.
        - Systemic heparinization is not required.

TREATMENT OF CELIAC TRUNK INJURIES

- Proximal and distal control of the aorta
  - Proximal control of the abdominal aorta
    - Transabdominal
    - Transthoracic
    - Through the lesser sac

- Distal control
  - Cross-clamping proximal to the bifurcation of the aorta
- Repair of the injury
  - Hemodynamically stable patients
    - Small nondestructive injury
      Repair with 4/0 polypropylene sutures.
    - Complex injury
      End-to-end anastomosis or interposition graft is not recommended.
      Ligation of the celiac trunk is well tolerated due to extensive collateral circulation.
      Cholecystectomy should be performed after celiac trunk ligation as it causes ischemia of the gallbladder.
  - Damage-control procedure for hemodynamically unstable patients
    - Ligation of celiac trunk
    - Cholecystectomy once hemodynamically stable

TREATMENT OF SUPERIOR MESENTERIC ARTERY INJURIES

- The SMA is divided into four zones for surgical management (Fullen zone classification).
  - Zone 1
    - SMA trunk proximal to the first branch of the SMA (inferior pancreaticoduodenal artery)
    - High risk of ischemia to jejunum, ileum, and right colon
  - Zone 2
    - SMA trunk between inferior pancreaticoduodenal artery and middle colic artery
    - Moderate risk of ischemia to major segment of small bowel and right colon
  - Zone 3
    - SMA trunk distal to middle colic artery
    - Mimimal risk of small segment ischemia of the small bowel and right colon
  - Zone 4
    - Involves segmental branches of the SMA (jejunal, ileal, colic)
    - No risk of bowel ischemia
- Exposure of the SMA
  - Proximal SMA (Fullen Zones 1 and 2) injuries may be exposed with one of the followings:
    - Left medial visceral rotation
    - Through the base of the transverse mesocolon
    - Through the lesser sac with or without the transection of the neck of the pancreas for direct exposure
  - Distal SMA injuries (Fullen Zone 3)
    - Exposure through the root of the mesentery
      Transverse mesocolon is reflected superiorly.
      Ligament of Treitz is divided at the duodenojejunal junction to expose the SMA.
    - From the right side
      Kocher maneuver by mobilizing the duodenum off the SMA.
  - Fullen Zone 4
    - Exposure of the injury site by opening the associated mesenteric hematoma or extending existing mesenteric lacerations.
- Proximal and distal control of the artery
  - Proximal control: Supraceliac cross-clamp of the abdominal aorta
  - Distal clamp: SMA distal to the injury
- Repair of the injury

- Hemodynamically stable patients
  - Small injury
    - Primary repair using 5-0 polypropylene sutures
  - Large or destructive injuries
    - Angioplasty with vein patch
    - Interposition graft
    - Reimplantation of SMA to the aorta
- Damage-control procedures in hemodynamically unstable patients
  - Ligation of the artery
    - High risk of bowel ischemia
  - TIVS
  - May be an alternative to ligation

TREATMENT OF IMA INJURIES

- Hemodynamically stable patient
  - Small laceration: Repair of laceration with 5-0 Polypropylene suture
  - Complex laceration: Ligation of IMA
- Hemodynamically unstable patients
  - Ligation of IMA as a damage-control procedure
    - It is well tolerated due to its good collateral circulation.
    - Colorectal ischemia is rare but may be seen in patients with atherosclerotic disease or poor collateral blood flow.

TREATMENT OF INFERIOR VENA CAVA INJURIES

- Classification based on the location of the IVC in relation to the liver:
  - Infrahepatic
    - Infrarenal
    - Suprarenal
  - Retrohepatic
  - Suprahepatic
    - Intraabdominal
    - Intrathoracic
- Infrahepatic IVC injury
  - Proximal and distal control of the IVC
    - Direct pressure against the spine proximal and distal to the injury using a sponge on sponge-holding forceps.
    - Direct pressure at the bifurcation using a sponge on sponge-holding forceps.
  - Hemodynamically stable patients
    - Repair using 4-0/5-0 polypropylene sutures for injury involving <50% circumference of the IVC.
    - Repair with patch angioplasty using PTFE or autologous vein saphenous vein patch.
      - Injury involving >50% circumference of the IVC
      - Concern of stenosis if >50 % narrowing of the IVC after the repair. Stenosis of IVC increases the risk of IVC thrombosis and pulmonary embolism.
    - Repair with interposition graft using Dacron or Gore-Tex graft.
      - Large anterior wall injury of the IVC
      - Large posterior wall injury of the IVC
      - Complete disruption of the IVC

- Hemodynamically unstable patients
  - Damage-control procedures
    - Ligation of infrahepatic IVC
      - Physiologically well tolerated
      - Transient bilateral leg edema.
      - High risk of bilateral lower extremities compartment syndrome requiring fasciotomies
    - Ligation of suprarenal IVC is not recommended.
      - Physiologically not tolerated because there is no collateral circulation due to lack of lumbar veins
      - Development of renal failure and very few long-term survivors
      - Attempt should be made to repair the injury whenever possible.
    - Shunt
      - Useful in complex suprarenal IVC injury
      - A chest tube is secured to the IVC using thick suture or vessel loop.
- Retrohepatic IVC injury
  - Suspected when dark venous bleeding is seen behind the liver that cannot be controlled by manual compression or the Pringle maneuver
  - Exploration is usually not recommended, it can result in worsening of bleeding due to loss of tamponade effect.
  - Usually best treated with liver packing without mobilizing the liver
  - Packing should be placed between the liver and anterior abdominal wall, and under the inferior surface of the liver to compress the liver against the IVC and to create a tamponade effect.
  - Packing should not be placed in the retrohepatic space.
  - Repair of injury
    - Recommended in patients with persistent bleeding after liver packing
    - May require total hepatic isolation (Heaney maneuver) or atriocaval shunt for the repair
    - Steps of total hepatic isolation and repair of vena cava injury
      - Control of supraceliac abdominal aorta (intraabdominal or transthoracic). It should be performed first to prevent the hypovolemic cardiac arrest.
      - Control of the infrahepatic IVC.
      - Control of the portal triad (Pringle maneuver).
      - Control of the suprahepatic IVC (intraabdominal or transthoracic).
      - Repair with 3-0/4-0 polypropylene running sutures.
      - High incidence of cardiac arrest
      - Very poor outcome
    - Steps of atriocaval shunt placement and repair of vena cava injury
      - Pringle maneuver
      - Exposure of the intrathoracic IVC with the left anterolateral thoracotomy and clamshell extension.
      - Placement of a thick suture around the intrapericardial IVC.
      - Placement of a purse string suture with 2-0 Silk in the right atrial appendage after occluding it with a vascular clamp.
      - Size 8 F endotracheal tube (ETT) or a size 36 chest tube may be used for the shunt.
      - A clamp is placed at the proximal end of the tube and side holes are cut in the tube about 8–10 cm distal to the clamp.
      - The shunt tube is then inserted through the right atrial appendage at the purse string site into the IVC and the purse string suture is tied.

If ETT is used for the shunt, the balloon is inflated just above the renal veins.
The intrapericardial IVC suture is tied to secure the tube.
If the chest tube is used for the shunt, another tie is placed around the suprarenal IVC to secure the tube.
Repair with 3-0/4-0 using Polypropylene running sutures.
Associated with extremely high (70%-90%) mortality
- Suprahepatic IVC injury
  - Intraabdominal suprahepatic IVC: Management is similar to retrohepatic IVC injury
  - Intrathoracic suprahepatic IVC
    - May present with cardiac tamponade or pericardial effusion
    - Pericardium is opened.
    - Bleeding is controlled with a vascular clamp.
    - Repair with 4/0 polypropylene running sutures.
- SMV Injuries
  - Procedures
    - Hemodynamically stable patients
      Smaller injury: Repair with 4-0/5-0 polypropylene sutures.
      Larger injury: Reconstruction using autologous saphenous vein.
    - Damage control in hemodynamically unstable patients
      Ligation
        May result in mesenteric venous congestion and reduced systemic venous return causing shock and possible cardiac arrest (syndrome of splanchnic hypervolemia/systemic hypovolemia)

Must-Know Essentials: Treatment of Zone 2 Vascular Injuries

INDICATIONS FOR EXPLORATION

- Source of retroperitoneal hematoma in Zone 2 injuries include:
  - renal arteries.
  - renal veins.
  - kidneys.
- All penetrating trauma with retroperitoneal hematoma should be explored.
- Blunt trauma with retroperitoneal hematoma should be explored if:
  - Expanding hematoma
  - Pulsatile hematoma
  - Ruptured hematoma
  - Hematoma with active bleeding

TECHNIQUES FOR EXPOSURE OF RENAL VESSELS

- Midline laparotomy.
- Ipsilateral medial visceral rotation.
- A vertical incision on the lateral aspect of the kidney to open Gerota's fascia.
- The kidney is elevated to expose the renal hilum.
- Renal vessels and the ureter is located at the hilum. The renal vein is situated anterior to the artery, and the ureter is the most posterior structure.
- Control of the hilar vessels with a vessel loop or vascular clamp.

TREATMENT OF RENAL VASCULAR INJURIES

- Renal artery injury
  - Hemodynamically stable patient
    - Small injury
      Primary repair with 5/0 polypropylene sutures
    - Large injury
      Tension free end-to-end anastomosis after mobilization
      Interposition graft with saphenous vein or PTFE
  - Stable patient with blunt renal artery injuries
    - Usually treated nonoperatively
    - May be treated with endovascular stents
  - Hemodynamically unstable patient
    - Extensive injury
      Nephrectomy
      Presence of contralateral kidney must be varified with manual palpation or CT scan
      before nephrectomy
- Renal venous injury
  - Hemodynamically stable patient
    - Small injury
      Primary repair with 5/0 polypropylene sutures
  - Hemodynamically unstable patients
    - Ligation of the renal vein
      Left renal vein receives branches from the left adrenal, left gonadal, and lumbar
      veins.
      If ligation of the left renal vein is performed between the left gonadal vein and the
      IVC, there is no risk of renal infarction, and a nephrectomy is not required.
      Nephrectomy is needed after ligation of the right renal vein.

Must-Know Essentials: Treatment of Zone 3 Vascular Injuries

SOURCES OF BLEEDING

- Iliac vessels: More common after penetrating trauma
- Soft tissue
- Venous plexus

UNSTABLE PATIENTS (PENETRATING/BLUNT): IMMEDIATE CONTROL OF BLEEDING

- Control of bleeding may be achieved with one of the followings methods:
  - ZoneIII: REBOA if available (see Chapter 9 for details) in the emergency room or the
    operating room.
  - Emergent exploratory laparotomy with pelvic packing (see Chapter 33 for details).
  - Preperitoneal pelvic packing (see Chapter 33 for details).

STABLE PATIENTS (PENETRATING/BLUNT)

- Post-REBOA management
  - Angiogram with angioembolization

- Angiogram with endovascular stent
- Exploratory laparotomy and repair of vascular injuries
- Post–pelvic packing management
  - Angiogram with embolization and removal of packing
  - Angiogram with endovascular stents and removal of packing
  - Exploratory laparotomy, removal of packing, and repair of vascular injuries
- Indications for exploration
  - Penetrating trauma
    - All penetrating vascular injuries must be explored.
  - Blunt trauma
    - Retroperitoneal hematoma must be explored if:
      Pulsatile hematoma
      Expanding hematoma
      Ruptured hematoma
      Hematoma with ipsilateral absent femoral pulse
- Management with endovascular stent
  - Stable blunt injury of the common and external iliac arteries without indications for an exploration
- Management with pelvic angiography and angioembolization
  - Pelvic hematomas or active extravasation of contrast in blunt trauma with pelvic fracture

EXPOSURE OF ZONE 3 VESSELS

- Exposure can be obtained with one of the following:
  - Direct dissection of the peritoneum over the vessel
    - Steps of direct dissection
      Evisceration of the small bowel to the patient's right side.
      Initial vascular control with sponge stick or digitally.
      Opening of the retroperitoneum over the aortic bifurcation to expose the common iliac artery.
  - Left medial visceral rotation for left-sided injury (see Chapter 24 for details)
  - Right medial visceral rotation for right-sided injury (see Chapter 24 for details)
- The ureter must be protected during exposure of the common iliac artery as it crosses anterior to bifurcation of the common iliac artery.
- Proximal control using a vessel loop or vascular clamp at the common iliac artery or aortic bifurcation.
- Distal control of the external iliac artery near the inguinal ligament.
- Distal control at the ipsilateral femoral artery below the inguinal ligament with a separate vertical incision if the injury extends into the ipsilateral femoral artery. Division of the inguinal ligament may be needed.
- Expose the iliac veins.
  - Exposure of the iliac veins may be difficult as the common iliac arteries lie anterior to the vein.
  - After exposure of the common iliac arteries, traction on the arteries after placement of vessel loops can expose the common iliac veins.

TREATMENT OF INJURIES

- Common iliac artery injury
  - Hemodynamically stable patients

- Small injury
  - Repair with 4-0 or 5-0 running polypropylene sutures
- Extensive injury
  - Primary end-to end anastomosis if possible
  - Reconstruction with size 6–8 PTFE graft or autologous saphenous vein
  - Iliac artery transposition to the contralateral common iliac artery or external iliac artery after ligation and division of the injured proximal common iliac artery
  - Ligation of the artery with subsequent extraanatomic (femoral-to-femoral or axillary-to-femoral) bypass in patients with gross contamination due to risk of anastomotic blowout
- Damage control in hemodynamically unstable patients
- TIVS
- External iliac artery injury
  - Hemodynamically stable patients
    - Small injury
      - Repair using a 4-0 or 5-0 polypropylene sutures
    - Larger injuries
      - End to end primary anastomosis if possible
      - Reconstruction with size 6 8 PTFE graft or autologous saphenous vein interposition graft
      - Iliac artery transposition to the contralateral common iliac artery or external iliac artery after ligation and division of the injured proximal common iliac artery
  - Damage control in hemodynamically unstable patients
    - TIVS
- Internal iliac artery injury
  - Ligation of the artery without any significant consequence due to the rich collaterals
- Common iliac vein and external iliac vein injury
  - Hemodynamically stable patients
    - Small injury
      - Repair the vein with 4-0 or 5-0 polypropylene sutures if no risk of stenosis (>50% narrowing after repair)
    - Larger injury
      - If concern of >50% narrowing, patch angioplasty with saphenous vein or PTFE.
      - Repair using reverse saphenous interposition grafts.
  - Damage control in hemodynamically unstable patients
    - Ligation of the iliac veins
      - Well tolerated
      - Risk of lower extremity edema
      - Risk of lower extremity compartment syndrome

Must-Know Essentials: Endovascular Stenting for Retroperitoneal Vascular Injuries

INDICATIONS

- Hemodynamically stable blunt trauma patients should be evaluated with angiogram for possible endovascular stents.
- Following injuries may be managed with endovascular stents:
  - traumatic aortic dissection.
  - SMA injury.
  - renal artery injury.
  - common iliac and external iliac injuries.

CHAPTER 32

Evaluation and Management of Vascular Injuries (Upper and Lower Extremities)

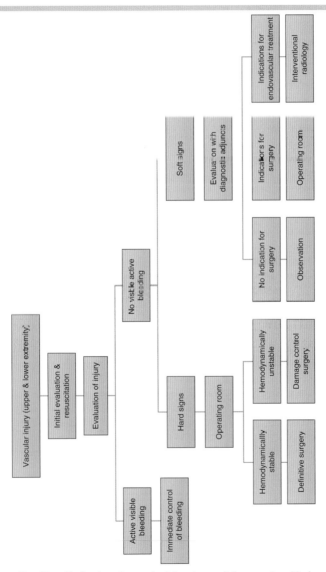

Algorithm: Evaluation of vascular injury (upper & lower extremities)

Must-Know Essentials: Vascular Anatomy of the Upper Extremities

AXILLARY ARTERY

- A continuation of the subclavian artery
- Extends from the lateral margin of the first rib to the lateral margin of the teres major muscle
- Externally origin of the axillary artery corresponds with mid clavicle, courses deep in the deltopectoral groove, and ends at the lateral border of the axilla
- Divided by the pectoralis minor into three parts
  - First part
    - Proximal to the muscle
    - One branch
      - Superior thoracic artery
  - Second part
    - Posterior to the muscle
    - Surrounded by the cords of the brachial plexus
    - Two branches
      - Acromiothoracic artery
      - Lateral thoracic artery
  - Third part
    - Distal to the muscle
    - Surrounded by the nerves of the brachial plexus
    - Three branches
      - Subscapular artery
      - Anterior circumflex humeral artery
      - Posterior circumflex humeral artery
- Injury to axillary artery has a high incidence of associated arteriovenous fistula and nerve injury due to its proximity to the axillary vein and brachial plexus.

BRACHIAL ARTERY

- Begins at the lateral margin of the teres major muscle as a continuation of the axillary artery.
- Terminates 2–3 cm below the elbow crease at its bifurcation.
- Course
  - Lies in the groove between the biceps and triceps muscles
  - The proximal part of the artery lies on the medial side of the humerus. It gradually travels to the lateral side of the humerus, and the distal part of the artery is situated anterior to the humerus.
  - In the antecubital fossa, the artery is located deep to the bicipital aponeurosis and bifurcates into the radial and ulnar arteries.
  - Two brachial veins (venae comitantes) run on either side of the artery.
- Branches
  - Profunda brachii artery: Large branch of brachial artery from posterior surface of proximal part of the artery
  - Superior ulnar collateral artery
  - Inferior ulnar collateral artery

- Terminal branches
  - Radial artery
  - Ulnar artery
- Important relations
  - Median nerve
    - Anterolateral to the artery in the upper arm
    - Crosses the artery anteriorly in the mid upper arm
    - Posteromedial to the artery in the distal upper arm
  - Ulnar nerve
    - Posterior to the artery in the upper half of the arm
    - Pierces the intermuscular septum in the mid arm and courses away from the artery posterior to the medial epicondyle
  - Radial nerve
    - Closely related to the profunda brachii artery

VEINS OF THE ARM

- Divided into:
  - deep veins, including the:
    - axillary vein
    - brachial vein.
  - Superficial veins, including the:
    - basilic vein.
    - cephalic vein.
- Axillary vein
  - Continuation of the brachial vein
  - The cephalic vein joins the terminal portion of the axillary vein just distal to the pectoralis minor muscle and continues as the subclavian vein.
  - The middle segment of the axillary vein lies inferior to the axillary artery under the pectoralis minor muscle.
  - The subclavian vein begins at the lateral border of the first rib.
- Brachial veins
  - Two brachial veins (venae comitantes) start in the elbow and run on either side of the brachial artery.
  - The lateral brachial vein is the continuation of the radial venae comitantes, and the medial brachial vein is the continuation of the ulnar venae comitantes.
  - The brachial veins join and continue as the axillary vein at the inferior border of the teres major muscle.
  - The basilic vein joins the terminal part of the brachial vein.
  - Brachial veins drain muscles of the anterior and posterior compartments of the arm by multiple venous perforators.
- Basilic vein
  - Superficial vein that runs in the subcutaneous tissue in the medial aspect of the arm
  - Drains the veins from the dorsal surface of the hand
  - Joins the terminal part of one of the brachial veins
- Cephalic vein
  - Superficial vein that runs in the subcutaneous tissue that extends from the hand to the deltopectoral groove and joins the terminal portion of the axillary vein

- Drains veins from the lateral aspect of the forearm and arm
- Joins the terminal portion of the axillary vein just distal to the pectoralis minor muscle and continues as the subclavian vein

ANATOMY OF THE ANTECUBITAL FOSSA

- Boundaries
  - Superior border: Formed by a line between the lateral and medial epicondyles
  - Lateral border: Brachioradialis muscle
  - Medial: Pronator teres muscle
- Contents from medial to lateral
  - Median nerve
  - Brachial vein and its terminal branches (ulnar and radial veins)
  - Brachial artery and its terminal branches (ulnar and radial veins)
  - Biceps tendon
  - Radial nerve and its branches (superficial and deep radial nerves)

RADIAL ARTERY

- One of the two terminal branches of the brachial artery
- Courses through the forearm and terminates as the deep palmar arch
- Runs under the brachioradialis muscle
- Distal part of the radial artery is subcutaneous and lies on the surface of the radius.
- Main branches
  - Radial recurrent artery
  - Palmar carpal branch
  - Dorsal carpal branch
  - Muscular branch

ULNAR ARTERY

- One of the two terminal branches of the brachial artery
- Courses through the forearm and terminates as the superficial palmar arch
- Larger than the radial artery
- Major source of blood supply to the digits
- The superficial palmar arch is incomplete in 20% of patients.
- When both the radial and ulnar arteries are injured, ulnar artery repair should be the priority because it is the dominant arterial supply to the hand.

RADIAL VEINS

- Radial veins are the deep venae comitantes of the radial artery.
- The deep palmar venous arch drains into the radial vein.
- The radial venae comitantes continue as one of the brachial veins at the elbow.
- The radial veins are smaller than the ulnar veins.
- The dorsal metacarpal veins drain in the radial vein.

ULNAR VEINS

- Ulnar veins are the deep venae comitantes of the ulnar artery.
- The superficial palmar venous arch drains into the ulnar vein.

- The ulnar veins receive the tributaries of the deep palmar venous arch.
- Superficial veins at the wrist also drain in the ulnar vein.
- The ulnar venae comitantes continue as one of the brachial veins at the elbow.

Must-Know Essentials: Vascular Anatomy of the Lower Extremities

FEMORAL TRIANGLE

- Triangular space in the anterior thigh below the inguinal ligament
- Borders
  - Lateral: Medial border of the sartorius muscle
  - Medial: Medial border of the adductor longus muscle
  - Base formed by the inguinal ligament
- The floor is formed by the iliacus, psoas major, pectineus, and adductor longus muscles.
- The roof is formed by the skin, superficial fascia, and deep fascia.
- From lateral to medial side, the femoral triangle contains:
  - the femoral nerve and its branches.
  - the femoral artery.
  - the femoral vein
  - the deep inguinal lymph nodes.
- Femoral sheath
  - A fascial sheath formed anteriorly by the extension of the transversalis fascia and posteriorly by the iliac fascia
  - Divided into lateral, intermediate, and medial compartments
  - Contents of the femoral sheath
    - Lateral compartment
      - Femoral artery
    - Intermediate compartment
      - Femoral vein
    - Medial compartment
      - Referred to as the femoral canal; contains the lymphatic tissue
      - Base of the femoral canal; called the femoral ring
      - Femoral hernia occurs due to weakness in the femoral ring.

ADDUCTOR CANAL (HUNTER'S CANAL)

- This aponeurotic tunnel extends from the apex of the femoral triangle to the opening in the adductor magnus.
- Boundaries
  - Anterior: Sartorius
  - Lateral: Vastus medialis
  - Posteromedial: Adductor longus and adductor magnus
- Contents
  - Superficial femoral artery
  - Femoral vein
    - The proximal part of the vein lies on the medial side of the artery, then lies posterior to the artery, and the distal femoral vein lies on the lateral side of the femoral artery.
  - Saphenous nerve
    - Crosses from the medial to the lateral side in the canal
  - Branches of the femoral nerve

COMMON FEMORAL ARTERY

- Continuation of the external iliac artery posterior to the inguinal ligament at the level of the mid-inguinal point.
- Approximately 4 cm long
- Located lateral to the femoral vein and medial to the femoral nerve in the femoral triangle
- Continues in the anteromedial aspect of the thigh as the superficial femoral artery after its profunda femoris artery branch
- In the middle third of the thigh, lies within the adductor canal (Hunter's canal)
- Continues as the popliteal artery after passing through the adductor magnus muscle
- Branches
  - Superficial epigastric artery
  - Superficial circumflex artery
  - External pudendal artery
  - Profunda femoris artery
    - Branch from the lateral side of the common femoral artery approximately 4 cm below the inguinal ligament
    - Branches
      - Lateral femoral circumflex artery
      - Medial femoral circumflex artery
      - Perforating branches

FEMORAL VEIN

- Deep vein of the thigh
- Originates at the opening of the adductor magnus muscle as a continuation of the popliteal vein
- Continues as external iliac vein posterior to the inguinal ligament
- Located in the intermediate compartment of the femoral sheath in femoral triangle
- Relations
  - Medial to the common femoral artery in the femoral triangle
  - Posterior to the superficial femoral artery in the proximal part of the adductor canal
  - Posterolateral to the superficial femoral artery in the distal adductor canal
- Tributaries
  - Profunda femoris vein
    - Joins the femoral vein posteriorly 5–10 cm distal to the inguinal ligament
  - Numerous muscular tributaries
  - Great saphenous vein
    - Joins the femoral vein anteriorly or anteromedially 3–4 cm below the inguinal ligament
  - Lateral and medial circumflex femoral veins

POPLITEAL FOSSA

- Diamond-shaped space behind the knee
- Boundaries
  - Superomedial: Semimembranosus and semitendinosus muscles
  - Inferomedial: Medial head of the gastrocnemius
  - Superolateral: Biceps femoris
  - Inferolateral: Lateral head of the gastrocnemius

- Floor is formed by the following:
  - Popliteal surface of the femur
  - Capsule of the knee
  - Oblique popliteal ligament
  - Popliteus muscle
- Roof is formed by the following:
  - Fascia lata
  - Skin and subcutaneous tissue
  - Small saphenous vein, and the posterior femoral cutaneous nerve pierces the roof
- Contents
  - Popliteal artery
    - Deepest structure
    - Situated in the upper medial side
    - Covered by the semimembranosus muscle
  - Popliteal vein
    - Superficial and lateral to the artery
  - Tibial nerve and common peroneal nerve
    - Two major branches of the sciatic nerve
    - Most superficial structure on the lateral side of the fossa
    - Situated under the margin of the biceps femoris muscle

POPLITEAL ARTERY

- Continuation of the superficial femoral artery in the popliteal fossa
- Begins at the opening in the adductor magnus muscle at the middle and lower thirds of the thigh and descends in the popliteal fossa
- Branches
  - Superior genicular artery
  - Inferior genicular artery
  - Anterior tibial artery
    - Continues under the extensor muscles of the anterior compartment of the leg and becomes the dorsalis pedis artery
  - Tibioperoneal trunk
    - Continuation of the popliteal artery after it gives rise to anterior tibial artery
    - It divides into the:
      fibular (peroneal) artery.
      posterior tibial artery.
      Situated under the gastrocnemius and soleus muscles
      Superficial behind the medial malleolus

Must-Know Essentials: Evaluation of Vascular Injuries (Upper and Lower Extremities)

ETIOLOGY

- Penetrating trauma
  - Most common cause of vascular injury.
  - Causes include:
    - gunshot wounds.
    - stab wounds.

- Blunt trauma
    - Vascular injuries are less common after blunt trauma.
    - Causes include:
        - motor vehicle collision.
        - falls.
        - crush injury.
        - injury from fracture or dislocations.
            - Common fractures/dislocations with associated vascular injuries include the following:
                - Posterior shoulder dislocation: Axillary artery and axillary vein
                - Supracondylar humerus: Brachial artery
                - Elbow dislocation: Brachial artery
                - Hip dislocation: Common femoral artery
                - Distal femur fracture: Superficial femoral artery
                - Tibial plateau fracture: Superficial femoral artery
                - Posterior knee dislocations: Popliteal artery

TYPES OF VASCULAR INJURIES

- Occlusive
    - Transection
    - Thrombosis
    - Reversible spasm
- Nonocclusive
    - Intimal flap
    - Dissection
    - Arteriovenous fistula
    - Pseudoaneurysm

PATHOPHYSIOLOGY OF VASCULAR INJURIES

- Vascular injury can result in ischemia or hemorrhage.
- Effects of ischemia
    - Nerve and muscle damage
        - Irreversible nerve and muscle damage after 6 hours of ischemia
        - Peripheral nerve damage can result after only 3 hours of ischemia.
    - Lactic acidosis
    - Rhabdomyolysis and renal failure
    - Compartment syndrome
- Hemorrhage
    - Can be visible or concealed (pelvis, gluteal soft tissue, and thigh)
    - May result in hemorrhagic shock

INITIAL EVALUATION AND RESUSCITATION

- Evaluation follows the same algorithm as for any other injuries that include the following:
    - Airway
    - Cervical spine protection
    - Breathing

- Circulation, including immediate control of bleeding
- Disability
- Exposure
- Management of life-threatening injuries takes precedence over the management of limb-threatening injuries.

TECHNIQUES OF CONTROL OF BLEEDING

- Direct pressure on the bleeding wounds
  - Constricts the blood vessels
  - Apply pressure using gauze pads for 5–10 minutes.
  - If bleeding stops, apply an elastic bandage over the gauze pad.
  - Wounds on the arms, shoulders, legs, and groin can be effectively controlled by direct pressure.
  - If available, may use topical coated hemostatic gauze.
- Wound packing
  - Indicated for cavitary wounds
  - Pack the wound tightly with rolled gauze
  - May use topical hemostatic agent coated gauze
- Foley catheter and inflation of balloon in a knife or gunshot wound (GSW) track
- Tourniquet
  - Indicated for uncontrolled external bleeding from either blunt or penetrating extremities injuries when direct pressure does not control the bleeding
  - Should be placed as distal as possible
  - It must occlude arterial inflow; occluding only the venous system can increase the bleeding.
  - Ongoing bleeding is suggestive of venous occlusion.
  - A second tourniquet above the first may be used if the first tourniquet does not control the bleeding.
  - Occlusion pressure: 100 mm Hg above the systolic blood pressure (SBP) of the patient
  - Tourniquet time should not exceed more than 2 hours.
  - It should be released to reassess for bleeding at 2 hour intervals.
  - Tourniquets properly applied in the prehospital setting should not be removed unless there is adequate team support is available to manage bleeding.
  - Complications
    - Rhabdomyolysis
    - Tissue ischemia
    - Nerve injury
    - Compartment syndrome
- Splints for fractures
  - Movement at fracture sites may cause significant bleeding.
- Blind clamping in the wound is not recommended.

CLINICAL EVALUATION OF VASCULAR INJURIES OF THE EXTREMITIES

- Examination for the following:
  - Soft tissue injuries
  - Fracture/dislocation

- Neurological deficit
- Hard signs of arterial vascular injury:
  - Pulsatile bleeding
  - Expanding hematoma
  - Absent distal pulses
  - Cold pale extremities
  - Palpable thrill
  - Audible bruits if arteriovenous fistula
- Soft signs of arterial vascular injury:
  - Peripheral nerve deficit
  - Moderate bleeding
  - Diminished pulses
  - Injury in the proximity of a major artery
  - Moderate hemorrhage occurring at the scene of the injury
  - Stable and nonpulsatile hematoma
  - Asymmetric extremity blood pressures
  - Presence of shock/hypotension
  - Associated fracture or dislocation
- Hypotensive patients should be reevaluated with clinical examination, arterial doppler, and arterial pressure index (API) after resuscitation to rule out vascular injury.

DIAGNOSTIC ADJUNCTS OF VASCULAR INJURIES

- Plain x-ray
  - Evaluation for suspected fracture or dislocation
  - Localize site of vascular injury in patients with GSWs or multiple fractures.
- Doppler ultrasound
  - Assessment of arterial flow
  - Measurement of API
    - Systolic pressure of the injured extremity (ankle or forearm) divided by the brachial systolic pressure in the uninjured upper extremity
    - Patient with API >0.9 is unlikely to have a vascular injury.
    - Patient with API <0.9 may have vascular injury and require further evaluation with CT angiogram or Doppler ultrasound.
- Duplex ultrasound
  - May detect occult arterial or partial arterial obstructions
  - Useful for the diagnosis of major venous injuries
  - Limitations
    - Operator dependent
    - Open wounds
    - Large hematomas
    - Bulky dressings/splints
- Angiogram
  - Indications
    - Diminished peripheral pulses
    - Absent Doppler signals in the artery
    - API <0.9
    - Injury in the proximity of a major vessel

- Types of angiograms
  - CT angiography (CTA)
    - Images comparable to conventional arteriograms
    - Provides detailed information of the bone and soft tissue
    - Useful for the diagnosis of certain injuries
      - Intimal injuries
      - Active bleeding by detecting extravasation of contrast
      - Thrombosis
      - Pseudoaneurysm
      - Arteriovenous fistula
  - Catheter angiogram
    - Useful for the diagnosis of the following:
      - Active bleeding by detecting extravasation of contrast
      - Thrombosis
      - Pseudoaneurysm
      - Arteriovenous fistula
    - Useful for endovascular treatment of vascular injuries during the angiogram. These conditions include the following:
      - Control of active bleeding
      - Pseudoaneurysm
      - AV fistula
    - Complications of catheter angiogram
      - Injury at vascular access site causing hematoma or pseudoaneurysm

Must-Know Essentials: Management of Vascular Injuries (Upper and Lower Extremities)

NONOPERATIVE MANAGEMENT

- Indications
  - Asymptomatic patients
  - Soft signs of vascular injury
  - Nonocclusive injuries diagnosed on CTA
    - Intimal flaps
    - Vessel narrowing
    - Small false aneurysms
    - Arteriovenous fistulas in which the artery and its runoff remain intact
- Treatment includes the following:
  - Frequent clinical examination
  - Measurement of API
    - CTA if API <0.9
  - Operating room if:
    - any hard signs of injury develop.
    - CTA findings are suggestive for vascular injury.

OPERATIVE MANAGEMENT

- Indications
  - Penetrating trauma
  - Blunt trauma with hard signs of injury

- Blunt trauma with soft signs of injury
  - Angiogram of upper-extremity, femoral, and popliteal arteries with:
    - pseudoaneurysms.
    - large arteriovenous fistulas.
    - intimal flaps.
    - focal lacerations.
- Timing of intervention
  - Surgical intervention within 3 hours of injury has the best outcome.
    - More than 3 hours of ischemia can result in peripheral nerve damage.
    - More than 6 hours of ischemia results in irreversible muscle and nerve damage.
- Surgical principles
  - Exposure of the vessel
  - Proximal and distal control of the vessel
  - Exploration of the injured area
  - Debridement of the devitalized tissue
  - Revascularization
    - Techniques
      - Primary repair
        - Small transverse injury involving small part of the circumference
      - Repair with a vein or synthetic patch
        - Large defect to avoid the risk of narrowing
      - End-to-end anastomosis
        - If divided ends can be approximated with or without mobilization
      - Repair with reverse saphenous or cephalic vein or polytetrafluoroethylene (PTFE) graft
        - If end-to-end anastomosis is not possible due to segmental loss
        - PTFE grafts should be avoided in the upper extremity due to the increased risk of infection and poor patency rate.
        - An autologous vein should be used for popliteal fossa reconstruction.
        - PTFE can be used for above-the-knee reconstructions.
    - Revascularization essentials
      - Assessment of inflow and outflow
      - Thrombectomy using a 3 F/4 F Fogarty proximally and distally if flow is poor
        - Overinflation with Fogarty balloon can cause intimal injury and thrombosis.
      - Heparinized saline (5000 units in 100 mL saline) injected proximally and distally in the vessel
      - Topical lidocaine or papaverine may be considered to relieve spasm, especially in the small vessels of the distal forearm and hand.
      - Systemic anticoagulation is not required.
      - Repair of concomitant venous injury should be performed first to avoid low-flow thrombosis after arterial repair.
      - Intraoperative angiogram for:
        - identification of an unknown injury.
        - evaluation of distal perfusion after repair.
        - completion angiogram should be performed.
      - Repairs should be covered with viable soft tissue.
      - External compression must be avoided at the vascular repair site.
- Damage-control procedures
  - Indications
    - Hemodynamically unstable patients

   Lack of vascular surgical expertise
   Unstable fractures
   Gustilo type IIIC fractures
   Mangled extremity
■ Ligation of the artery
   The following arteries can be ligated without the risk of limb ischemia:
      Isolated radial or ulnar artery
      Profunda femoris artery
   The following arteries should never be ligated due to risk of limb ischemia:
      Axillary artery
      Brachial artery
      Common femoral artery
      Superficial femoral
■ Ligation of veins
   Ligation of a venous injury is typically well tolerated due to extensive collaterals.
   All veins in the upper and lower extremities can be ligated.
   Ligation of the axillary vein and femoral vein is well tolerated.
   Ligation of the popliteal vein is poorly tolerated.
■ Temporary intravascular shunt (TIVS)
   Technique
      Debridement of arterial edges should not be performed.
      Many types of shunts are available. Argyle shunt is commonly used, and it comes in various sizes.
      An appropriate size of the shunt is secured proximally and distally using a 0 silk suture.
      Distal blood flow must be checked with Doppler.
   Definitive vascular reconstruction should be performed within <6 hours if possible after:
      hemodynamic stability
      availability of vascular surgical expertise.
      stabilization of an unstable fracture/dislocation.

ENDOVASCULAR MANAGEMENT

■ Transcatheter embolization with coils
   ■ Indications
      ■ Low-flow arteriovenous fistulas
      ■ Active bleeding from noncritical arteries
■ Endoluminal stent graft
   ■ Indications
      ■ Anterior tibial or tibioperoneal arterial injures with:
         Pseudoaneurysms
         Large arteriovenous fistulas
         Intimal flaps
         Focal lacerations

MANAGEMENT OF COMPLICATIONS

■ Reperfusion syndrome
   ■ Occurs after revascularization of an ischemic limb

- Causes
  - Microvascular dysfunction and increased capillary and arteriolar permeability due to activation of the inflammatory mediators in circulation
  - Lactic acidosis
- Manifestations
  - Myocardial depression
  - Hypotension due to vasodilatation
  - Multisystem organ dysfunction
  - Compartment syndrome
- Treatment
  - Supportive care
  - Fasciotomy for compartment syndrome
- Compartment syndrome (see Chapter 34 for details)
  - Risk factors
    - Combined arterial and venous injury
    - Post-revascularization
    - Higher incidence after lower-extremity and upper-extremity vascular injuries
    - Prolonged ischemia time (>3–4 hours)
    - Significant preoperative hypotension
    - Associated crush injury
    - Major venous ligation such as in the popliteal or femoral area
  - Monitoring
    - Clinical examination
    - Serial creatine kinase (CK) enzyme measurement
  - Fasciotomy
    - Prophylactic fasciotomy is usually not recommended but may be considered in high-risk patients.
    - For established compartment syndrome based on clinical examination or compartment pressure measurement
- Rhabdomyolysis (see Chapter 34 for details)
  - Risk factors
    - Limb ischemia
    - Compartment syndrome
    - Post-revascularization
  - Monitoring
    - Serial CK enzyme measurement
    - Amber-colored urine, positive for hemoglobin
    - Myoglobinuria
    - Renal function test for acute kidney injury (AKI)
  - Treatment
    - Aggressive IV crystalloid solution infusion
    - 0.9% normal saline solution preferred

Must-Know Essentials: Exposure of the Vessels for Vascular Injuries (Upper and Lower Extremities)
FEMORAL ARTERY

- Position
  - Supine with hip and knee joints slightly flexed and externally rotated
  - Incision

- Make a vertical skin incision from a point midway between the pubic tubercle and the anterior iliac spine and extend it downward along the anterior border of the sartorius muscle toward the medial femoral condyle.
- Extend the incision superiorly through the inguinal ligament for proximal vascular control at the external iliac artery for a very proximal common femoral artery injury.
- Extend the incision superiorly and parallel to the inguinal ligament for exposure of the iliac vessels.
- Extend the incision longitudinally along the anterior border of the sartorius muscle for exposure of the superficial femoral artery.
- Exposure
  - Open the subcutaneous tissue, superficial fascia, and deep fascia.
  - Open the femoral sheath directly over the femoral artery.
  - Identify the femoral vein located medial to the artery.
  - Identify and protect the greater saphenous vein in the subcutaneous tissue along the medial edge of the incision.
  - Dissect the common and superficial femoral arteries circumferentially and place vessel loops.
  - Expose the profunda femoris artery and place a vessel loop after retracting the common femoral and superficial femoral arteries.
  - For exposure of the superficial femoral artery in the mid-thigh
    - Open the aponeurosis of the adductor canal.
    - Retract the medial and lateral muscles to expose the artery.
    - Open the adductor magnus opening for distal exposure of the artery.

POPLITEAL ARTERY

- Position
  - Supine with knee slightly flexed and supported, hip abducted and externally rotated
  - Incision
  - Make a skin incision 10–15 cm long starting at the level of the tubercle 1 cm posterior to the femur between the vastus medialis and sartorius muscles, extending across the knee fold to distal lower extremity 1 cm posterior to tibia.
- Exposure
  - Identify and preserve the great saphenous vein and saphenous nerve during mobilization of the skin flaps.
  - Divide the subcutaneous tissue and fascia.
  - Enter the space between the vastus medialis superiorly and the sartorius muscle inferiorly.
  - Retract the sartorius muscle posteriorly and the vastus medialis muscle superiorly to identify the popliteal artery that is covered in the fatty tissue under the distal shaft of the femur.
  - The sartorius, semimembranosus, semitendinosus, and gracilis muscles may be divided just proximal to their tibial attachments for better exposure of the artery; muscles are repaired after the vascular injury repair.
  - Identify and expose the neurovascular structures in the popliteal fossa:
    - Popliteal artery is the most medial and posterior.
    - Popliteal vein is lateral to the artery.
    - Tibial nerve most lateral.
  - Extend the incision proximally and enter the adductor canal to expose the supragenicu-late portion of the popliteal artery if better proximal control is required.
  - Extend the incision distally, retract the gastrocnemius muscle posteriorly, and divide the origin of the soleus muscle medially to expose the infrageniculate portion of the popliteal artery if better distal vascular control is required.

EXPOSURE OF THE AXILLARY VESSELS

- Position
  - Patient supine with arm 30 degree abducted and head turned to opposite side
- Incision
  - Make a skin incision below the middle of the clavicle and extend it over the deltopectoral groove.
  - Extend the incision over the clavicle up to the sternoclavicular junction; the clavicle may be divided for very proximal axillary artery exposure.
- Exposure
  - Ligate and divide the cephalic vein in the subcutaneous tissue of the deltopectoral groove.
  - Mobilize the skin and expose the pectoralis major muscle.
  - Split or divide the pectoralis major muscle distal to its attachment with the humerus to expose the pectoralis minor muscle.
  - If divided, the pectoralis major muscle should be repaired after completion of the vascular procedure.
  - Retract or divide the pectoralis minor muscle distal to its attachment with the cricoid process or retract the pectoralis minor muscle to expose the axillary vein, axillary artery, and brachial plexus.
  - If divided, the pectoralis minor muscle should be repaired after completion of the vascular procedure.
  - The axillary vein lies anterior and inferior to the artery.
  - The brachial plexus roots surround the axillary artery.

EXPOSURE OF THE BRACHIAL ARTERY

- Position
  - Supine patient with arm on an arm board, 90 degrees abducted and externally rotated
- Incision
  - Make a skin incision in the medial side of the arm in the groove between the biceps and triceps muscles.
  - Extend the incision proximally in the deltopectoral groove to expose the axillary artery if required.
  - Extend the incision distally in the antecubital fossa below the tendon of the biceps muscle, curving toward the radius to expose the bifurcation of the brachial artery.
- Exposure
  - Retract the biceps and triceps muscles to expose the neurovascular structures.
  - Neurovascular structures are covered with fascia.
  - Open the fascia longitudinally to expose the neurovascular structures.
  - During exposure of the artery, identify and protect the following structures:
    - Median nerve
      - Anterior and lateral to the artery in the proximal arm
      - Crosses the artery anteriorly in the mid arm, then lies medial to the artery

- Ulnar nerve
  - Posterior and medial to the artery
  - Basilic vein
  - Medial and outside the brachial artery sheath in the proximal arm
- Profunda brachial artery
  - Medial branch of the brachial artery in the proximal arm
  - Radial nerve
  - Accompanying the profunda brachial artery
- Divide the bicipital aponeurosis to expose the bifurcation of the brachial artery

SECTION IX

Musculoskeletal Trauma

Evaluation and Management of Pelvic Fracture Emergencies

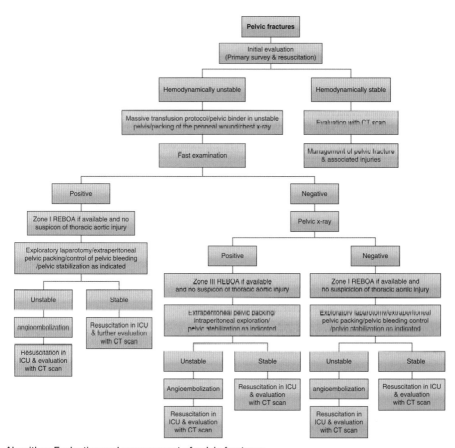

Algorithm: Evaluation and management of pelvic fractures

Must-Know Essentials: Classification of Pelvic Fractures

ISOLATED FRACTURES WITH INTACT RING

- Avulsion fractures
  - Caused by violent contraction of muscles

- Types of fractures and specific muscles involved
- Anterior superior iliac spine: Sartorius muscle
- Anterior inferior iliac spine: Rectus femoris
- Pubis: Adductor longus
- Part of the ischium: hamstrings (Biceps femoris, semimembranosus, semitendinosous)
- Direct fractures
  - Caused by local injury
  - Types
  - Fracture of the iliac blade
  - Fracture of the ischium
- Fractures of the pubic rami in osteoporosis

FRACTURES WITH BROKEN PELVIC RING (YOUNG-BURGESS CLASSIFICATION)

- Anteroposterior compression (APC) fractures (open book fracture of the pelvis)
  - APC I
    - Pubic symphysis diastasis <2.5 cm
    - No sacro-iliac (SI) joint diastasis due to intact anterior and posterior SI joints ligaments.
    - Stable fracture
  - APC II
    - Pubic symphysis diastasis >2 cm
    - Diastasis of one or both anterior SI joint due to disruption of anterior SI joint ligaments causing SI joints rotational instability
    - Intact posterior SI ligaments. Disruption of sacrospinous and sacrotuberous ligaments. No vertical instability.
    - High incidence of vascular injury with hemodynamic instability
    - Unstable fracture
  - APC III
    - Complete disruption of both anterior and posterior SI ligaments causing SI joint dislocation. Disruption of sacrospinous and sacrotuberous ligaments
    - High incidence of vascular injury with hemodynamic instability
    - Vertically and rotationally unstable pelvic fracture
- Lateral compression (LC) fractures
  - LC I
    - Ipsilateral horizontal pubic rami fractures
    - Ipsilateral sacral ala fracture
    - Less common: disruption of pubic symphysis with overlap of pubic bones
    - Intact posterior ligaments
    - Stable fracture
  - LC II
    - Internal rotation of the hemipelvis
    - Pubic rami fracture associated with ipsilateral iliac wing fracture or disruption of the ipsilateral posterior SI joint
    - Severely unstable injury associated with soft tissue injuries, intraabdominal injuries, and retroperitoneal hemorrhage
    - Rotationally unstable, vertically stable pelvis
  - LC III
    - Type I or II injury with internal rotation of pelvis and external rotation of contralateral pelvis on the side of the injury

- May have contralateral vertical pubic rami fractures or disruption of the ligaments
- Rotationally unstable pelvis, vertically stable pelvis
- Associated with soft tissue injuries, intraabdominal injuries, and retroperitoneal hemorrhage
- Unstable injury
- Vertical shear (VS) fractures
  - Anterior vertically oriented fractures of the pubic rami
  - Vertical displacement of the innominate bone (hemipelvis) on one side with fracture of the pubic rami
  - Disruption of the SI joint ligaments on the side of the displaced hemipelvis
  - Occasional disruption of contralateral SI joint ligaments
  - Associated with soft-tissue injuries, intraabdominal injuries, and retroperitoneal hemorrhage
  - Unstable fracture
- Combination mechanism (CM) fractures
  - Combination of any injury patterns
  - Results in severe injury
  - Associated with soft tissue, intraabdominal, and vascular injuries
  - Associated with hemodynamic instability
  - Unstable fracture

PELVIC FRACTURES (TILE CLASSIFICATION)

- Type A: Stable fractures
  - A1: Fractures of the pelvis not involving the ring
  - A2: Minimally displaced fractures of the ring
- –Type B: Rotationally unstable, vertically stable
  - B1: Open book
  - B2: Lateral compression; ipsilateral
  - B3: Lateral compression; contralateral (bucket handle)
- Type C: Rotationally and vertically unstable
  - C1: Rotationally and vertically unstable
  - C2: Bilateral injury
  - C3: Associated with an acetabular fracture

ACETABULAR FRACTURES (JUDET-LETOURNEL CLASSIFICATION)

- Both columns (anterior and posterior) fracture
  - Most common acetabular fracture
  - Fracture pattern
    - Disruption of obturator ring
    - Extension of fracture line into the iliac wing
- T-shaped fracture
  - Fracture pattern
    - Disruption of obturator ring
    - No extension of fracture line into the iliac wing
- Transverse fracture with posterior wall involvement
  - Fracture pattern
    - No disruption of obturator ring
    - Disruption of ilioischial and ischiopectineal line
    - Fracture of the posterior wall

- Transverse fracture
  - Fracture pattern
    - No disruption of obturator ring
    - Disruption of ilioischial and ischiopectineal line
    - No fracture of the posterior wall
- Isolated posterior wall fracture
  - No disruption of obturator ring
  - No disruption of ilioischial and ischiopectineal line

SACROCOCCYGEAL FRACTURES

- AO classification of sacral injuries
  - Type A: Lower sacrococcygeal injuries
  - Type B: Posterior pelvic injuries
  - Type C: Spinopelvic injuries
- Denis classification
  - Commonly used
  - Types
    - Zone 1: Fracture of involves the sacral ala lateral to the neural foramina
    - Zone 2: Fracture of the sacrum involving the neural foramina (but not the spinal canal)
    - Zone 3: Fracture of the sacrum medial to the neural foramen involving the spinal canal
      - Fracture lines may be transverse or longitudinal.
      - Subclassified into four types
        - Type 1: Only kyphotic angulation at the fracture site, no displacement of the fracture fragments
        - Type 2: Kyphotic angulation with anterior displacement of the distal sacrum
        - Type 3: Kyphotic angulation with complete displacement of the fracture fragments
        - Type 4: Comminuted S1 segment, usually caused by axial compression
- Isler classification
  - Used for fractures involving the lumbosacral articulation
  - Isler 1: Fracture lateral to the L5-S1 facet
  - Isler 2: Fracture involving the L5-S1 facet
  - Isler 3: Fracture medial to the L5-S1 facet

Must-Know Essentials: Pelvic Vessels

ARTERIES IN THE PELVIS

- Abdominal aorta bifurcates into the two common iliac arteries at the L4-L5 vertebra level.
- Ureters cross anterior to the bifurcation of the common iliac artery.
- Common iliac artery divides into the external and internal (hypogastric) iliac arteries.
- Internal iliac artery divides into the anterior and posterior branches at the level of the greater sciatic foramen.
- Superior gluteal artery
  - Branch from the posterior division of the internal iliac artery
  - Most common source of arterial bleeding in pelvic fractures
  - Gives off the iliolumbar and lateral sacral arteries
  - Exits the pelvis through the greater sciatic notch
- Branches of the anterior division of the internal iliac artery
  - Superior vesical artery

- Obturator artery: Courses along the lateral pelvic wall and exits the pelvis through the obturator canal
- Inferior vesical artery
- Middle rectal artery
- Internal pudendal artery
  - Source of bleeding in anterior ring fracture
  - Passes through the greater sciatic foramen, courses around the sciatic spine, and enters the perineum through the lesser sciatic foramen
- Inferior gluteal artery
- Median sacral artery (middle sacral artery): A branch from the posterior aspect of the abdominal aorta superior to its bifurcation
- External iliac artery
  - Becomes the femoral artery posterior to the inguinal ligament
  - Branches
    - Inferior epigastric artery
    - Deep circumflex artery

VEINS IN THE PELVIS

- Common iliac veins are located posterior and to the right of the right common iliac artery.
- Branches of the common iliac vein
  - External iliac vein, a continuation of the femoral vein
  - Internal iliac vein. It divides into anterior and posterior divisions.
- Branches of the posterior division of the internal iliac vein
  - Superior gluteal vein: Branches include the iliolumbar and lateral sacral veins.
  - Branches of the anterior division of the internal iliac vein
    - Obturator vein
    - Inferior gluteal vein
    - Internal pudendal vein
    - Vesical plexus
    - Rectal plexus
- Median sacral vein (or middle sacral vein): a branch from the left common iliac vein, or sometimes from the junction of the two iliac veins

Must-Know Essentials: Evaluation of Pelvic Fractures
INITIAL EVALUATION AND RESUSCITATION

- Pelvic fracture should be suspected in patients with severe abdominal or lower extremity injuries.
- Pelvis injuries from high-energy trauma are frequently associated with the following:
  - Hemorrhagic shock
  - Intraabdominal injuries
  - Bladder/urethral injuries
  - Nerve deficits secondary to disruption of sacral and lumbar plexus injury
- Initial evaluation and resuscitation
  - Assessment and management of airway
  - Assessment and management of breathing
  - Assessment and management of circulation

- Persistent hypotension (SBP <90 mm Hg/transient responders)
  - Complex unstable pelvic fractures associated with vascular or pelvic visceral injuries
  - Open pelvic fracture with complex perineal soft laceration
  - Open pelvic fractures associated with vascular or pelvic visceral injuries
  - Associated intraabdominal or other injuries
- Clinical evaluation for unstable pelvis
  - Gross motion of the pelvis ring on palpation of both iliac crests with internal and external rotation stress, anteroposterior stress, and superior inferior stress

CLINICAL EVALUATION FOR ASSOCIATED INJURIES

- High index of suspicion of associated injuries
  - Severe lower abdominal pain and tenderness
  - Bruises in the lower abdomen
  - Bruising of scrotum
  - Bruising of vulva
- Features of specific injuries
  - Colon and rectal injury: Rectal bleeding
  - Vaginal injury: Vaginal bleeding
  - Bladder or ureteral injury:
    - Blood at urethral meatus
    - Hematuria
    - High-riding prostate in men
- Open pelvic fractures are usually associated with the following:
  - Soft-tissue perineal lacerations
  - Rectal injury
  - Vaginal injury
  - Bladder and urethral injury
- Neurological examination of the lower extremities for sacral and lumbar plexus injury

OTHER TESTS FOR DETAILED EVALUATION IN A HEMODYNAMICALLY STABLE PATIENT

- Imaging
  - Plain x-rays
  - CT abdomen and pelvis
- Evaluation of specific injuries
  - Urological injury: Cystoscopy
  - Rectal injury: Proctoscopy/colonoscopy
  - Vaginal injury: Gynecological evaluation

Must-Know Essentials: Management of Hemodynamically Unstable Fractures

SOURCES OF BLEEDING IN PELVIC FRACTURES

- Presacral venous plexus
- Fractured bones
- Branches of the internal iliac artery (hypogastric artery), in descending order:

- Superior gluteal artery
- Internal pudendal artery
- Obturator arteries
- Any other branches
- Rarely from injuries to external iliac arteries and veins
- Associated injuries
  - Most commonly with bladder and urethral injuries
  - Intraabdominal injuries

PREDICTORS OF SEVERE HEMORRHAGE IN PELVIC FRACTURES

- Persistent hypotension
- Transient response to resuscitation with crystalloids or blood transfusion
- CT findings
  - Contrast extravasation
  - Large pelvic sidewall hematoma
  - SI joint disruption
  - Symphysis diastasis >2.5 cm
  - Bilateral and concomitant superior and inferior pubic rami fractures (butterfly fracture)
- Anteroposterior compression fracture (open-book pelvic fractures)

RESUSCITATION FOR HEMORRHAGIC SHOCK

- Balanced resuscitation
  - Limited use of crystalloid infusion
  - Blood transfusion
    - Massive transfusion protocol
- Correction of coagulopathy
- Prevention of hypothermia
- Reduction of pelvic volume and pelvic stabilization
  - Pelvic retroperitoneal space can accommodate 3–4 liters of blood before venous tamponade occurs.
  - Significant pubic symphysis diastasis (>2.5 cm) increases the pelvic volume and reduces the effectiveness of tamponade.
  - Reduction of pelvic volume and stabilization of the pelvis helps obtain bleeding control in a fractured pelvis.
  - Techniques of pelvis stabilization
    - Pelvic binder
      - Indicated in diastasis of pubic symphysis and open-book fractures
      - Contraindicated in fractures of the iliac wing
      - Should be applied over the greater trochanters to appropriately reduce pelvic volume and allow laparotomy and femoral artery access for catheter-based angiographic embolization
    - Pelvic C-clamp
      - Device for rapid reduction and stabilization of unstable pelvic ring fractures
    - External fixator
- Control bleeding with the following techniques:
  - Packing of the perineal wounds
  - Resuscitative Endovascular Balloon Occlusion of the Aorta (REBOA)

- Preperitoneal pelvic packing
- Exploratory laparotomy
  - Direct control of bleeding vessels
  - Pelvic packing
  - Ligation of hypogastric arteries

REBOA

- (See Chapter 9 for details.)
- Not recommended in patients with a high clinical/radiological suspicion of thoracic aortic injury
- Location of REBOA balloon in pelvic fracture:
  - Zone I REBOA
    - Positive Focused Assessment with Sonography in Trauma (FAST) suggestive for intraabdominal hemorrhage
    - Negative FAST and pelvic x-ray negative for fractures
  - Zone III REBOA
    - Negative FAST and pelvic x-ray positive for fractures

PREPERITONEAL PELVIC PACKING

- Helps control the venous and bony bleeding from pelvic fractures
- Indications
  - During exploratory laparotomy after Zone I REBOA placement
  - After Zone III REBOA placement
  - During exploratory laparotomy for intraabdominal injury with associated pelvic bleeding
  - Failed angioembolization
  - Nonavailability of angioembolization
- Technique
  - Make a midline incision 6–8 cm long and below the umbilicus.
  - May make two separate incisions for a combined exploratory laparotomy and preperitoneal pelvic packing:
    - A laparotomy incision from the xiphoid process to just below the umbilicus and
    - A preperitoneal packing incision approximately 6 cm away in the suprapubic area.
  - Incise the fascia down to the peritoneum.
  - Stay in the extraperitoneal space and expose the prevesical space of Retzius.
  - After removal of blood clots from the prevesical space, swipe the bladder and peritoneum posteriorly and laterally to expose the space along the lateral wall of the pelvis bilaterally for the packing.
  - Place the first laparotomy pad by using ringed forceps all the way down onto the presacral space in the midline posterior to the bladder.
  - Then pack the extraperitoneal space with three laparotomy pads along the pelvic sidewall on both sides of the bladder toward the SI joint and internal iliac vessels to control any bleeding originating from the internal iliac arteries and vein plexuses.
  - Typically, six or seven laparotomy pads are needed to complete the packing, but up to nine pads may be necessary to complete the tamponade.
  - Close the fascia with running monofilament sutures.
  - Close the skin with staples.

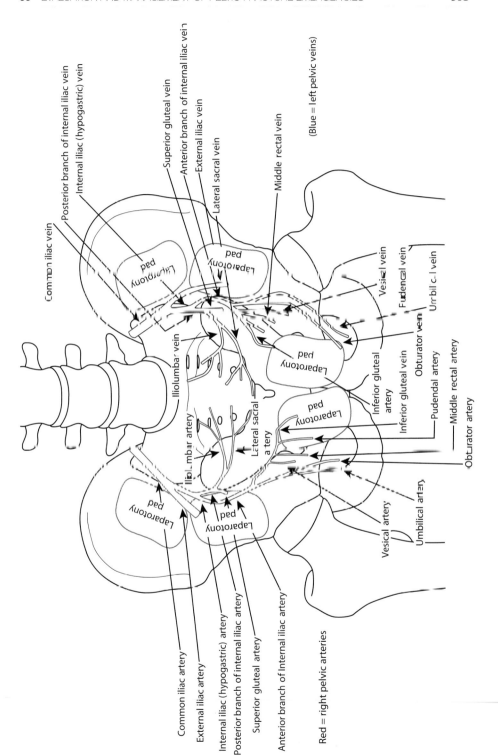

Illustration: Pelvic vessels and pelvic packing

EXPLORATORY LAPAROTOMY AND CONTROL OF PELVIC BLEEDING

- Indications
  - Pelvic bleeding with associated intraabdominal injuries
  - Exploratory laparotomy after Zone I REBOA placement
  - For direct evaluation of major vessels and areas of bleeding in the pelvis
- Technique
  - Perform an exploratory laparotomy.
  - May make two separate incisions for an effective tamponade of the pelvic space if possible.
    - A laparotomy incision from the xiphoid to just below the umbilicus and
    - A preperitoneal packing incision approximately 6 cm away in the suprapubic area.
  - Identify and treat any associated intraperitoneal injuries.
  - Reflect the sigmoid colon laterally to expose the retroperitoneal hematoma, distal aorta, iliac artery bifurcations, and ureters.
  - Open the retroperitoneum by medial mobilization of the left or the right colon or by incising the retroperitoneum directly over the common iliac artery bifurcation.
  - Evacuate the hematoma and control any obvious major bleeding with sutures, ligation, or repair.
  - Ligation of the hypogastric artery
    - Dissect the common iliac arteries bilaterally.
    - Identify and isolate the internal iliac arteries using right-angle clamps.
    - Avoid injury to the ureters, which cross over the bifurcation of the common iliac artery into the external and internal iliac arteries.
    - Ligate the internal iliac arteries using sutures or surgical clips in a damage control situation.
  - Pelvic packing
    - Retract the bladder to the contralateral side to allow introduction of three standard surgical laparotomy pads.
    - Place the first laparotomy pad by using ringed forceps all the way down onto the presacral space in the midline posterior to the urinary bladder.
    - Typically, six or seven pads are needed to complete the packing, but up to nine pads may be necessary to complete the tamponade.
  - If a bladder injury is identified, perform the primary repair of the bladder.
  - If a suprapubic cystostomy is required, bring the tube through a separate stab incision rather than bringing it through the midline fascial incision.
  - Fascia may be closed with running monofilament sutures for tamponade effect.
  - Close the skin with staples.
- Removal of packing
  - Usually after 24-48 hours if the patient meets the followings criteria:
    - Hemodynamically stable
    - No base deficit
    - Stable hemoglobin
    - No coagulopathy
    - No hypothermia
  - May require repacking for ongoing bleeding
  - Repacking has a high risk of infection.

ANGIOEMBOLIZATION

- Indications
  - Unstable patients after preperitoneal packing with ongoing bleeding after correction of coagulopathy

- Bleeding control with selective angioembolization after Zone III REBOA placement
- Unstable patient after pelvic stabilization with ongoing bleeding after correction of coagulopathy
- CT scan with blush or large pelvic hematoma may predict arterial bleeding.

Must-Know Essentials: Management of Hemodynamically Stable Patients

MANAGEMENT OF FRACTURES

- Nonoperative
  - Pubic rami fractures with no posterior displacement
  - Diastasis of pubic symphysis <2.5 cm
  - Lateral impaction type fractures with minimal displacement
  - Isolated fractures
  - Options
    - Traction
    - Protected weight bearing
- Operative
  - Open book fracture and vertically unstable fractures
  - Diastasis of pubic symphysis >2.5 cm
  - SI joint displacement >1 cm
  - Leg length discrepancy >1.5 cm
  - Rotational deformity
  - Open pelvic fracture with visceral injury
  - Operative techniques
    - External fixation
    - Posterior ring fixation with plates and screws
    - Percutaneous fixation of pubic ram

MANAGEMENT OF ASSOCIATED INJURIES

- Open fractures
  - Open wound may extend to perineum involving colon, rectum, scrotum, vagina
  - Evaluation
    - Clinical examination of the rectum, vagina, perineal laceration
    - Proctoscopy/sigmoidoscopy
  - Management
    - Early diverting colostomy
    - Repair of vaginal laceration
    - Repair of scrotal laceration
    - Debridement of soft-tissue laceration
    - Management of fractures
- Management of bladder/urethral injury (see Chapter 30 for details)
  - More common in men
  - Urethral injuries are more common after pubic diastasis or inferomedial pubic bone fractures.
  - Clinical features
    - Hematuria
    - Blood at the ureteral meatus

- High-riding prostate in men
- Further evaluation
  - CT cystogram
  - Cystourethrogram
  - Cystoscopy
- Management
  - No urethral catheter if bleeding at the meatus
  - Intraperitoneal bladder injury
    - Bladder repair
  - Extraperitoneal bladder injury/urethral injury
    - Suprapubic cystostomy
    - Cystoscopy/Foley catheter
    - Repair of the bladder
    - High risk of hardware infection in patients treated with suprapubic cystostomy
    - Bladder repair preferred over the suprapubic catheter
- Large and small bowel injury
  - Clinical examination, including rectal examination with proctoscopy under anesthesia
  - Further evaluation
    - CT abdomen/pelvis
    - Evaluation of colon and rectum with rectal contrast x-ray
    - Endoscopic evaluation as indicated
  - Management
    - Depends on the injury
    - Colostomy in patients with colorectal injury with complex pelvic fractures
- Vascular injury
  - Vascular injuries include the following:
    - Intraosseous vessels
    - Intramuscular vessels
    - Intrapelvic vessels
    - Intraabdominal vessels
    - External bleeding from open wounds
  - Evaluation
    - CT angiogram
  - Management: Depends on the injury
- Neurological injury
  - May include the following:
    - Lumbosacral plexus
    - Presacral plexus
    - Sciatic nerve
    - Genitofemoral nerve
    - Ilioinguinal nerve
    - Lateral cutaneous nerve of thigh
  - Management: Depends on the injury

MANAGEMENT OF COMPLICATIONS

- Early complications
- Infection
- Thromboembolism

- Latc complications
  - Fixation failure
  - Malunion of fractures
  - Nonunion of fractures
  - Chronic pain
  - Decubitus ulcers
  - Urinary incontinence
  - Sexual dysfunction

CHAPTER 34

Evaluation and Management of Extremity Fracture Emergencies

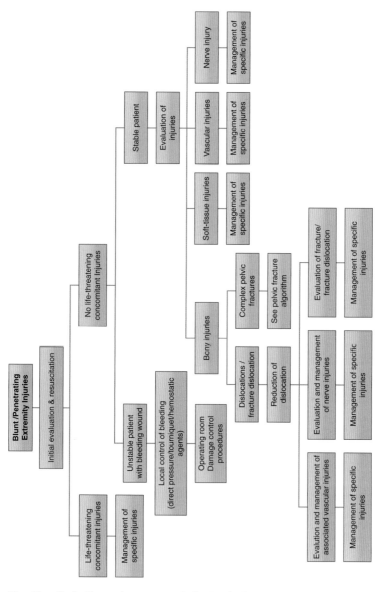

Algorithm: Evaluation and management of extremity fracture emergencies

Must-Know Essentials: Emergencies in Extremity Injuries

POTENTIALLY LIFE-THREATENING INJURIES

- Major arterial hemorrhage
- Crush injury (rhabdomyolysis)
- Fat embolism

POTENTIALLY LIMB-THREATENING INJURIES

- Open-fracture and joint injury
- Vascular injury
- Traumatic amputation
- Compartment syndrome
- Neurologic injuries

Must-Know Essentials: Extremity Vascular Injuries

FRACTURES WITH HIGH INCIDENCE OF VASCULAR INJURIES

- Distal femur fracture
- Open femur fracture
- Tibial plateau fractures
- Floating knee (ipsilateral tibia and femur fractures) injury
- Knee dislocations
- Elbow fracture/dislocation
- Ankle fracture/dislocation

HARD SIGNS OF VASCULAR INJURIES

- Expanding hematoma
- Pulsatile hematoma
- Cold, pale, and pulseless extremities

INDICATIONS FOR ANGIOGRAM IN SUSPECTED ARTERIAL INJURIES

- Diminished peripheral pulses
- Absent Doppler in the artery
- Ankle brachial index <0.9 in lower-extremity injuries
- Injury in the proximity of a major vessel

MANAGEMENT OF VASCULAR INJURIES

- Patients with hard signs of vascular injury require emergent surgical exploration and revascularization.
- Revascularization must be performed as soon as possible.
- Muscle ischemia for >6 hours results in irreversible injury and muscle necrosis.
- Unstable fractures should be stabilized with an external fixation before revascularization.

- Revascularization procedures
  - Vascular repair
  - Vein grafting
  - Arterial stents
  - Temporary shunts indicated in the following:
    - Unstable patients with concomitant life-threatening injuries
    - >3-4 hours of delay in arterial revascularization
- Fasciotomy should be performed in high-risk patients with vascular injury:
  - Prolonged ischemia time (>3-4 hours)
  - Significant preoperative hypotension
  - Associated crush injury
  - Combined arterial and venous injury
  - Major venous ligation in the popliteal or femoral area

Must-Know Essentials: Crush Injuries (Rhabdomyolysis)

ETIOLOGY

- Direct muscle injury
- Muscle ischemia
- Myoglobin release

PATHOPHYSIOLOGY

- Disruption of the sarcolemma of the muscle cells
- Cellular adenosine triphosphate (ATP) depletion
- Cellular sodium-potassium pumps failure
- Generation of oxidative free radicals

DIAGNOSIS

- Elevated creatine kinase (CK)
- Amber-colored urine, positive for hemoglobin
- Myoglobinuria
- Renal function test for acute kidney injury (AKI)

MANAGEMENT

- Aggressive IV crystalloid solution infusion
  - 0.9% normal saline solution preferred
  - Infusion rate may range from 200 mL/hr to 1000 mL/hr based on the response.
- Renal protection
  - Use of sodium bicarbonate is controversial.
  - Sodium bicarbonate may cause hypocalcemia.
  - Alkalinization of the urine and diuresis are considered renal protective in myoglobinuria because myoglobin is more soluble in alkaline solution.
  - IV fluid with bicarbonate may be considered in patients with significant myoglobinuria.
  - May consider mannitol 1 g/kg after resuscitation with crystalloid.

- Close monitoring of urine output with a goal of 1–2 mL/kg/hr
- Monitor for complications including the following:
  - Acute renal failure
  - disseminated intravascular coagulation (DIC)
  - Hyperkalemia
  - Hypocalcemia
- Compartment syndrome

Must-Know Essentials: Fat Embolism Syndrome
ETIOLOGY

- Long bone fractures
- Pelvic fractures

PATHOPHYSIOLOGY

- Fat globules release in peripheral circulation.
- Interaction of fat globules with platelets and clotting cascades, causing intravascular coagulation.
- Leukocyte activation
- Intravascular endothelial damage
- Increased capillary permeability
- Decreased level of functional surfactant leading to pulmonary edema and acute respiratory distress syndrome (ARDS)

MANIFESTATIONS

- Early persistent tachycardia
- Acute respiratory failure/ARDS
- High temperature
- Petechial rash
  - Over the upper body, especially in the axillae
  - Usually develops 24–36 hours after the injury
  - Seen in in 20%–50% of patients
- Subconjunctival hemorrhage
- Mental status changes
  - Agitation
  - Delirium
  - Seizures
  - Stupor or coma
- Retinal hemorrhages with intraarterial fat globules seen in fundoscopy

DIAGNOSIS

- High index of suspicion
- No specific tests
- Lipiduria
- Fat globules in alveolar macrophage on bronchoalveolar lavage

MANAGEMENT

- Supportive care
- Management of respiratory distress, including mechanical ventilation
- Corticosteroid: Controversial
- Early (<24 hours after injury) fixation of long bone fractures are associated with decreased incidence of fat embolism syndrome.

Must-Know Essentials: Mangled Extremities

MANGLED EXTREMITY SEVERITY SCORE (MESS)

- Skeletal/soft-tissue injury Points
  - Low energy   1
    - Stab wound
    - Simple closed fracture
    - Low velocity gunshot wound
  - Medium energy   2
    - Open or multiple fractures
    - Dislocation
    - Moderate crush injury
  - High energy   3
    - Close-range gunshot wound
    - Military gunshot wounds
    - High-speed motor vehicle collision (MVC) wound
    - Severe crush injury
  - Very high energy   4
    - High-speed MVC wound with gross contamination
    - Soft-tissue avulsion
- Limb ischemia
  - Pulse reduced with normal perfusion   1
  - Pulseless, paresthesia, diminished capillary refill   2
  - Cool, paralyzed, insensate/numb   3
- Shock
  - Systolic BP constantly >90 mm Hg   0
  - Transient hypotension   1
  - Persistent hypotension   2
- Age (years)
  - <30   0
  - 30–50   1
  - >50   2

Score doubled for limb ischemia >6 hours. MESS score of 7 or more has a 100% predictability of amputation

MANAGEMENT OF MANGLED EXTREMITIES

- Indications for Amputation
  - Injury of three of the four major components of a limb including the following:
    - Soft tissues (muscle, fascia, skin)

- Nerves
- Vascular supply
- Bones
- Significant physiologic derangement including the following:
  - Hemodynamic instability
  - Acidosis
  - Coagulopathy
  - Concomitant life-threating injuries
- Limb salvage
  - Multidisciplinary approach including orthopedics, vascular, plastics, and trauma surgery
  - Patient- and injury-specific factors should be taken into account before planning for the limb salvage, including the following:
    - Patient's age
    - Comorbidities
    - Occupation
    - Associated injuries

Must-Know Essentials: Compartment Syndrome

PATHOPHYSIOLOGY

- Compartment syndrome is a manifestation of nerve and muscle ischemia when the tissue pressure within a closed muscle space (compartment) exceeds the perfusion pressure.
- It can occur in any fascial compartment of the extremities, including the hand, forearm, upper arm, deltoid, buttocks, thigh, calf, and foot.
- Increase in compartment pressure results in the following:
  - Impairment of venous outflow
  - Impairment of sensation due to lack of oxygenated blood and accumulation of waste products in the peripheral nerve of the muscle compartment
  - Impairment of arterial flow
    - Absent distal pulse
    - Extremity paresis
    - Ischemic necrosis of the muscles and nerve within the compartments
    - Limb contracture (Volkmann contracture)
    - Rhabdomyolysis and renal failure
- Clinical symptoms may occur within 2–4 hours after an increase in compartment pressure.
- Increased compartment pressure results in irreversible tissue damage after 6 hours due to impaired perfusion.

COMPARTMENTS OF THE UPPER ARM

- Anterior compartment
  - Flexor muscles: biceps brachii, brachialis
  - Musculocutaneous nerve (C5-C7)
- Posterior compartment
  - Extensor muscles: triceps brachii, anconeus
  - Radial nerve

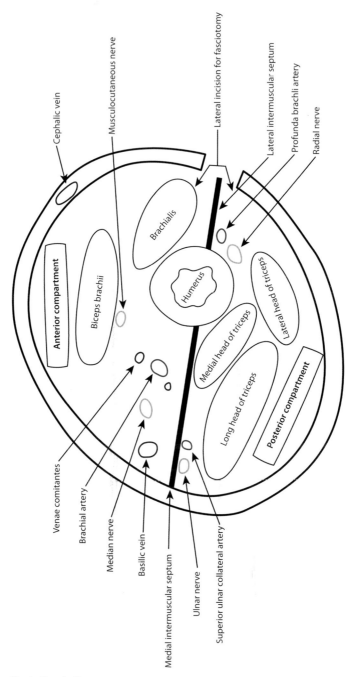

Illustration: Left upper arm compartments

COMPARTMENTS OF THE FOREARM

- Superficial volar
  - Pronator teres, flexor carpi radialis, flexor digitorum superficialis, and flexor carpi ulnaris muscles
  - Ulnar artery
  - Ulnar nerve
  - Median nerve
- Deep volar
  - Flexor digitorum profundus, flexor pollicis longus, and pronator quadratus muscles and tendons
  - Median nerve
- Mobile wad compartment
  - Brachioradialis, extensor carpi radialis longus, and Extensor carpi radialis brevis muscles
  - Radial artery
  - Radial nerve
- Dorsal (extensor) compartment
  - Supinator, abductor pollicis longus, extensor pollicis brevis, extensor pollicis longus and extensor indicis muscles
  - Extensor carpi ulnaris, extensor digitorum communis, and extensor digiti minimi

COMPARTMENTS OF THE WRIST

- Volar compartments
  - Carpal tunnel
    - Thumb and finger flexor tendons
    - Median nerve
  - Separate compartments for tendons of the following:
    - Flexor carpi radialis
    - Flexor carpi ulnaris
    - Palmaris longus
- Dorsal compartments
  - Dorsal extensor tendons pass under the extensor retinaculum
  - Six compartments
    - Radial wrist abductor
      - Abductor pollicis longus tendon
      - Extensor pollicis brevis tendon
    - Radial wrist extensors
      - Extensor carpi radialis longus tendon
      - Extensor carpi radialis brevis tendon
    - Extensor pollicis longus tendon
    - Common finger extensors (extensor digitorum communis tendon).
    - Extensor digiti minimi tendon
    - Ulnar wrist extensor (extensor carpi ulnaris tendon)

COMPARTMENTS OF THE HAND

- Four dorsal interossei compartments
- Three palmar interossei compartments

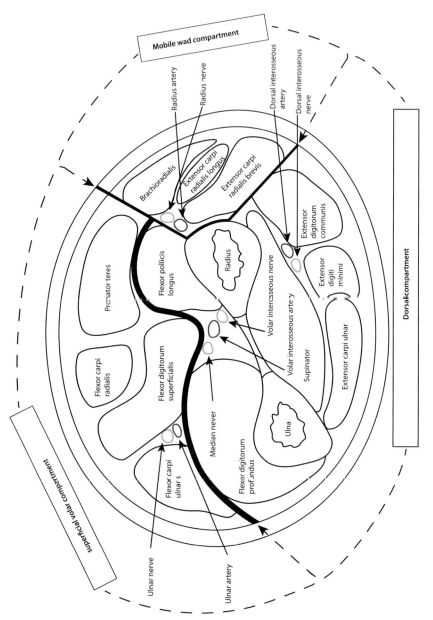

Illustration: Left forearm compartments

- Adductor pollicis compartment
- Thenar compartment
- Hypothenar compartment

COMPARTMENTS OF THE BUTTOCK

- Three compartments
  - Gluteus maximus compartment
  - Gluteus medius/minimus compartment
  - Tensor fascia lata compartment
- Nerve: Sciatic nerve is the only major structure in the compartments of the buttock.

COMPARTMENTS OF THE THIGH

- Anterior compartment
  - Muscles
    - Extensors of knee: quadriceps femoris muscles (rectus femoris, vastus lateralis, vastus medialis, vastus intermedius), and sartorius muscle
    - Flexors of hip: sartorius, pectineus, psoas major, and iliacus
  - Nerve: femoral nerve
- Posterior compartment
  - Muscles
    - Flexors of knee: hamstrings (semitendinosus, semimembranosus, biceps femoris), gracilis, sartorius, gastrocnemius, plantaris, and popliteus
    - Extensors of hip: biceps femoris, semitendinosus, semimembranosus
  - Nerve: sciatic nerve
- Medial compartment
  - Muscles
    - Adductors of hip: adductor longus, adductor brevis, adductor magnus, gracilis
  - Nerve: obturator nerve

COMPARTMENTS OF THE LEG

- Anterior compartment
  - Muscles: tibialis anterior, extensor digitorum longus, extensor hallucis longus, peroneus tertius
  - Deep peroneal nerve
  - Anterior tibial artery
  - Anterior tibial vein
- Lateral compartment
  - Muscles: peroneus longus and peroneus brevis
  - Superficial peroneal nerve
- Superficial posterior compartment
  - Muscles: gastrocnemius, soleus, and plantaris
  - Sural nerve
- Deep posterior compartment
  - Muscle: flexor digitorum longus, flexor hallucis longus, popliteus, tibialis posterior
  - Posterior tibial artery
  - Posterior tibial vein
  - Tibial nerve

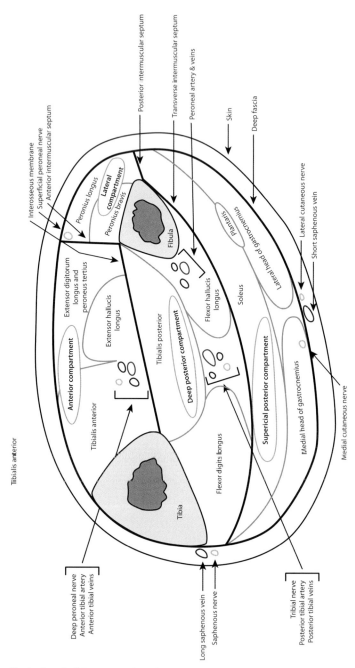

Illustration: Left leg compartments

COMPARTMENTS OF THE FOOT

- Four interosseous compartments
  - Muscles: dorsal interossei, plantar interossei
  - Lateral planter vessels
  - Lateral planter nerve
- Medial compartment
  - Muscles: abductor hallucis, flexor hallucis brevis
  - Tendon of flexor hallucis brevis
  - Medial plantar vessels
  - Medial planter nerve
- Lateral compartment
  - Muscles: adductor digiti minimi, flexor digiti minimi, opponens digiti minimi
  - Branches of lateral planter vessels
  - Branches of lateral planter nerve
- Central compartment
  - Three levels
    - First level: adductor hallucis
    - Second level: quadratus plantae muscle, lumbrical muscles, tendons of flexor digitorum longus
    - Third level: flexor digitorum brevis
  - All levels of the central compartment contain the following:
    - Deep branches of the lateral plantar vessels
    - Branches of the lateral planter nerve

ETIOLOGY OF ACUTE COMPARTMENT SYNDROME

- Fractures: Most common after leg and the forearm fractures
- Crush injuries
- Burns
- Envenomation
- Gunshot injury to extremities
- Overly tight bandage
- Prolonged compression of a limb during a period of unconsciousness
- Revascularization of vascular injury of the arm or leg
- Deep vein thrombosis (DVT) in arm or leg

DIAGNOSIS OF COMPARTMENT SYNDROME

- Clinical
  - High index of suspicion in patients with extremity injuries
  - Pain out of proportion is the most reliable early clinical finding.
  - Pain with passive stretch of the muscle within the involved compartment
  - Tightness of the compartment with tenderness
  - Paresthesias in the distribution of the involved nerve running through the compartment
  - Late findings
    - Anesthesia in the distribution of the involved nerve due to ischemic nerve injury
    - Paralysis
    - Pallor
    - Pulselessness
- Measurement of compartment pressure

- Compartment pressure measurement should be performed in patients with an unreliable or unobtainable clinical exam (unconsciousness, altered sensorium, distracting injuries, pediatric patients)
- Absolute compartment pressures >30–45 mm Hg in patient with normal blood pressure is suggestive of compartment syndrome.
- Delta P (difference between the diastolic blood pressure and compartment pressure) is more predictive of tissue perfusion. Pressure <30 mm Hg is diagnostic of compartment syndrome.
- Technique of compartment pressure measurement
  - Compartment pressure measurement using a transducer connected to a catheter in the muscle compartment. It is the most accurate method of compartment pressure measurement.
  - Injection technique: Stryker device, a handheld manometer for direct measurement of compartment pressure.

TREATMENT OF COMPARTMENT SYNDROME

- Fasciotomy
  - Compartment syndrome is a surgical emergency.
  - Treated with emergent fasciotomy
  - Fasciotomy performed >6 hours of diagnosis results in irreversible muscle ischemia and muscle necrosis.
- Supportive management
  - Supplemental oxygen
  - Removal of any restrictive casts, dressings, or bandages to relieve pressure
  - Elevation is contraindicated as it decreases arterial flow and narrows the arterial-venous pressure gradient.
  - Renal protection
    - Aggressive IV crystalloid solution infusion
      - 0.9% normal saline solution is preferred.
      - Infusion rate may range from 200 mL/hr to 1000 mL/hr based on the response.
    - Use of sodium bicarbonate is controversial.
    - Sodium bicarbonate may cause hypocalcemia.
    - Alkalization of the urine and diuresis are considered renal protective in myoglobinuria because myoglobin is more soluble in alkaline solution.
    - IV fluid with bicarbonate may be considered in patients with significant myoglobinuria.
    - May consider mannitol 1 g/kg after resuscitation with crystalloid.
  - Close monitoring of urine output with a goal of 1–2 mL/kg/hr
- Postfasciotomy wound management
  - Negative pressure wound therapy (NPWT)
  - Delayed closure
  - Skin grafts

PROGNOSIS OF COMPARTMENT SYNDROME

- Fasciotomy performed within 6 hours results in complete recovery of limb function.
- Delay in management results in muscle necrosis and healing with fibrosis and contracture (Volkmann contracture).
- Acute renal failure is secondary to myoglobinuria.
- Permanent nerve damage
- Chronic pain
- Calcific myonecrosis.
- May require amputation

STEPS OF THIGH FASCIOTOMY

- Anterior and posterior compartment fasciotomy
    - Make a lateral skin incision beginning just distal to the intertrochanteric line and extending to the lateral epicondyle.
    - Expose the iliotibial band and make a straight incision through the iliotibial band.
    - Reflect the vastus lateralis off the lateral intermuscular septum.
    - Make a 1- to 2-cm transverse incision in the lateral intermuscular septum.
    - Using a Metzenbaum scissors, cut the fascia proximally and distally along the length of the incision to release the anterior and posterior compartments.
    - Obtain hemostasis.
    - Apply a dressing or a negative pressure wound therapy (NPWT).
- Medial compartment fasciotomy
    - Decompression of the anterior and posterior compartments also reduces medial compartment pressure.
    - A medial fasciotomy is rarely required.
    - Make a longitudinal skin incision approximately 20 cm long extending 5 cm above the medial condyle of the femur along the long saphenous vein.
    - Protect and avoid injury to the long saphenous vein.
    - Expose the fascia.
    - Open the fascia using Metzenbaum scissors.
    - Obtain hemostasis.
    - Apply a dressing or a NPWT.

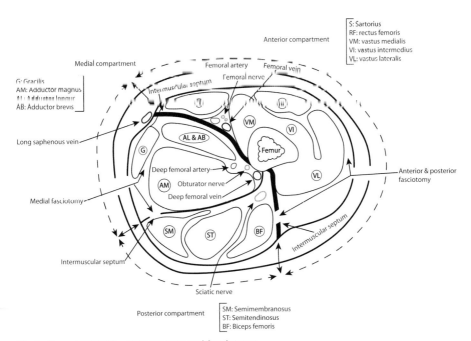

Illustrations: Left thigh compartments and fasciotomy

STEPS OF LEG FASCIOTOMY

- Anterior and lateral fasciotomy
    - Make a skin incision approximately 15–20 cm long over the anterior intermuscular septum, centered halfway between the fibular shaft and the crest of the tibia and extending proximally approximately 3 cm distal to the level of the tibial tuberosity and distally just above the lateral malleolus.
    - Dissect the subcutaneous tissue to expose the fascia overlying the lateral and anterior compartments.
    - Identify the intermuscular septum of the anterior and lateral compartments.
    - Make a transverse incision to expose the lateral intermuscular septum. Identify and protect the superficial peroneal nerve, which is located just deep to the septum.
    - Release the anterior compartment.
        - Make a small incision in the anterior fascia overlying the anterior compartment midway between the intermuscular septum and tibial crest.
        - Using Metzenbaum scissors, cut the fascia longitudinally and proximally up to the lateral border of the patella and distally up to the center of the ankle.
    - Release the lateral compartment.
        - Make a small transverse incision in the lateral compartment fascia.
        - Incise the fascia longitudinally using Metzenbaum scissors parallel to the shaft of the fibula.
        - To minimize the risk of injury to the common peroneal nerve, proximally extend the fascial incision approximately 5 cm distal to the fibular head.
        - To minimize the risk of injury to the superficial peroneal nerve, distally extend the fascial incision toward the lateral malleolus.
    - Posterior compartment (superficial and deep) fasciotomy:
        - Make a longitudinal skin incision 2 cm posterior to the medial margin of the tibia and extending proximally to the level of 3 cm distal to the tibial tuberosity and distally at the level of the medial malleolus.
        - Dissect the subcutaneous tissue to identify the fascia.
        - Identify and protect the saphenous vein and nerve situated anterior to the incision.
        - Make a transverse incision to identify the septum between the deep and superficial posterior compartments.
        - Release the fascia over the entire length of the superficial posterior compartment.
        - Make another fascial incision over the flexor digitorum longus (FDL) muscle and release the entire deep posterior compartment.
        - Obtain hemostasis.
        - Apply a dressing or NPWT.

STEPS OF UPPER ARM FASCIOTOMY (SEE ILLUSTRATION OF UPPER ARM COMPARTMENTS)

- Make a lateral skin incision extending from the insertion of the deltoid muscle to the lateral epicondyle of the humerus.
- Mobilize the skin flaps to expose the fascia.
- Identify the intermuscular septum of the anterior and posterior compartments.
- Incise the fascia of the anterior and posterior compartments longitudinally.
- Avoid radial nerve injury as it passes through the intermuscular septum from the posterior compartment to the anterior compartment just under the fascia.

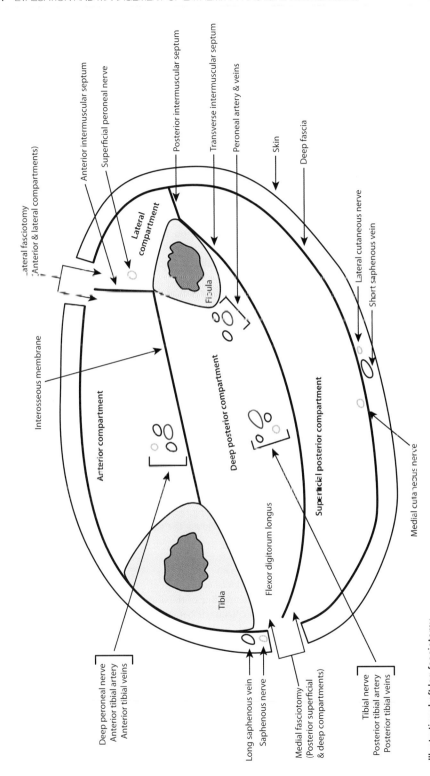

Illustration: Left leg fasciotomy

STEPS OF FOREARM FASCIOTOMY (SEE ILLUSTRATION OF FOREARM COMPARTMENTS)

- Approach for forearm decompression
  - Volar
  - Dorsal
  - Combination of volar and dorsal
- Fasciotomies of all three compartments may be unnecessary because they are interconnected.
- A volar fasciotomy should decompress the dorsal compartment.
- Volar (anterior) forearm fasciotomy
  - Volar incision is used to decompress the volar and mobile wad compartments.
  - Lazy-S-shaped volar incision
    - Make a skin incision starting just proximal to the antecubital fossa on the medial side in the groove between the biceps and triceps.
    - Extend the incision in a curvilinear fashion toward the radial aspect of the mid forearm.
    - Extend the incision distally in a curvilinear fashion toward the ulnar aspect of the wrist crease.
    - Extend the incision transversely to the center of the wrist and then extend it approximately 3 cm distal to the flexion crease between the thenar and hypothenar eminences.
  - Expose the fascia of the flexor compartment.
  - Proximally divide the lacertus fibrosus (bicipital aponeurosis) during this procedure, and identify and protect the brachial artery and median nerve.
  - Open the entire length of the fascia longitudinally using scissors to release the volar (anterior) and mobile wad (lateral) compartments.
  - Incise the fascia overlying the flexor carpi ulnaris longitudinally.
  - Expose the deep compartment of the forearm by retracting the flexor carpi ulnaris medially and the flexor digitorum superficialis laterally.
  - Incise the fascia overlying the deep muscles of the forearm longitudnally.
  - Incise the fascia overlying the mobile wad muscles.
  - Distally incise the palmar fascia to expose the transverse carpal ligament.
  - Divide the transverse carpal ligament (flexor retinaculum) along the ulnar side to perform a carpal tunnel release.
  - Identify and protect the median nerve during the carpal tunnel release.
  - Incise the flexor retinaculum of the hand along the thenar aspect of the palm.
  - Obtain hemostasis.
  - Apply a dressing or NPWT.
- Dorsal forearm fasciotomy
  - It is performed to decompress the dorsal compartment.
  - Make a longitudinal incision in the midline of the dorsal surface of the forearm extending from 2 cm distal to the lateral epicondyle between the extensor digitorum communis and the extensor carpi radialis brevis to the wrist.
  - Dissect the subcutaneous tissue to expose the fascia of the dorsal compartment.
  - Incise longitudinally the fascia overlying the extensor digitorum communis muscle.
  - Dissect the deep fascia between the extensor digitorum communis and the extensor carpi radialis muscles.
  - Incise longitudinally the deep fascia overlying the deep dorsal compartment muscles.
  - Obtain hemostasis.
  - Apply a dressing or NPWT.

Must-Know Essentials: Extremity Nerve Injuries

SCIATIC NERVE

- Etiology: Posterior dislocation of hip
- Motor: Weakness planter/dorsiflexion of the ankle
- Sensory: Loss of sensation of the foot

OBTURATOR NERVE

- Etiology: Obturator ring fracture
- Motor: Weakness of adduction of the hip
- Sensation: Impaired sensation in the medial thigh

SUPERIOR GLUTEAL NERVE

- Etiology: Fracture of the acetabulum
- Motor: Weakness of abduction of the hip
- Sensory: Loss of sensation in the upper buttocks

INFERIOR GLUTEAL NERVE

- Etiology: Fracture of the acetabulum
- Motor: Weakness of extension of the hip
- Sensory: Impaired sensation in the lower buttocks

FEMORAL NERVE

- Etiology: Pubic rami fractures
- Motor: Weakness of the knee extension
- Sensory: Numbness over distal 1/3 of the anteromedial aspect of the thigh

PERONEAL NERVE

- Etiology
  - Fractured neck of fibula
  - Posterior knee dislocation
  - Leg compartment syndrome
- Motor
  - Common peroneal nerve
    - Foot drop (weakness or inability of dorsiflexion of the foot or toes as well as eversion of the foot)
  - Deep peroneal nerve
    - Commonly seen after fracture of the neck of the fibula and compartment syndrome of the leg
    - Weakness or inability of the dorsiflexion of the ankle or toes
  - Superficial peroneal nerve
    - Common after fracture of the neck of the fibula and posterior dislocation of the knee
    - Inability of eversion of the foot

- Sensory
  - Deep peroneal nerve
    - Impaired or absent sensation on the dorsal aspect of foot between first and second toes
  - Superficial peroneal nerve
    - Impaired or absent sensation on the dorsal aspect of the foot except for between the first and second toes

POSTERIOR TIBIAL NERVE

- Etiology: Knee dislocation
- Motor: Weakness in flexion of the toes
- Sensory: Impaired sensation in sole of the foot

AXILLARY NERVE

- Etiology
  - Anterior shoulder dislocation
  - Fracture of the proximal humerus
- Motor: Weakness of the deltoid muscle
- Sensory: Impaired sensation in the lateral shoulder area

RADIAL NERVE

- Etiology
  - Fracture of the distal shaft of the humerus
  - Anterior dislocation of the shoulder
- Motor
  - Weakness or absent dorsiflexion of the wrist and/or thumb
  - Weakness of the metacarpophalangeal joint extension
- Sensory
  - Decreased or absent sensation in the dorsal web space between the thumb and index fingers

MEDIAN NERVE

- Etiology
  - Injury at the wrist and elbow joints
  - Supracondylar fracture of the humerus
- Motor
  - Weak or absent flexion of the thumb and index finger interphalangeal (IP) joints
- Sensory
  - Decreased or absent sensation in the palmar surface of the thumb, index finger, and middle finger

ULNAR NERVE

- Etiology
  - Elbow injury

- Motor
  - Weakness or absence of abduction and adduction of fingers, abduction of index and little finger
- Sensory
  - Decreased or absent sensation in the palmar surface of the little finger and the ulnar half of the ring finger

Must-Know Essentials: Management of Fractures

CLASSIFICATION OF FRACTURES

- Open fracture (compound fracture)
- Closed fracture
- Simple fracture
- Comminuted fracture

GUSTILO-ANDERSON CLASSIFICATION OF OPEN FRACTURES

- Type I
  - Skin laceration <1 cm long with minimal soft-tissue injury
  - Clean wound
  - Simple bone fracture with minimal communication
- Type II
  - Skin laceration >1 cm long with moderate soft-tissue injury
  - No associated flap or avulsion
  - Minimal crushing
  - Moderate communication and contamination
- Type III
  - Laceration >10 cm long
  - Exposed bones
  - Missing soft tissue
  - Neurovascular involvement
  - High-speed crush injury
  - Segmental diaphyseal loss
  - Wound from high-velocity weapon
  - Extensive contamination of the wound bed
  - Any size open injury with farm contamination
- Type IIIA
  - Extensive laceration of soft tissues with covered bone fragments
  - Usually, high-speed traumas with severe comminution or segmental fractures
  - Soft-tissue coverage facilitated by primary closure despite soft tissue laceration and flap
- Type IIIB
  - Extensive loss of soft tissues with periosteal stripping, exposed bones, and contamination
  - Severe comminution due to high-speed trauma
  - Usually requires replacement of exposed bone with a local or free flap as a cover
- Type IIIC
  - Extensive fracture with arterial damage that requires repair for limb salvage

ANTIBIOTICS IN OPEN FRACTURES

- Intravenous antimicrobials should be given to patients with open fractures within 1 hour of presentation.
- Gustilo-Anderson Types I and II
  - Antibiotics to cover gram-positive organisms for 24 hours after the surgical procedure
  - First-generation cephalosporin (eg, cefazolin)
    - Dose
      - 1 g IV Q 8 hours for patients <50 kg weight
      - 2 g IV Q 8 hours for patients 50–100 kg weight
      - 3 g IV Q 8 hours for patients >100 kg weight
  - Clindamycin for patients with penicillin allergy
    - Dose
      - 600 mg IV Q 8 hours for patients <80 kg weight
      - 900 mg IV Q 8 hours for patients >80 kg weight
- Gustilo-Anderson Type III
  - Antibiotics coverage for both gram-positive and gram--negative organisms for 72 hours after closure of the wound
  - First-generation cephalosporin (eg, cefazolin)
    - Dose
      - 1 g IV Q 8 hours for patients <50 kg weight
      - 2 g IV Q 8 hours for patients 50–100 kg weight
      - 3 g IV Q 8 hours for patients >100 kg weight
  - Clindamycin for patients with penicillin allergy
    - Dose
      - 600 mg IV Q 8 hours for patients <80 kg weight
      - 900 mg IV Q 8 hours for patients >80 kg weight
  - Gentamicin for gram-negative coverage
    - Dose
      - Loading dose: 2.5 mg/kg body IV for patients <50 kg weight
      - Loading dose: 5 mg/kg IV for patients >50 kg weight
      - Maintenance dose: Based on gentamicin level
  - Penicillin should be added in the presence of severe contamination, impaired vascularity, or potential clostridia contamination such as from farm injuries.
  - Piperacillin/tazobactam
    - Dose
      - 3.375 g IV Q 6 hours for patients <100 kg weight
      - 4.5 g IV Q 6 hours for patients >100 kg weight

DAMAGE CONTROL MANAGEMENT OF FRACTURES

- Indications for damage-control procedures in extremity injuries
  - Hemodynamically unstable patients
    - Ongoing bleeding
    - Acidosis
    - Base deficit

- Coagulopathy
- Hypothermia
- Severe traumatic brain injury
- Chest injury with respiratory distress requiring significant ventilatory support
- Open or closed fractures with the following:
  - Soft-tissue loss
  - Significant contamination
  - Severe closed soft-tissue injury
- Damage-control procedures
  - Skeletal stabilization
    - Minimizes ongoing soft-tissue damage
    - Decrease risks of fat embolism
    - Controls hemorrhage
    - Helps in pain control
    - Maintains bone length, rotation, and alignment of the extremities in unstable fractures
    - Techniques of skeletal stabilization
      - Skeletal traction
      - External fixation
  - Control of bleeding
  - Vascular injury repair
  - Fasciotomy if indicated
  - Debridement of soft tissue to decrease contamination

DEFINITIVE MANAGEMENT OF FRACTURES

- Optimal timing for definitive management of fractures is controversial.
- It should be considered after the following:
  - Hemodynamic stability
  - Resolution of coagulopathy, acidosis, and hypothermia
  - Stable intracranial pressure (ICP), cerebral perfusion pressure (CPP), and mean arterial pressure (MAP) in patients with severe traumatic brain injury
- Early (<24 hours after injury) fixation of long-bone fractures are associated with decreased incidence of the following:
  - Respiratory distress syndrome (ARDS)
  - Fat embolism syndrome (FES)
  - Pneumonia
  - ICU and hospital length of stay
- Open fractures requiring wound coverage with skin grafting or soft-tissue transfers should be completed within 7 days of injury.

Must-Know Essentials: Amputations
INDICATIONS OF AMPUTATIONS

- Total or "near total" after trauma
- Warm ischemia time >6 hours
- Complete anatomic sciatic or tibial nerve transection
- Loss of plantar skin and soft tissue
- Inability to revascularize an extremity (and unsuccessful attempts at revascularization)
- Mangled extremities

- Failed limb salvage
- Inability to salvage limb based on the injury pattern or physiological derangements

BELOW-KNEE AMPUTATION: STEPS

- Place a tourniquet in the thigh and inflate to a pressure about 100 mm Hg above the systolic pressure.
- Prep and drape the leg.
- Make an anterior incision at 10–12 cm or one handbreadth below the tibial tuberosity and extend the incision up to the middle of the calf circumference bilaterally.
- From the middle of the calf circumference, extend the incision vertically downward in a slightly curved fashion to a length approximately 1.5 times the length of the anterior incision.
- Identify and ligate the saphenous vein on the medial side of the calf.
- Divide the muscles of the anterior compartment down to the interosseous membrane.
- Ligate and divide the anterior tibial artery and anterior tibial vein using 2-0 silk sutures.
- Ligate and divide the deep peroneal nerve as high as possible after applying traction on the nerve.
- Divide the anterior interosseus membrane.
- Clear the muscle attachments circumferentially from the tibia.
- Elevate the periosteum of the tibia using a periosteal elevator, and transect the tibia using a power saw/Gigli saw 5–10 cm proximal to the skin incision.
- Divide the lateral compartment muscles to expose the fibula at the level of the anterior skin incision.
- Elevate the periosteum of the fibula using a periosteal elevator and transect the fibula 2–3 cm proximal to the tibial osteotomy site using a power saw/Gigli saw.
- Divide the posterior compartment muscles distal to the divided distal tibia and fibula using a sharp amputation knife to create the posterior myocutaneous flap. Proper thickness of the soleus muscle is important in creating the posterior myocutaneous flap.
- Ligate and divide the posterior tibial artery, posterior tibial vein, peroneal artery, and peroneal vein using 2-0 silk sutures.
- Ligate and divide the tibial nerve and the peroneal nerve as high as possible after applying traction on the nerve.
- Release the tourniquet to check for bleeding and achieve hemostasis.
- Smoothe the bone edges using a bone rasp or file.
- Approximate the anterior and posterior muscular fascia to cover the bone stump with interrupted 1-0 Polyglactin absorbable sutures.
- Close the skin with staples.
- Apply a dressing and place a knee immobilizer.

ABOVE-KNEE AMPUTATION: STEPS

- The ideal length of the femoral shaft for a functional prosthesis is 15–20 cm from the greater trochanter or proximal two-thirds of the shaft.
- Place a tourniquet in the thigh proximal to the amputation site and inflate it to a pressure of about 100 mm Hg above the systolic pressure.
- Prep and drape the leg.
- Make a fish-mouth incision with an equal anterior and posterior flap at a level 15 cm distal to the selected amputation site.
- Divide the skin and subcutaneous tissue circumferentially.

- Ligate and divide the long saphenous vein on the medial side of the incision.
- Create skin flaps.
- Divide the anterior compartment muscles down to the bone 5 cm distal to the planned osteotomy site.
- Identify, ligate, and divide the femoral artery and vein separately using 2-0 silk sutures on the medial side of the thigh situated deep to the sartorius muscle.
- Divide the medial compartment muscles.
- Elevate the periosteum from the femur.
- Transect the femur using a power saw/Gigli saw at the planned osteotomy site.
- Identify the sciatic nerve between the medial posterior compartments.
- Ligate and divide the sciatic nerve after applying traction.
- Identify, ligate, and divide the profunda femoris artery, which lies posterolateral to the superficial femoral vessels, using 2-0 Silk suture.
- Divide the posterior compartment muscles distal to the femoral osteotomy.
- Perform three unicortical holes on the medial side of the femur using a drill and perform myodesis by attaching the fascia of the adductor and medial hamstring muscles using 1-0 Polyglactin absorbable sutures.
- Approximate the anterior and posterior fascia to cover the bone stump with 1-0 Polyglactin absorbable sutures.
- Close the skin with staples.

PART 3

Miscellaneous

Pediatric Trauma, Trauma in Pregnancy, Scoring and Grading, Medications

CHAPTER 35

Evaluation and Management of Pediatric Trauma

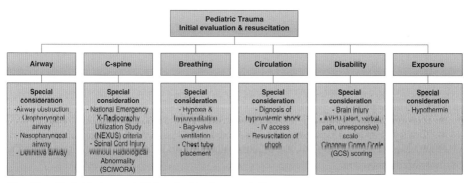

Algorithm: Pediatric trauma initial evaluation & resuscitation

Must-Know Essentials: Pediatric Trauma Evaluation and Management

ANATOMICAL AND PHYSIOLOGICAL FACTORS IN PEDIATRIC TRAUMA

- Trauma is the leading cause of death among children >1 years of age.
- Small body size
  - Multiple injuries can result from a single impact due to the proximity of multiple organs and the wide transmission of energy.
- Small blood volume
  - Hemorrhagic shock can result even from small blood loss.
- Large surface-area-to-body-mass ratio
  - High risk of hypothermia due to larger heat loss
  - High risk of hypovolemia due to larger insensible fluid loss
  - Higher caloric requirement
- Cartilaginous skeleton, less fat, and more elastic connective tissue
  - Severe pulmonary injury can result without any rib fracture.
  - Severe brain injury can result without skull fracture.
  - There is less risk of extremities fractures.
- Larger solid organs with thin abdominal wall with less subcutaneous fat predisposes to the following:
  - Liver injury
  - Spleen injury
- High risk of head injury is due to the proportionately larger size of the head.

INITIAL EVALUATION AND RESUSCITATION

- Follows the same algorithm as in adults, which includes the following:
  - Airway
  - Cervical spine protection
  - Breathing
  - Circulation
  - Disability
  - Exposure
- Leading causes of cardiopulmonary arrest in children
  - Lack of airway resulting in hypoxia and hypoventilation
  - Tension pneumothorax
  - Hypovolemia
  - Cardiac tamponade
  - Cardiac contusion
  - Severe head injury
  - Cervical spinal cord injury
  - Hypothermia
- Hypotension is a sign of significant blood loss
- The Broselow Pediatric Emergency Tape is an essential adjunct in pediatric resuscitation. It provides weight- and length-based information on the following:
  - Medication dose
  - Fluid volume
  - Equipment size
- Pediatric vital functions depend on age and weight, as shown in the illustration.

Pediatric Vital Functions

Vital Functions	Infant (0–12 months)	Toddler (1–2 years)	Preschool age (3–5 years)	School age (6–12 years)	Adolescent > 13 years
Weight Range (kg)	0–10	10–14	14–18	18–30	30–70
Heart Rate (beats/min)	>160	<150	<140	<120	<100
Blood pressure (mm Hg)	>60	>70	>75	>80	>90
Respiratory rate (breaths/min)	<60	<40	<35	<30	<30
Urine output (mL/kg/hour)	2.0	1.5	1.0	1.0	0.5

- Imaging in children
  - Potential risk of radiation-induced malignancy should be considered when evaluating with computerized tomography scan (CT).
  - Radiation must be kept as low as reasonably possible.
  - Selective CT is recommended to reduce radiation exposure.
  - Plain films are the initial imaging of choice.

AIRWAY: SPECIAL CONSIDERATIONS

- High risk of airway obstruction
  - Smaller diameter of airway

- Large occiput causing flexion of the neck
- Larger tongue
- Funnel-shaped larynx in children <8 years of age: High risk of aspiration as secretions accumulate in the retropharyngeal area.
- Characteristics of respiratory distress
  - Tachypnea
  - Nasal flaring
  - Use of accessory muscles
  - Inspiratory retractions (suprasternal, substernal, and intercostal)
- Oropharyngeal airway
  - Should be inserted only in unconscious children because the intact gag reflex can result in vomiting and aspiration.
  - Correct size of the tube
    - Flange at the level of incisors and distal end at the angle of the mandible
  - Insertion technique
    - Gently and directly into the oropharynx
    - A tongue blade to depress the tongue may be helpful.
    - Inserting the airway backward and rotating it to 180 degrees, as in adults, is not recommended due to risk of injury to soft-tissue structures.
- Nasopharyngeal airway
  - Correct size
    - Diameter of the patient's little finger
  - Insertion depth
    - Nose to the tragus of the ear
- Indications for definitive airways
  - Respiratory failure or arrest
  - Airway obstruction
  - Potential of airway obstruction
  - Severe brain injury (Glasgow Coma Scale [GCS] 8 or less)
  - Intrathoracic injury
  - Severe or multiple injuries
  - Shock
- Types of definitive airways
  - Endotracheal tube
  - Surgical airway
    - Needle cricothyroidotomy
    - Open cricothyroidotomy
- Rescue airway
  - Laryngeal mask airway (LMA)
  - Intubating LMA
- Endotracheal intubation
  - Considerations during intubation
    - Larger tongue and tonsils may occlude visibility of the airway during intubation.
    - There is risk of injury with bleeding to the prominent nasopharyngeal adenoids.
    - The larynx is placed anteriorly and higher at the level of C2-C3 in young children and at the level of C6-C7 in older children and adults.
    - A very narrow airway at the level of the cricoid ring may make intubation difficult.
    - The epiglottis is floppy, narrow, and angled posteriorly.
      - A straight-bladed laryngoscope should be used during intubation in smaller children.

A short trachea may result in intubation in the right mainstem bronchus causing the following:
- Inadequate ventilation
- Hypoxia
- Barotrauma

- Steps of drug-assisted/rapid sequence (orotracheal) intubation (RSI)
  - Evaluation for difficult intubation
    - Examination of the mouth
    - Examination of the neck for range of movement
    - Examination for any loose teeth
  - Selection of the endotracheal tube (ETT)
    - Cuffed ETTs
    - Diameter of the ETT
      - Approximate diameter of the ETT should correspond to the diameter of the child's external nares or the tip of the little finger.
      - ETT diameter: Age/4 + 4 or Age + 16/4
  - Preoxygenation
    - 100% oxygen using face mask for 3 minutes
    - Displaces nitrogen from the lungs and replaces it with oxygen
    - An increased amount of oxygen in the lung during intubation prevents apneic hypoxia during the procedure.
  - Medications
    - Atropine
      - 0.1–0.5 mg in children <1 year
      - Infants have a pronounced vagal response to endotracheal intubation, more so than do children and adults.
      - Helps prevent bradycardia due to direct laryngeal stimulation
      - Not required for children >1 year of age
    - Sedation
      - Hypovolemic: etomidate 0.1 mg/kg or midazolam 0.1 mg/kg
      - Normovolemic: etomidate 0.3 mg/kg or midazolam 0.1 mg/kg
    - Paralytics
      - Succinylcholine: <10 kg weight: 2 mg/kg, >10 kg weight: 1 mg/kg *or*
      - Vecuronium: 0.1 mg/kg *or*
      - Rocuronium: 0.6 mg/kg
  - Intubation
    - May be performed using a video laryngoscope or a regular laryngoscope
    - Straight laryngoscope blade is preferred in smaller children.
    - In-line stabilization of the neck
    - Cricoid pressure (Sellick maneuver)
      - Compression of the esophagus between the cricoid cartilage and the vertebral body to prevent regurgitation of stomach content into the oropharynx
      - Also helps by moving the larynx during intubation
    - Position of the ETT
      - Depth (in cm) of the ETT from the level of the gum: approximately the size of the tube × 3. For example, a size 4.0 ETT should be positioned 12 cm from the gums.
  - Confirmation of the ETT position
    - Auscultation
      - Presence of bilateral breath sounds
      - Absence of breath sound over the epigastrium (stomach)

Capnography
Sensitive and specific to detect ETT placement
Colorimetric end-tidal carbon dioxide detector
Color change from purple to yellow
Chest x-ray
- Secure the tube in position
Because of the short trachea, any movement of the head can result in displacement of the ETT leading to the following:
Inadvertent extubation
Right mainstem bronchial intubation
- Surgical airways
  - Indications
    - Failed endotracheal intubation
  - Needle cricothyroidotomy
    - Steps
      Cricothyroid membrane is punctured with a large IV catheter with needle.
      Puncture is confirmed with aspiration of air in the syringe.
      Needle is withdrawn and catheter is advanced in the trachea.
      Cannula is connected to the high pressure oxygen source (needle-jet insufflation).
    - It does not provide adequate ventilation and leads to progressive hypercarbia.
  - Open cricothyroidotomy
    - Rarely indicated for infants or small children
    - Can be performed in older children (>12 years of age) where cricothyroid membrane is easily palpable
- Recue airway
  - Used for failed ETT
  - Performed with:
    - laryngeal mask airway LMA.
    - intubating LMA.
  - Selection of LMA size

Size of LMA in Children

LMA Size	Patient's Weight
1	0–5 kg
1.5	5–10 kg
2	10–20 kg
2.5	20–30 kg
3	30–50 kg
4	50–70 kg

CERVICAL SPINE: SPECIAL CONSIDERATIONS

- The cervical spine injury must be suspected and immobilized in severe pediatric trauma patients, especially with head injury and multiple injuries.
- Techniques of cervical spine immobilization
  - Appropriate-size cervical collar (C-collar)
  - Towel rolls or IV fluid bag on both sides of the head may be an alternative if proper size of the C-collar is not available.

- Cervical spine clearance
  - Challenging in pediatric trauma patients
  - National Emergency X-Radiography Utilization Study (NEXUS) clinical criteria are most reliable for cervical spine clearance in pediatric blunt trauma patients.
  - The C-collar can be removed if the NEXUS clinical criteria are met:
    - No neck pains.
    - No midline cervical spine tenderness.
    - No altered mental status.
    - No focal neurological deficit.
    - No intoxication.
    - No painful, distracting injury.
  - If the NEXUS criteria are not met, further evaluation should be performed with the following:
    - Plain film
    - CT scan
- Spinal cord injury without radiographic abnormality (SCIWORA)
  - Spinal cord injury can result without fracture due to flexible spine in children.
  - Seen in approximately 30%-40% of the pediatric patients with spinal cord injury

BREATHING: SPECIAL CONSIDERATIONS

- Hypoxia and ventilation problems are common in children due to the following:
  - The smaller diameter of the pediatric airway causes increased airway resistance and work of breathing.
  - High oxygen consumption and low functional residual capacity
  - Limited tidal volume during inspiration due to horizontal position of the ribs in small children
- Hypoxia and hypoventilation are leading causes of pediatric cardiac arrest.
- Bag-valve-mask (BVM) ventilation
  - Used to assist ventilation in patients with apnea or poor respiratory effort
  - BVM ventilation for a short period of time is as effective as ventilation via an ETT.
  - Minimal force and tidal volume should be used.
  - Excessive volume and pressure can cause:
    - gastric inflation and increase in risk of aspiration. Cricoid pressure may reduce gastric inflation.
    - barotrauma due to fragile tracheobronchial tree and alveoli.
- Tube thoracostomy
  - Indications
    - Hemothorax
    - Pneumothorax
  - Selection of chest tube size
    - 0–6 months: 12–18 Fr
    - 6–12 months: 14–20 Fr
    - 1–3 years: 14–24 Fr
    - 4–7 years: 20–28 Fr
    - 8–10 years: 28–32 Fr
  - Site of chest tube insertion is the same in children as in adults: the fifth intercostal space, just anterior to the midaxillary line.
  - Tunneling of the chest tube is recommended because of the thinner chest wall in children.

CIRCULATION: SPECIAL CONSIDERATIONS

- Blood volume in children
  - Infant: 80 mL/kg
  - 1–3 years: 75 mL/kg
  - >3 years: 70 mL/kg
- Blood pressure in children
  - Normal systolic blood pressure (SBP) = 70–90 mm Hg + 2 × age in years
  - Normal diastolic blood pressure (DBP) = 2/3 of the SBP
- Systemic response of hemorrhage in children (see illustration)
  - Hemorrhagic shock can result even from a small blood loss due to low circulating blood volume.
  - SBP and pulse pressure (PP) may be normal despite 25%–30% of blood volume loss due to physiologic reserve.
  - Hypotension in children is a sign of significant blood loss.
  - Early features of hemorrhagic shock
    - Tachycardia
    - Poor skin perfusion
    - Mental status changes.

Systemic Response of Blood Loss in Children

Approximate Blood Loss	Cardiovascular System	Mental Status	Skin Changes	Urine Output
Mild (<30%)	Tachycardia Weak thready peripheral pulses Normal SBP & PP	Anxious, irritable, very confused	Cool, mottled Prolonged capillary refill	Normal or low
Moderate (30%–45%)	Tachycardia Weak, thready central or absent peripheral pulses Low-normal SBP and narrow PP	Lethargic	Cyanotic Markedly prolonged capillary refill	Minimal
Severe (>45%)	Tachycardia followed by bradycardia Very weak or absent central pulses Absent peripheral pulses Hypotension Narrow PP Absent DP	Comatose	Pale and cold	None

- Special-consideration pediatric IV access sites
  - Smaller vessels and increased subcutaneous tissue make IV access difficult.
  - Peripheral IV sites
    - Antecubital fossa or dorsal surface of the hand
    - Saphenous vein
    - External jugular vein
  - Intraosseous access if IV access is difficult to obtain
    - Can be used to infuse fluid, blood products, and drugs

- Sites
  - Noninjured tibia
    - 1–2 cm below and medial to tibial tuberosity
  - Distal femur
- Central venous access sites
  - If unable to obtain a peripheral vein or intraosseous access
  - Sites
    - Femoral vein
    - Subclavian vein
    - Internal jugular vein
- Saphenous venous cutdown
  - If failed peripheral IV access, intraosseous access or central venous access
- Resuscitation of hemorrhagic shock
  - Should be started based on early features of shock
  - Resuscitation fluid
    - Initial isotonic crystalloids (normal saline/lactated Ringer's) bolus 20 mL/kg
    - Blood transfusion
      - Transient responders or nonresponders after two boluses of crystalloids
      - Packed red blood cells (RBCs) 10 mL/kg
      - Activation of massive transfusion protocol
  - Control of bleeding
- Urine output in resuscitation
  - Measurement of adequate resuscitation
  - Urine output goal
    - Infants: 1–2 mL/kg/hr
    - Children: 1–1.5 mL/kg/hr
    - Adolescent: 0.5 mL/kg/hr
- Cardiopulmonary resuscitation (CPR) in pediatric trauma
  - Field CPR and return of spontaneous circulation may have 50% chance of neurologically intact survival.
  - CPR in the emergency department (ED) has a uniformly dismal prognosis.
  - Field CPR for more than 15 minutes before arrival to an ED or fixed pupils on arrival are uniformly nonsurvivors. Prolonged CPR is not beneficial.

DISABILITY: SPECIAL CONSIDERATIONS

- High risk of head injury due to proportionally larger size of the head
- High risk of brain injury due to:
  - larger brain size.
  - smaller subarachnoid space making the children prone to parenchymal injury.
  - pattern of cerebral blood flow making the children susceptible to cerebral hypoxia and hypercarbia.
  - Children are more susceptible to secondary brain injury from hypovolemia and hypoxia.
- Infants can tolerate an increase in intracranial volume (bleeding/swelling) due to open fontanelles and mobile cranial sutures.
- Decreased level of consciousness in pediatric trauma patients may be due to:
  - traumatic brain injury (TBI).
  - hypoxia.
  - hypovolemia.

- Neurological evaluation
  - AVPU Pediatric Response Scale
    - **A:** Alert
    - **V:** Verbal stimulus response
    - **P:** Painful stimulus response
    - **U:** Unresponsive
  - Pediatric Glasgow Coma Scale (GCS) (see illustration)

Pediatric Glasgow Coma Scale

Criteria	Features	Scores
Best Eye Response (E)	Spontaneous	4
	To sound	3
	To pain	2
	None	1
Best Verbal Response (V)	Age-appropriate vocalization, smile or orientation to sound; interacts (coos, babbles); follow objects	5
	Cries, Irriatable	4
	Cries to pain	3
	Moans to pain	2
	None	1
Best Motor Response (M)	Spontaneous movements (obeys verbal command)	6
	Withdraws to touch (localizes pain)	5
	Withdraws to pain	4
	Abnormal flexion to pain (decorticate posture)	3
	Abnormal extension to pain (Decerebrate posture)	2
	None	1

- Grading of brain injury based
  - Mild brain injury   GCS 13–15
  - Moderate brain injury   GCS 9–12
  - Severe brain injury: GCS 3–8

EXPOSURE: SPECIAL CONSIDERATIONS

- High risk of hypothermia (core body temperature <35°C [95°F]) from greater heat loss due to the following:
  - Larger surface area to body mass ratio
  - Increased metabolic rate
  - Thin skin
  - Lack of substantial subcutaneous tissue
- Mechanism of heat loss
  - Conduction: Physical contact with a cold object
  - Convection: Flow of cold air or water on the skin
  - Evaporation: From water vaporizing from the skin
  - Radiation: Loss of heat generated from the body to the environment
- Predisposing factors
  - Exposure to cold
  - Exposure to cooler ambient air
  - Burns
  - Drowning

- Traumatic brain injury
- Spinal cord injury
- Effects
  - Cardiac arrhythmias
  - Coagulopathy
  - Acidosis
  - Hypoxia due to increase in oxygen consumption from shivering
- Methods of hypothermia prevention
  - Removal of wet clothes
  - Warm blanket
  - Increase in ambient room temperature >27°C (80°F)
  - Convective heating air blanket (e.g., Bair Hugger)
  - Increase temperature of the humidified supplemental oxygen to 37°C (98.6°F).
  - Infusion of warm (temperature 40°C–44°C [104°F–111.2°F]) IV fluids and blood products

PEDIATRIC HEAD INJURY

- Blunt head injury accounts for 50% of trauma-related deaths in children.
- Causes of blunt head injury
  - Motor vehicle collision (MVC)
  - Fall
  - Bicycle accident
- Factors contributing to brain injury outcome
  - Children are susceptible to more parenchymal injury due to their smaller subarachnoid space.
  - Cerebral hypoxia and hypercarbia are more common due to the pattern of cerebral blood flow.
  - Optimal cerebral perfusion pressure (CPP) in children is unknown and may depend on the age.
  - CPP <40 mm Hg is associated with poor outcome.
  - Children are more susceptible to secondary brain injury from hypovolemia, hypoxia, reduction in cerebral perfusion, seizures, and/or hyperthermia.
  - Bleeding in the subgaleal space, intraventricular space, and epidural space in infants can result in significant hypovolemia.
  - Infants can tolerate an increase in intracranial volume (bleeding/swelling) due to having open fontanelles and mobile cranial sutures without manifestations.
- Evaluation
  - Pediatric Glasgow Coma Scale
    - Mild brain injury   GCS 13–15
    - Moderate brain injury   GCS 9–12
    - Severe brain injury   GCS 3–8
  - AVPU Pediatric Response Scale
    - **A:** Alert
    - **V:** Verbal stimulus response
    - **P:** Painful stimulus response
    - **U:** Unresponsive
  - CT head is not recommended for patients with low risk of severe head injury based on the Pediatric Emergency Care Applied Research Network (PECARN) criteria.
  - PECARN criteria for low risk of severe head injury

- Age <2 years
  - Normal mental status
  - Normal behavior per routine caregiver
  - No loss of consciousness (LOC); LOC for <5 seconds is not considered as LOC.
  - No severe mechanism of injury. Severe mechanism of injury includes the following:
    - Fall >0.9 m (3 ft)
    - Head struck by high-impact object
    - MVC with patient ejection, death of another passenger, rollover
    - Unhelmeted pedestrian or bicyclist struck by a motorized vehicle
  - No nonfrontal scalp hematoma
  - No evidence of palpable skull fracture
- Age >2–18 years
  - Normal mental status. Signs of altered mental status include the following:
    - Agitation
    - Somnolence
    - Repetitive questioning
    - Slow response to verbal questioning
  - No LOC
  - No severe mechanism of injury. Severe mechanism of injury includes the following:
    - Fall >1.5 m (5 ft)
    - Head struck by high-impact object
    - MVC with patient ejection, death of another passenger, rollover
    - Unhelmeted pedestrian or bicyclist struck by a motorized vehicle
  - No vomiting
  - No severe headache
  - No signs of basilar skull fracture such as the following:
    - Hemotympanum
    - Cerebrospinal fluid (CSF) rhinorrhea
    - CSF otorrhea
    - Raccoon eyes
    - Postauricular hematoma (Battle sign)
- Management
  - As described for adult head injury (see Chapter XII for details)
- Outcome after severe brain injury
  - Better than that in adults
  - Worse in younger children (<3 years) than in older children

PEDIATRIC SPINE INJURIES

- Pediatric spine injury is uncommon.
- It is commonly due to blunt trauma.
  - MVC
  - Fall
- Cervical spine injuries are more common than other spine injuries due to anatomical characteristics:
  - Larger head compared with neck results in higher fulcrum in the cervical spine.
  - Fulcrum of cervical mobility progressively moves downward with age.
  - Level of fracture location with age:
    - Children <8: –C1-C3

- Children 8–12 years: C3-C5
- Children >12 years: C5-C6
- Chance fracture
  - Flexion-distraction fracture of the lumbar spine
  - Seen in patients restrained by lap belt only
  - High risk of associated bowel injury
- Evaluation of injury
  - Plain x-ray is the initial imaging of choice.
  - Pseudosubluxation of cervical spine
    - Anterior displacement of C2 on C3, less commonly at C3 on C4
    - Seen in 20% of children <7 years of age
  - Spinal cord injury without radiographic abnormality (SCIWORA)
    - Spinal cord injury results without fracture due to flexible spine.
    - Seen in approximately 30%–40% of pediatric spinal cord injuries
  - Indications of CT scan and MRI in spinal cord injury
    - SCIWORA
    - Pseudosubluxation
    - Spinal cord injury
- Neurological outcome in children after spinal cord injury is better than in adults.

PEDIATRIC THORACIC INJURIES

- The majority of serious pediatric thoracic injuries result from blunt trauma, such as an MVC or fall.
- Compliant noncalcified thoracic cage contributes to the following:
  - Significant chest injury without external signs of injury
  - Low incidence of rib fractures and flail chest
  - High incidence of pulmonary contusions and hematomas
  - Increased mobility of the mediastinal structures contributes to the following:
    - Higher incidence of tension pneumothorax
    - Lower incidence of aortic transection, major tracheobronchial tears, and cardiac contusions
- High incidence of hypoxemia refractory to oxygen therapy due to high oxygen consumption and low functional residual capacity
- Diaphragmatic rupture is uncommon.
- Pneumomediastinum is rare and mostly benign.
- Life-threatening thoracic injuries
  - Airway obstruction
  - Tension pneumothorax
  - Massive hemothorax
  - Cardiac tamponade
- Evaluation of thoracic injury
  - Clinical examination
  - Chest x-ray
  - CT of the chest
- Management of thoracic injuries for children is the same as for adults.

PEDIATRIC ABDOMINAL TRAUMA

- The majority of pediatric abdominal injuries are due to blunt trauma.
- Common causes
  - MVC
  - Fall
  - Bicycle handlebars
- Liver and spleen injuries are common due to the following:
  - Less protection by the abdominal wall and thoracic cage
  - Thin abdominal wall
  - Proportionally larger solid organs in children than in adults
- Assessment
  - Clinical examination
  - CT abdomen
    - Preferred imaging
    - Risk of radiation
  - Focused Assessment with Sonography for Trauma (FAST)
    - Low sensitivity and high false-negative rates
    - Avoids ionizing radiation
    - Can identify intraabdominal blood
  - Diagnostic peritoneal lavage (DPL)
    - Not commonly used
    - Rapid identification of intraabdominal bleeding in hemodynamic unstable patients
    - Criteria for a positive DPL test are the same in children as in adults.
- Specific visceral injuries in children
  - Bicycle handlebar injury
    - Seen in 15%–20 % of blunt abdominal trauma
    - Injuries include the following:
      - Spleen laceration
      - Bowel perforation
      - Mesenteric injury
      - Abdominal wall hernia
  - Lap belt injuries
    - Injuries include the following:
      - Pancreatic injury
      - Small bowel perforations at or near the ligament of Treitz
      - Mesenteric avulsion injury
      - Small bowel avulsion injury
  - Bladder rupture
    - More common in children than in adults because of the shallow depth of the pelvis
  - Penetrating straddle perineal injury
    - Occurs from fall onto a prominent object
    - Usually associated with intraperitoneal injuries due to the proximity of the peritoneum to the perineum
- Management
  - Specific injuries are managed in children as in adults.

DOSAGES OF COMMONLY USED MEDICATIONS IN PEDIATRICS

- Midazolam
  - 0.02–0.2 mg/kg IV as required every 30–90 min

- Ketamine
  - 1–2 mg/kg IV as required every 10–20 min
- Fentanyl
  - 1–2 mcg/kg IV as required every 0.5–1 hr
- Morphine
  - 0.03–0.1 mg /kg IV as required every 1–2 hrs
- Lorazepam
  - 0.05–0.1 mg/kg IV as required
- Mannitol
  - 20% mannitol: 0.25 gm/kg per dose, repeated as needed. Maintain serum Na between 155–160 mEq/L, osmolality between 310–320 mOsm/L.
- Propofol
  - 1–3 mg/kg
- Etomidate
  - 0.2–0.3 mg/kg
- Succinylcholine
  - 1–2 mg/kg
- Rocuronium
  - 0.6–1 mg/kg

PEDIATRIC TRAUMA SCORE

- Predicts pediatric trauma mortality
- A higher trauma score is associated with lower trauma mortality.
- Score >8 has an estimated mortality of 9%.
- Score ≤ 0 has an estimated mortality of zero.

Pediatric Trauma Score

Factors	+2	+1	−1
Weight (kg)	>20	10–20	<10
Airway	Patent	Oral/nasal airway Oxygen	Need for airway
Systolic pressure	>90 mm Hg	50–90 mm Hg	<50 mm Hg
Mental status	Awake	Obtunded	Comatose
Skin injury	None	Contusion, abrasion Laceration <7 cm not involving fascia	Tissue loss Penetrating wound involving fascia
Fracture	None	Single closed	Open or multiple

CHAPTER 36

Evaluation and Management of Trauma in Pregnancy

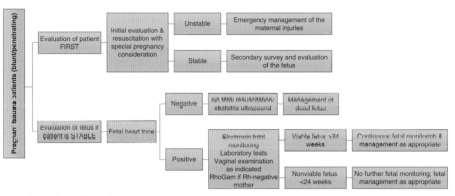

Algorithm: Evaluation of pregnant trauma patients

Must-Know Essentials: Evaluation of Pregnant Trauma Patients

TRAUMA BASICS

- Trauma involves approximately 6%–7% of all pregnancies.
- Trauma results in maternal and fetal injuries
- Causes
  - Motor vehicle collision (MVC)
    - Most common cause in the United States
    - Unrestrained drivers have a higher risk of fetal and maternal injuries.
    - Use of seat belt in pregnancy
      Shoulder restraints in conjunction with a lap belt reduce the incidence of direct and indirect fetal injuries.
      Shoulder restraints should be placed between the breasts and to the side of the abdomen.
      Shoulder belts alone without lap belts are associated with risk of uterine rupture or abruptio placentae (placental abruption). Lap belt should be placed in the lower abdomen touching the thighs and hip bones.
      High placement of a lap belt (over the uterus) may cause uterine rupture due to transmission of direct force to the uterus.
  - Assault
    - May be due to blunt or penetrating trauma to the abdomen
  - Falls
    - More common in the latter half of pregnancy

- Increase in lumbar lordosis moves the center of gravity forward, contributing to an increased incidence of falls.
  - Penetrating injury
    - Gunshot wounds (GSWs) and stab wounds
- Maternal injury pattern:
  - Bowel injury in penetrating trauma
    - Intestine is pushed up and shielded by the uterus after midpregnancy.
    - Lower incidence of bowel injuries in penetrating abdominal trauma
    - Higher incidence of bowel injuries in thoracoabdominal penetrating trauma
  - Solid organ injury
    - Patterns of blunt abdominal injury remain the same as in nonpregnant patients because the location of these organs do not change in pregnancy.
  - Urinary bladder
    - Urinary bladder is displaced anteriorly and superiorly by the gravid uterus after 12 weeks of gestation, making it an extrapelvic organ with increased risk of injury.
    - High risk of retroperitoneal bleeding in patients with pelvic fracture due to engorgement of the pelvic vessels surrounding the gravid uterus.
- Fetal injury pattern:
  - Direct fetal injury
    - Commonly due to direct blunt abdominal wall trauma
    - Abdominal wall, uterine myometrium, and amniotic fluid may act as protective barriers.
  - Indirect injury may be due to:
    - rapid compression.
    - deceleration resulting in shearing force.

INITIAL EVALUATION AND RESUSCITATION: SPECIAL CONSIDERATIONS

- Maternal evaluation and resuscitation are the priorities.
- Maternal resuscitation is important to prevent fetal hypoxia and death.
- Unstable patients should be identified and managed emergently.
- Evaluation of the fetus should be performed after maternal assessment and resuscitation.
- Evaluation follows the same algorithm as in nonpregnant patients:
  - Airway
  - Cervical spine protection
  - Breathing
  - Circulation
  - Disability
  - Exposure
- Airway
  - Fetus is very sensitive to maternal hypoxia.
  - Pregnant patients have a high-risk of hypoxia due to the following:
    - Decrease in functional residual capacity
    - Decrease in total lung capacity
    - Reduced respiratory compliance
    - Decrease in oxygen reserve
    - Marked increase (15%–20%) in basal oxygen consumption
    - Normal PaO_2: <60 mm Hg
    - Normal oxygen saturation: <95%
  - High risk of aspiration due to poor gastric emptying and relaxed lower esophageal sphincter. Early nasogastric tube placement is recommended.

- Special considerations during intubation of pregnant patients
  - Risk of bleeding due to mucosal engorgement of the nasal passage, oropharynx, larynx, and trachea
  - To avoid intubation trauma, during intubation, consider an endotracheal tube (ETT) 0.5–1 mm smaller than for nonpregnant patient to avoid intubation- related trauma.
- Spine immobilization
  - Spine immobilization technique:
    - Cervical collar for C-spine immobilization
    - Back board for spine immobilization
      - Patients with >20 weeks of gestation should be immobilized in the left lateral decubitus position with 30-degree to 50-degree tilt to avoid pressure on the inferior vena cava (IVC).
      - Pressure on the IVC can cause supine hypotensive syndrome.
- Breathing and ventilation
  - Adequate maternal breathing is essential to maintain fetal oxygenation.
  - Goal is to maintain maternal oxygen saturation >95% and PCO_2 ≤30 mm Hg.
  - Ventilatory parameters require adjustment based on the following physiological changes in pregnancy:
    - Increase in tidal volume
    - Increase in minute ventilation by 50%
    - Decrease in residual volume due to diaphragmatic elevation
    - Increased airway resistance
    - Reduced respiratory compensation for metabolic acidosis
    - Baseline respiratory alkalosis due to hyperventilation
    - Normal blood gases in pregnancy
      - pH range: 7.40–7.45
      - Bicarbonate range: 17–22 mEq/L
      - Base excess range: 3–4 mEq/L
  - Chest tube placement
    - Chest tube should be placed 1–2 intercostals higher than usual due to displacement of the diaphragm during pregnancy.
- Circulation and control of bleeding
  - Effective maternal circulatory volume is essential for fetal placental circulation.
  - Hemorrhagic shock results in uterine vasoconstriction causing fetal hypoxia.
  - High risk of fetal distress with:
    - 50% decrease in maternal hematocrit.
    - 20% decrease in maternal mean blood pressure.
  - Causes of hemorrhagic shock
    - External or internal injuries
    - Concealed uterine bleeding
  - Clinical manifestations of hemorrhagic shock are not reliable:
    - Patients may remain hemodynamically stable despite significant blood loss due to the following physiological changes in pregnancy:
      - Increase in heart rate 10–15 beats/min
      - Increase in blood volume by 45%
      - Increase in red cell mass by 25%
      - Decrease in systolic blood pressure (SBP) by 2–4 mm Hg and diastolic blood pressure (DBP) by 5–15 mm Hg in the second trimester, and it returns to normal in the third trimester.
      - Increase in cardiac output by 30%–45%

- Resuscitation of hemorrhagic shock
  - High risk of pulmonary edema from crystalloid infusion and blood transfusion due to decrease in colloid osmotic pressure in pregnancy
  - Vasopressors in pregnancy
    - Norepinephrine and epinephrine (Adrenalin) are not recommended due to the risk of fetal hypoxia from uteroplacental vasoconstriction.
    - Ephedrine
    - Safe in pregnancy
    - Increases alpha- and beta-adrenergic activities
    - Mephentermine
    - Safe in pregnancy
    - No effect on uterine perfusion
    - Inotropic effect on the myocardium
  - Supine hypotensive syndrome
    - Compression on the IVC by the gravid uterus after >20 weeks of pregnancy in supine position can result in reduced venous return causing reduced cardiac output and hypotension.
    - Pressure on the vena cava can be prevented by placement of the patient in the left lateral decubitus position with 15-degree to 30-degree tilt.
  - Blood transfusion
    - O-negative blood is recommended in Rh-negative patients to avoid Rh sensitization.
  - Patients with preeclampsia
    - Blood pressure monitoring is not a reliable sign.
    - May be associated with reduced intravascular volume
    - Risk of pulmonary edema from crystalloid infusion due to increased capillary permeability
- Disability (neurological status)
  - Differential diagnosis in pregnant patients with head injury
    - Postural hypotension with dizziness due to vasodilation in pregnancy
    - Eclampsia
      - Grand mal seizures
      - Loss of consciousness
      - Hyperreflexia
      - Headache
      - Vision changes

SECONDARY SURVEY: SPECIAL CONSIDERATIONS

- Evaluation follows the same algorithm as in nonpregnant patients.
- Detailed obstetric history is important:
  - Last menstrual period (LMP)
  - Previous pregnancies
    - Miscarriages
    - Premature deliveries
    - Abortions
    - History of delivery including complications
- Abdominal examination
  - Stretching of the abdomen and increase in intraabdominal pressure results in a desensitivity to peritoneal irritation.

- Fluid or blood in the peritoneal cavity may not show signs of peritoneal irritation as tenderness, rebound tenderness, or guarding.
- Irregular abdominal examination during palpation due to palpable fetal parts in uterine rupture.
- Assessment of the uterus
  - Height of the fundus
  - Shape of the uterus
  - Tone and tenderness
  - Uterine tenderness is an important sign of placental abruption.
- Pelvic examination
  - Pregnancy >24 weeks gestation with vaginal bleeding
    - May be due to disruption of the placenta.
    - Ultrasound should be performed first to exclude placenta previa.
    - Vaginal examination with speculum should be performed to assess the following:
      - Cervical dilatation
      - Presentation of the fetus
      - Amniotic fluid
      - Vaginal or cervical lacerations
      - Expulsion of gestational tissue
      - Ruptured membrane
- Interpretation of laboratory results
  - Anemia is normal. It is caused by an increase in plasma volume relative to the increase in red cell mass.
  - Leukocytosis is a normal. It may not be an indicator of infection.
  - Blood urea nitrogen (BUN) and creatinine decrease by half of the prepregnancy level. Normal BUN and creatinine is abnormal in normal pregnancy.
  - Normally calcium and magnesium levels are low in pregnancy.
  - Glycosuria is often physiological during pregnancy.
  - Fibrinogen level
    - Normally elevated in pregnancy
    - Hypofibrinogenemia (<2 g/L) may be due to disseminated intravascular coagulation (DIC) from placental abruption.
  - Alkaline phosphatase
    - It is secreted by the placenta.
    - Elevated levels, even twice the upper limit for nonpregnant patients, may be normal in pregnancy.
- Imaging for maternal trauma evaluation
  - Radiological evaluation of the mother is the priority despite the risk to the fetus of radiation exposure (Eastern Association for the Surgery of Trauma Guidelines (EAST], 2010).
  - The fetus should be protected with a shield whenever possible.
  - Repeat imaging should be avoided.
- Ultrasound
  - No risk of radiation exposure to the fetus
  - Intraperitoneal blood may be detected with Focused Assessment with Sonography in Trauma (FAST).
  - FAST exam becomes less accurate with increased gestational age because the gravid uterus occupies the abdominal cavity.

- Plain films
  - Low radiation exposure to the fetus
- CT scan
  - Recommended if there is significant concern for intraabdominal injury
  - Associated with fetal radiation exposure
  - Usually radiation exposure <5 rad (50 mGy) does not have any fetal adverse effect.
  - Radiation exposure
    - CT head: <0.05 rad
    - CT chest: <0.1 rad
    - CT abdomen/pelvis: <2.6 rad
  - Effects of radiation
    - Increased risk of miscarriage: Exposure before 5 weeks of gestation
    - Teratogenic effect: Exposure during the period of organogenesis (5–10 weeks of gestation)
    - Growth retardation
    - Central nervous system (CNS) effects: Exposure even after 10 weeks of gestation
    - Malignancy: Exposure even after 25 weeks of gestation
- Magnetic resonance imaging (MRI)
  - No adverse fetal effects
- Diagnostic peritoneal lavage (DPL) in pregnancy
  - May be used for the rapid detection of intraabdominal injury
  - Sensitivity: 96%–100%
  - Does not provide information about specific organ injury
  - Open technique with catheter placement above the umbilicus is recommended to minimize injury to the gravid uterus.

Must-Know Essentials: Evaluation of the Fetus in Trauma

MECHANISM OF FETAL INJURIES

- Direct injury
  - Commonly due to direct blunt abdominal wall trauma
  - Abdominal wall, uterine myometrium, and amniotic fluid may act as protective barriers.
- Indirect injury
  - Rapid compression
  - Deceleration resulting in shearing force
  - Fetal hypoxia
    - Maternal hypovolemic shock leading to fetal hypoxia
    - Maternal hypoxia
  - Fetomaternal hemorrhage (FMH)
- Risk of fetal injury increases with gestational age:
  - Less risk of injury in the first trimester due to thick-walled intrapelvic uterus
  - High risk of injury in second and third trimester due to:
    - thin-walled intraabdominal uterus.
    - thinning of the maternal abdominal wall.
    - direct contact of the uterus with the abdominal wall.

COMMON FETAL INJURIES

- Preterm delivery
- Spontaneous abortion (miscarriage)
- Direct fetal injury
- Placental abruption
- Uterine rupture
- Uteroplacental injury
- Rh isoimmunization

ULTRASOUND IN FETAL EVALUATION

- Ultrasound is used for:
  - determination of the gestational age.
  - demonstration of the fetal cardiac rate and rhythm.
  - localization of the placenta and exclusion of placenta previa.
  - determination of placental abruption:
    - Ultrasound can miss 50%–80% of traumatic placental abruption
    - Electronic fetal monitoring (EFM) is more sensitive than ultrasound in diagnosing placental abruption.
  - diagnosis of the fetal injury.
  - confirmation of fetal death.

ESTIMATION OF GESTATIONAL AGE

- May be estimated from the first day of the pregnant woman's last menstrual cycle
- Fetal gestational age may be estimated from the height of the fundus:
  - First trimester: Uterus remains in the pelvis.
  - Second trimester: At the level of the umbilicus
  - Third trimester: At the level of the costal margin
- Ultrasound: Most accurate way to determine fetal age

ESTIMATION OF FETAL VIABILITY

- Criteria for fetal viability
  - Age of the fetus: >24 weeks of gestation
  - Weight of the fetus based on ultrasound: ≥500 g
  - Presence of fetal heart tone (FHT)

ELECTRONIC FETAL MONITORING

- EFM is also called cardiotocography (CTG).
- Involves recording of the FHT and the uterine contractions
- Fetal heart tone
  - Instability of the FHT reflects maternal hemodynamic instability
  - Audible by Doppler at 10–14 weeks of gestation
  - Audible with conventional stethoscope at 20 weeks of gestation
  - Normal fetal heart rate: 120–160 beats per minute

- Nonreassuring patterns of FHT include:
  - bradycardia.
  - tachycardia.
  - deceleration.
  - loss of beat-to-beat variability.
  - recurrent decelerations.
- Uterine contractions monitoring (tocodynamometry)
  - Measures the frequency, strength, and duration of uterine contractions
  - More sensitive than ultrasound to predict placental abruption, fetal hypoxia, and preterm labor compared
  - Occasional uterine contractions are common after trauma in pregnancy, and the majority of these contractions resolve spontaneously without any adverse fetal outcome.
  - Normal uterine contraction: 1 contraction every 2–3 min or <5 contractions in 10 min
  - Abnormal uterine contraction pattern
    - Elevated basal uterine tone
    - Absent uterine contraction
    - Sustained contractions (1 contraction lasting for 10 min)
    - Less frequent contractions (1 contraction every 15 min)

INDICATION OF ADMISSION AND CONTINUOUS FETAL MONITORING

- Viable fetus after >24 weeks of gestation
- High-risk factors for fetal injury
  - Injury mechanism
    - High-speed MVC
    - Pedestrian hit by a vehicle
    - Ejection during an MVC
  - Injury Severity Score (ISS) > 9
  - Injury associated with:
    - significant maternal injury.
    - maternal injury with hypotension.
    - significant abdominal pain.
    - vaginal bleeding.
    - leakage of amniotic fluid.
    - uterine tenderness.
    - rupture of the membranes.
    - frequent uterine activity.
  - EFM with:
    - nonreassuring FHT pattern.
    - abnormal uterine contraction pattern.
  - Serum fibrinogen <200 mg/dL
- Duration of continuous EFM
  - Minor maternal injury without fetal injury: 4–6 hrs
  - High-risk factors for fetal injury: 24 hrs

Must-Know Essentials: Management of Specific Problems after Trauma in Pregnancy

EXPLORATORY LAPAROTOMY IN PREGNANCY

- Indications are the same as in nonpregnant patients.
- Cesarean section during exploratory laparotomy
  - Viable fetus with:
    - uteroplacental compromise causing fetal distress in EFM.
    - uterine injury.
  - Not indicated for a dead or injured fetus because they usually abort spontaneously or can be delivered vaginally

PERIMORTEM CESAREAN SECTION

- Defined as cesarean section during maternal cardiac arrest to resuscitate the mother and improve fetal survival
- Also called resuscitative hysterotomy
- Emptying the uterus results in improved maternal circulation.
- The fetus may survive if the procedure is performed within 4 min of maternal cardiac arrest (EAST guideline, 2005).
- Recommended if fetus is viable based on:
  - pregnancy >24 weeks of gestation.
  - fundus of the uterus at the level of the umbilicus.
  - presence of FHT.
- A neonatologist should be available at bedside.
- The procedure should be performed using a midline, vertical incision.
- Skin-to-fetus time of the procedure should not exceed >1 min.

PRETERM LABOR

- Defined as labor occurring before the 38th week of gestation
- Causes
  - Placental abruption
  - Prostaglandin release due to:
    - extravasation of blood at the placental margin causing decidual necrosis.
    - direct uterine trauma.
  - Premature rupture of membranes
- Evaluation
  - EFM
    - Nonassuring fetal heart rate
    - Frequent uterine contractions
  - Rupture of the membranes in speculum examination
- Survival of the fetus depends on the gestational age.
- Fetus with gestational age >24 weeks can survive outside the uterus.

SPONTANEOUS ABORTION (MISCARRIAGE)

- Delivery of the fetus before the 20th week of gestation
- Manifestations
  - Abdominal pain/cramp
  - Vaginal bleeding
- Evaluation
  - EFM
  - Ultrasound

PLACENTAL ABRUPTION

- Defined as partial or complete placenta–uterine separation
- Causes
  - Commonly due to direct blunt trauma to the uterus
  - Indirect trauma: Shearing force due to sudden deceleration
- Manifestations
  - Placental abruption with >50% placental separation increases the risk of:
    - fetal death.
    - preterm labor.
  - Intrauterine bleeding and fetal hypoxia
  - Vaginal bleeding in up to 70% of patients
  - Maternal hypovolemic shock
  - Uterine tenderness
  - Frequent uterine contractions
  - Occult or concealed abruption
    - Major maternal bleeding with hemorrhagic shock
    - Hypofibrinogenemia
    - DIC
- Evaluation
  - EFM
    - More sensitive than ultrasound to predict placental abruption
    - Nonreassuring pattern of FHT
    - Sustained uterine contraction in tocodynamometry
  - Uterine ultrasonography
    - May be helpful in diagnosis, but not definitive
    - Specific sonographic findings are uncommon; retroplacental hematoma is seen in 2% to 25% of abruptions.
  - CT scan
    - May show placental abruption
    - Much more sensitive than ultrasound
- Management
  - Emergent cesarean section
    - Severe placental abruption
    - Fetal or maternal distress
    - Deterioration in fetal condition
    - Maternal hemodynamic instability
  - Vaginal delivery
    - Placental abruption is often associated with rapid cervical dilation and delivery.

- Induction or augmentation of labor with a trial of vaginal birth
  - Hemodynamically stable patient
  - Near-term fetus with a normal FHT
- Nonviable fetus
  - Vaginal birth is preferable.
- Maternal bleeding and coagulation abnormalities should be aggressively treated to optimize maternal and fetal outcomes.
- Continuous fetal monitoring
  - Hemodynamically patient with viable fetus

UTERINE RUPTURE

- Uterine rupture after trauma in pregnancy is rare.
- Associated with high maternal and fetal mortality
- More common after direct abdominal trauma during the latter half of pregnancy
- Common after MVC
- Risk factors
  - Uterine scarring from:
    - cesarean section,
    - uterine surgeries
  - Uterine malformation
  - Uterine overdistention
    - Polyhydramnios
    - Multiple gestation
- Uterine fundus is the common site of rupture.
- Types of rupture
  - Complete avulsion of the uterus
  - Serosal hemorrhage
  - Uterine abrasions
  - Disruption of placenta, fetus, or umbilical cord
- Evaluation
  - Manifestations
    - Severe abdominal pain
    - Maternal hypovolemic shock
    - Abdominal tenderness, rigidity, or guarding
    - Abnormal (oblique or transverse) fetal lie
    - Irregular uterine contour
    - Easily palpable fetal parts because of their extrauterine location
  - CT abdomen
    - Abnormal fetal position
    - Free intraperitoneal air
  - Nonreassuring FHT in EFM
- Management
  - Emergent laparotomy and evacuation of the fetus with C-section

DIRECT FETAL INJURY

- Rare
- Usually after a blunt trauma
- Most common injuries

- Fetal head injury
- Fracture of the clavicle
- Associated with maternal pelvic injury
- Evaluation
  - CT scan to assess the fetus
- Management
  - C-section if viable fetus

DISSEMINATED INTRAVASCULAR COAGULATION IN PREGNANCY

- Causes of DIC
  - Placental abruption
  - Amniotic fluid embolization
- Effects
  - Consumptive coagulopathy causing:
    - hypofibrinogenemia.
    - thrombocytopenia.
    - depletion of other coagulation factors.
    - elevation of D-dimer.
- Associated with high maternal mortality
- Treatment
  - Uterine evacuation
  - Platelet transfusion
  - Fresh frozen plasma transfusion
  - Transfusion of cryoprecipitate

FETOMATERNAL HEMORRHAGE

- Fetomaternal hemorrhage (FMH) is defined as transfer of fetal blood to maternal circulation.
- FMH occurs in 10%–30% of blunt trauma patients after >12 weeks of gestation.
- Usually due to placental injury resulting in placental abruption
- Majority of FMH is small and subclinical.
- FMH from Rh-positive fetus to Rh-negative mother results in alloimmunization and risk of newborn developing hemolytic disease.
- Blood volume as little as 0.01 mL can cause isoimmunization in 70% of Rh-negative mothers.
- Massive volume transfer (>30 mL) can cause significant fetal morbidity and mortality.
- Fetal manifestations of isoimmunization
  - Decreased movements
  - Cardiac rhythm changes
  - Anemia
  - Fetal anomalies
  - Stillbirth
  - Fetal hydrops
  - Postpartum infant death
  - Massive FMH is rare and results in fetal mortality due to sudden fetal anemia and cardiac failure.
- Kleihauer-Betke (KB) test

- Quantifies FMH in patients where >30 mL of fetal blood is suspected in maternal circulation, especially in patients with placental abruption or blunt abdominal trauma after >12 weeks of gestation
- Rh immune prophylaxis
  - A single dose of anti-D IgG (RhoGAM) 300 mg IM should be given within 72 hours of injury in all Rh-negative trauma patients.
  - Provides protection against sensitization for up to 30 mL of fetal blood in the maternal circulation
  - An additional dose of RhoGAM if the KB test indicates >30 mL of transplacental hemorrhage

HEMOLYSIS, ELEVATED LIVER ENZYMES, AND LOW PLATELETS

- Acronym: HELLP syndrome
- Life-threatening condition associated with preeclampsia
- Manifestations
  - Hemolysis
  - Elevated liver enzymes
  - Low platelets
- Treatment
  - Delivery of fetus and placenta

AMNIOTIC FLUID EMBOLISM

- Manifestations
  - Dyspnea
  - Hypoxia
  - Profound hypotension
  - DIC in 50% of patients
- Cardiac echo: Right heart strain
- Treatment
  - Supportive care

CHAPTER 37

Commonly Used Scoring and Grading Systems in Trauma

Must-Know Essentials: Injury Severity Scores for Trauma Assessment

ABBREVIATED INJURY SCALE (AIS)

- An anatomical scoring system
- Each injury is ranked on a scale of 1 to 6 based on the severity of the injury.

AIS Score	Injury severity
1	Minor
2	Moderate
3	Serious
4	Severe
5	Critical
6	Unsurvivable

INJURY SEVERITY SCORE (ISS)

- An anatomical scoring system
- Provides an overall score for patients with multiple injuries
- Is the only anatomical scoring system that correlates linearly with mortality, morbidity, hospital stay, and other measures of severity
- The AIS for the following six body regions is used to calculate the ISS:
  - Head and neck
  - Face
  - Chest
  - Abdomen
  - Extremity including the pelvis
  - External
- AIS scores of the three most severely injured body regions are added and squared to calculate the ISS.
- ISS scores range from 0 to 75.
- An AIS score of 6 (unsurvivable injury) is assigned an ISS score of 75.

PEDIATRIC TRAUMA SCORE (PTS)

- Predicts pediatric trauma mortality
- A higher trauma score is associated with lower mortality.
  - A score >8 has an estimated mortality rate of 9%.

- A score ≤0 has an estimated mortality rate of 100%.
- Calculated by using weight (kg), airway, systolic blood pressure (SBP), mental status, skin injury, and fracture with a minimal score of −6 and the maximum score of +12.

Factors	+2	+1	−1
Weight (kg)	>20	10–20	<10
Airway	Patent	Oral/nasal airway Oxygen	Need for airway
Systolic blood pressure	>90 mm Hg	50–90 mm Hg	<50 mm Hg
Mental status	Awake	Obtunded	Comatose
Skin injury	None	Contusion, abrasion, laceration <7 cm not involving fascia	Tissue loss, penetrating wound involving fascia
Fracture	None	Single closed	Open or multiple

Must-Know Essentials: The American Association for the Surgery of Trauma (AAST) Grading for Traumatic Injuries

BACKGROUND FOR AAST GRADING

- Commonly used for severity of traumatic organ injuries
- Injuries grading are based on the following:
  - Imaging findings
  - Operative findings
  - Pathological criteria
- The highest grade is assigned to the most severe injury.
- Injuries are advanced by one grade up to Grade III for multiple injuries.
- Grading helps to guide the management and prognosis of the injuries.
- Commonly used for AAST grading

AAST GRADING OF SPLENIC INJURIES

Grade I	• Subcapsular hematoma: <10% surface area • Capsular tear • Laceration: <1 cm parenchymal depth
Grade II	• Subcapsular hematoma: 10%–50% surface area • Intraparenchymal hematoma: <5 cm diameter • Laceration: 1–3 cm parenchymal depth, not involving a parenchymal vessel
Grade III	• Subcapsular hematoma: >50% surface area or expanding • Ruptured subcapsular or parenchymal hematoma • Intraparenchymal hematoma: >5 cm diameter • Laceration: ≥3 cm parenchymal depth • Laceration involving trabecular vessels
Grade IV	• Laceration: Segmental or hilar vessels producing major devascularization (>25% of spleen)
Grade V	• Completely shattered spleen • Hilar vascular injury with devascularized spleen

AAST GRADING OF LIVER INJURIES

Grade I	• Subcapsular hematoma: <10% surface area • Capsular tear or parenchymal laceration <1 cm deep
Grade II	• Subcapsular hematoma: 10%–50 % surface area • Intraparenchymal laceration <10 cm diameter • Capsular tear or parenchymal laceration 1–3 cm deep, <10 cm in length
Grade III	• Subcapsular hematoma: >50% surface area • Ruptured subcapsular or parenchymal hematoma • Intraparenchymal hematoma >10 cm or expanding hematoma • Parenchymal laceration ≥3 cm deep
Grade IV	• Parenchymal laceration with disruption of 25%–75% hepatic lobe or 1–3 Couinaud's segments
Grade V	• Parenchymal laceration with disruption of >75% hepatic lobe or >3 Couinaud's segments within a single lobe • Juxtahepatic venous injury (retrohepatic vena cava/central major hepatic veins)
Grade VI	• Hepatic avulsion

AAST GRADING OF PANCREATIC INJURIES

Grade I	• Minor contusion without duct injury • Superficial laceration without duct injury
Grade II	• Major contusion without duct injury or tissue loss • Major laceration without duct injury or tissue loss
Grade III	• Distal transection (left of the superior mesenteric vessels) • Distal parenchymal injury with duct injury (left of the mesenteric vessels)
Grade IV	• Proximal transection (right of superior mesenteric vein) • Parenchymal injury involving ampulla
Grade V	• Massive disruption of the pancreatic head

AAST GRADING OF KIDNEY INJURIES

Grade I	• Subcapsular hematoma and /or parenchymal contusion without laceration
Grade II	• Perirenal hematoma confined to Gerota's fascia • Renal parenchymal laceration ≤1 cm depth without urinary extravasation
Grade III	• Renal parenchymal laceration >1 cm depth without collecting system rupture or urinary extravasation • Any injury in the presence of a kidney vascular injury or active bleeding contained within Gerota's fascia
Grade IV	• Parenchymal laceration extending into urinary collecting system with urinary extravasation • Renal pelvis laceration and/or complete ureteropelvic disruption • Segmental renal vein or artery injury • Active bleeding beyond Gerota's fascia into the retroperitoneum or peritoneum • Segmental or complete kidney infarction due to vessel thrombosis without active bleeding
Grade V	• Main renal artery or vein laceration or avulsion of hilum • Devascularized kidney with active bleeding • Shattered kidney with loss of identifiable parenchymal renal anatomy

AAST GRADING OF STOMACH INJURIES

Grade I	• Contusion /intramural hematoma • Partial thickness laceration
Grade II	• Laceration <2 cm in gastroesophageal (GE) junction or pylorus • Laceration <5 cm in proximal one-third of stomach • Laceration < 10 cm in distal two-thirds of stomach
Grade III	• Laceration >2 cm in GE junction or pylorus • Laceration >5 cm in proximal one-third of stomach • Laceration >10 cm in distal two-thirds of stomach
Grade IV	• Tissue loss or devascularization in less than two-thirds of stomach
Grade V	• Tissue loss or devascularization less than two-thirds of stomach

AAST GRADING OF DUODENAL INJURIES

Grade I	• Hematoma involving single portion of the duodenum • Partial thickness laceration, no perforation
Grade II	• Hematoma involving more than one portion of the duodenum • Laceration with disruption <50% of the circumference of the duodenum
Grade III	• Laceration with disruption of 50%–75% circumference of D2 segment of the duodenum • Laceration with disruption of 50%–100% circumference of D1, D3, D4 segment of the duodenum
Grade IV	• Laceration with disruption of >75% circumference of D2 segment of the duodenum • Laceration involving ampulla or intrapancreatic portion (distal) common bile duct
Grade V	• Laceration with massive disruption of duodenopancreatic complex • Devascularization of the duodenum

AAST GRADING OF SMALL BOWEL INJURIES

Grade I	• Minor hematoma • Partial thickness laceration
Grade II	• Full thickness laceration involving <50% of the circumference
Grade III	• Full thickness laceration involving >50 % of the circumference without complete transection
Grade IV	• Complete transection without devascularization
Grade V	• Mesenteric disruption causing devascularized bowel • Transection with segmental tissue loss

AAST GRADING OF COLON INJURIES

Grade I	• Contusion or hematoma without devascularization • Partial thickness laceration, no perforation
Grade II	• Laceration with <50 % of circumference
Grade III	• Laceration with >50% of circumference without transection
Grade IV	• Transection of colon
Grade V	• Transection of the colon with segmental tissue loss • Devascularized segment

AAST GRADING OF RECTAL INJURIES

Grade I
- Hematoma: Contusion or hematoma without devascularization
- Partial thickness laceration, no perforation

Grade II
- Laceration with <50 % of circumference

Grade III
- Laceration with >50% of circumference

Grade IV
- Full-thickness laceration with extension into the perineum

Grade V
- Devascularized segment

AAST GRADING OF URETERIC INJURIES

Grade 1
- Contusion or hematoma without devascularization

Grade II
- Transection <50%

Grade III
- Transection ≥50%

Grade IV
- Complete transection with <2 cm of devascularization

Grade V
- Avulsion with >2 cm of devascularization

AAST GRADING OF BLADDER INJURIES

Grade I
- Contusion, intramural hematoma
- Partial thickness laceration

Grade II
- Extraperitoneal bladder wall laceration <2 cm

Grade III
- Extraperitoneal (>2 cm) or intraperitoneal (<2 cm) bladder wall laceration

Grade IV
- Intraperitoneal bladder wall laceration >2 cm

Grade V
- Intraperitoneal or extraperitoneal bladder wall laceration extending into the bladder neck or ureteral orifice (trigone)

AAST GRADING OF URETHRAL INJURIES

Grade I
- Contusion: Blood at urethral meatus; urethrography normal

Grade II
- Stretch injury: Elongation of urethra without extravasation on urethrography

Grade III
- Partial disruption: Extravasation of urethrography contrast at injury site with visualization in the bladder

Grade IV
- Complete disruption: Extravasation of urethrography contrast at injury site without visualization in the bladder; <2 cm of urethra separation

Grade V
- Complete disruption: Complete transaction with >2 cm urethral separation, or extension into the prostate or vagina

Must-Know Essentials: Scoring for Evaluation of Shock

AMERICAN COLLEGE OF SURGEONS (ACS) CLASSIFICATION OF HEMORRHAGIC SHOCK

- Grading of hemorrhagic shock based on the following:
  - Approximate blood loss
  - Heart rate
  - Pulse pressure
  - Respiratory rate

- Urine output (mL/hr)
- Glasgow Coma Score
- Base deficit
- Need for blood products

Factors	Class I	Class II (Mild)	Class III (Moderate)	Class IV (Severe)
Approximate blood loss	<15%	15%–30%	30%–40%	>40%
Heart rate	Normal	Normal/High	High	High
Blood pressure	Normal	Normal	Normal/Low	Low
Pulse pressure	Normal	Low	Low	Low
Respiratory rate	Normal	Normal	Normal/Increased	Increased
Urine output (mL/hr)	Normal	Normal	Low	Very Low
Glasgow Coma Scale score	Normal	Normal	Low	Low
Base deficit	0 to −2 mEq/L	−2 to −6 mEq/L	−6 to −10 mEq/L	−10 mEq/L or less
Need for blood products	Monitor	Possible	Yes	Massive transfusion

SEQUENTIAL (SEPSIS RELATED) ORGAN FAILURE ASSESSMENT (SOFA) SCORE IN SEPTIC SHOCK

- Quick SOFA score (qSOFA)
  - 1 point for each of the following:
    - Alteration in mental status (GCS <15)
    - Systolic blood pressure ≤100 mm Hg
    - Respiratory rate ≥22 minute
  - q SOFA score of ≥2 suggests sepsis.
- The SOFA score measures organ dysfunction and predicts mortality in the ICU.
- The SOFA score should be calculated on admission to the ICU and then every 24 hrs.
- The baseline SOFA score can be assumed to be 0 in patients without preexisting organ dysfunction.
- A SOFA score ≥2 reflects an overall mortality risk of approximately 10% in a general hospital population with suspected infection.

Systems	0	1	2	3	4
Respiratory (PaO$_2$/FiO$_2$ mm Hg)	>400	<400	<300	<200 with respiratory support	<100 with respiratory support
Coagulation (platelets)	>150	<150	<100	<50	<20
Liver (bilirubin mg/dL)	<1.2	1.2–1.9	2–5.9	6–11.9	>12
Cardiovascular (mean arterial pressure [MAP] mm Hg)	>70	<70	Dopamine <5 or dobutamine any dose	Dopamine (Intropin) 5.1–15 or epinephrine <0.1 or norepinephrine <0.1	Dopamine >15 or epinephrine >0.1 or norepinephrine >0.1

Systems	0	1	2	3	4
Central nervous systems (GCS)	15	13–14	10–12	6–9	<6
Renal (creatinine mg/dL)	<1.2	1.2–1.9	2.0–3.4	3.5–4.9	>5
Urine output (mL/day)				<500	<200

Must-Know Essentials: Scoring for Chronic Liver Disease

MODEL FOR END-STAGE LIVER DISEASE (MELD) SCORE

- Used for estimation of severity and prognosis of patients with chronic liver disease
- MELD scores range from 6–40 and are calculated using the following:
  - International normalized ratio (INR)
  - Creatinine
  - Bilirubin
  - Serum sodium
- 3 months mortality based on MELD score:

MELD Score	Mortality
≥40	71.3%
30–39	52.6%
20–29	19.6%
10–19	6.0%
<9	1.9%

CHILD-PUGH SCORE

- Used for assessment of the severity of chronic liver disease
- Severity of the disease is classified based on scores that range from 5–15:
  - Class A: 5–6
  - Class B: 7–10
  - Class C: 11–15

Criteria	1 Point	2 Points	3 Points
Total bilirubin	<2 mg/dL	2–3 mg/dL	>3 mg/dL
Albumin	>3 g/dL	2–3 g/dL	≤3 g/dL
INR	<1.7	1.7–2.2	>2.2
Ascites	Absent	Slight	Moderate
Encephalopathy	Absent	Grades 1–2	Grades 3–4

Must-Know Essentials: Scoring System for Head Injury

ADULT GLASGOW COMA SCALE (GCS)

- The Glasgow Coma Scale (GCS) is used to describe the extent of impaired consciousness.
- Assessment is based on eye-opening, motor, and verbal responses.
- GCS has a total score of 15.
- Based on the GCS score, traumatic brain Injury (TBI) can be classified thus:
  - Mild TBI score: 13–15
  - Moderate TBI score: 9–12
  - Severe TBI score: 3–8

Adult Glasgow Coma Scale (GCS) Criteria	Features	Scores
Best eye-opening response (E)	Spontaneous	4
	To speech	3
	To Pain	2
	None	1
Best verbal response (V)	Oriented	5
	Confused conversation	4
	Inappropriate words	3
	Incomprehensible	2
Best motor response (M)	Obeys commands	6
	Localizes pain	5
	Flexion withdrawal to pain	4
	Abnormal flexion (decorticate)	3
	Extension (Decerebrate)	2
	None (flaccid)	1

PEDIATRIC GLASGOW COMA SCALE (GCS)

Pediatric Glasgow Coma Scale (GCS) Criteria	Features	Scores
Best eye-opening response (E)	Spontaneous	4
	To sound	3
	To pain	2
	None	1
Best verbal response (V)	Age-appropriate vocalization, smile, or orientation to sound; interacts, follows objects	5
	Cries, irritable	4
	Cries to pain	3
	Moans to pain	2
	None	1
Best motor response (M)	Spontaneous movements (obeys verbal command)	6
	Withdraws to touch (localizes pain)	5
	Withdraws to pain	4
	Abnormal flexion to pain (decorticate posture)	3
	Abnormal extension to pain (decerebrate posture)	2
	None	1

FULL OUTLINE OF UNRESPONSIVENESS (FOUR) SCORE

- Useful for assessing consciousness in intubated trauma patients where components of GCS cannot be assessed
- Has a good correlation with GCS
- Low score <4 has better predictive value of mortality and morbidity compared to GCS.

Criteria	Features	Scores
Eye response (E)	Eyelids open or opened, tracking, or blinking to command	4
	Eyelids open but not tracking	3
	Eyelids closed but open to loud voice	2
	Eyelids closed but open to pain	1
	Eyelids remain closed to pain	0
Motor response (M)	Follows commands (thumbs up, fist, or peace sign)	4
	Localizes pain	3
	Flexion response to pain	2
	Extension response to pain	1
	No response to pain or generalized myoclonus status	0
Brainstem reflexes (B)	Pupillary and corneal reflexes present	4
	One pupil wide and fixed to light	3
	Pupillary or corneal reflexes absent	2
	Pupillary and corneal reflexes absent	1
	Pupillary, corneal, and cough reflexes absent	0
Respiration (R)	Not intubated; regular breathing pattern	4
	Not intubated; Cheyne-Stokes breathing pattern	3
	Not intubated; irregular breathing pattern	2
	Intubated (endotracheal or tracheostomy tube); breathing faster than ventilator rate	1
	Breathing at ventilator rate or is apneic	0

Must-Know Essentials: Grading for Spine Injuries

AMERICAN SPINAL INJURY ASSOCIATION (ASIA) IMPAIRMENT SCALE

- Commonly used for spinal cord injury
- Defines the extent and severity of the spinal cord injury
- Should be completed within 72 hours after the initial injury
- Scores are based on motor function grades from 0–4 and sensory function grades from 0–2:
  - Motor Scores
    - Grade 0: Total paralysis
    - Grade 1: Palpable or visible contraction
    - Grade 2: Active movement, gravity eliminated
    - Grade 3: Active movement against gravity
    - Grade 4: Active movement against some resistance
    - Grade 5: Normal, corrected for pain or disuse
  - Sensory Scores
    - Grade 0: Absent sensation
    - Grade 1: Altered
    - Grade 2: Normal sensation

ASIA Impairment Scale	Neurological deficit
A	• Complete: No motor or sensory function including sacral segments (S4–S5) below the level of injury.
B	• Incomplete: Some sensory function including sacral segments (S4-S5) but not motor function below the level of injury.
C	• Incomplete: Motor function is preserved below the neurological level, and more than half of key muscles below the neurological level have a muscle grade less than 3 (no movements against the gravity).
D	• Incomplete: Motor function is preserved below the neurological level, and at least half of key muscles below the neurological level have a muscle grade of 3 or more (can move against gravity).
E	• Normal: Motor and sensory functions are normal.

THORACOLUMBAR INJURY CLASSIFICATION AND SEVERITY (TLICS) SCALE

- Scoring system is based on the following:
  - Injury mechanism
  - Fracture morphology
  - Integrity of the posterior ligamentous complex
  - Presence of neurological injury
- Treatment recommendation based on TLICS scale
  - Scale <4: Nonsurgical management
  - Scale 4: Indeterminate (both nonsurgical and surgical) managements acceptable
  - Scale >4: Surgical management

Criteria	Features	Scores
Injury mechanism/fracture morphology (based on CT scan)	Compression	1
	Burst	2
	Translation/rotation	3
	Distraction	4
Integrity of the posterior ligamentous complex (based on MRI)	Intact	0
	Suspected/indeterminate	2
	Injured	3
Neurological status (physical exam)	Intact	0
	Nerve root	2
	Complete cord injury	2
	Incomplete cord injury	3
	Cauda equina	3

Must-Know Essentials: Scoring and Grading for Musculoskeletal Injuries

MANGLED EXTREMITY SEVERITY SCORE (MESS)

- Used for prediction for amputation after lower- or upper-extremity injuries
- Score doubled for limb ischemia >6 hrs

- MESS score of 7 or more has a 100% predictability of amputation and is used as a cutoff point for amputation.

Injuries	Features	Scores
Skeletal /Soft tissue injury	Low energy (stab wound/simple closed fracture/civilian gunshot wound)	1
	Medium energy (open or multiple fractures/dislocation/ moderate crush injury)	2
	High energy (close-range gunshot wound/military gunshot wounds/high-speed motor-vehicle-collision [MVC] wound) Severe crush injury	3
	Very high energy (high-speed MVC wound with gross contamination/soft-tissue avulsion	4
Limb ischemia	Pulse reduced with normal perfusion	1
	Pulseless/paresthesia/diminished capillary refill	2
	Cool/paralyzed/insensate/numbness	3
Shock	Systolic blood pressure (SBP) constantly >90 mm Hg	0
	Transient hypotension	1
	Persistent hypotension	2
Age (Years)	<30	0
	30–50	1
	>50	2

GUSTILO-ANDERSON CLASSIFICATION OF OPEN FRACTURES

- Useful for the treatment guidelines and prediction of outcome

Type	Description
Type I	• Skin laceration <1 cm with minimal soft tissue injury • Clean wound • Simple bone fracture with minimal communication
Type II	• Skin laceration >1 cm with moderate soft tissue injury • No associated flap or avulsion • Minimal crushing • Moderate communication and contamination
Type III	• Laceration >10 cm long • Exposed bones • Missing soft tissue • Neurovascular involvement • High-speed crush injury • Segmental diaphyseal loss • Wound from high-velocity weapon • Extensive contamination of the wound bed • Any size of open injury with farm contamination
A	• Extensive laceration of soft tissues with covered bone fragments • Usually, high-speed traumas with severe comminution or segmental fractures • Soft-tissue coverage facilitated by primary closure despite soft tissue-laceration, and flap
B	• Extensive loss of soft tissues with periosteal stripping, exposed bones, and contamination • Severe comminution due to high-speed traumas • Usually requires coverage of exposed bone with a local or free flap
C	• Extensive fracture with arterial damage that requires repair for limb salvage

Must-Know Essentials: Grading and Scoring for Operative Management Outcome

AMERICAN SOCIETY OF ANESTHESIOLOGISTS (ASA) PHYSICAL STATUS CLASSIFICATION SYSTEM

- Used for the assessment of patient's preanesthesia medical comorbidities
- Based on multiple factors

ASA Class	Definition	Comorbidities
I	Normal healthy patient	No acute/chronic disease, no smoking, minimal alcohol, normal BMI
II	Mild systemic disease	Mild disease without substantive functional limitation, current smoker, social alcohol, well-controlled diabetes/hypertension (HTN), obesity (body mass index [BMI] <40), mild lung disease
III	Severe systemic disease	Moderate to severe disease with substantive functional limitation, poorly controlled diabetes/HTN/ chronic obstructive pulmonary disease (COPD), obesity (BMI >40), alcohol dependence, implanted pacemaker, renal disease on dialysis, >3 months history of myocardial infarction (MI), cerebrovascular accident (CVA), coronary stents
IV	Severe systemic disease with constant threat to life	Recent history (<3 months MI, CVA, coronary stents), ongoing cardiac ischemia, severe valve dysfunction, severe reduction of ejection fraction, shock, sepsis, acute respiratory distress syndrome (ARDS)
V	Moribund patient not expected to survive without operation	Massive trauma, ruptured abdominal/thoracic aneurysm, intracranial bleeding with mass effect, ischemic bowel with significant cardiac pathology or multiple systems/organ dysfunction
VI	Declared brain dead, organs being removed for donor purposes	

FRAILTY SCORE

- Frailty is a measurement of physiological reserve in older patients.
- Frailty in older patients (>65) predicts postoperative outcomes such as the following:
  - Postoperative complications
  - Length of stay
  - Discharge to a skilled nursing or assisted living facility
- A frailty score has been recommended by the American College of Surgeons and American Geriatric Society for an optimal preoperative assessment in patients >65 years.
- The frailty score is calculated based on weakness, weight loss, exhaustion, low physical activity, and slowed walking speed. One point is assigned for each abnormality.

- Frailty is scored on a scale of 0–5:
  - Nonfrail score: 0–1
  - Intermediate or prefrail score: 2–3
  - Frail score: 4–5

Frailty criteria	Measurement	Score
Shrinking (weight loss)	• ≥10 pounds weight loss in past year	1
Weakness	• Grip strength <20th percentile adjusted for gender and BMI	1
Exhaustion	• Exhaustion measurement based on response to questions about effort and motivation	1
Slowness	• Walking speed for 15 feet <20th percentile adjusted for gender and height	1
Low activity	• Low physical activity based on leisure time <20th percentile	1

CLAVIEN-DINDO CLASSIFICATION

- Used to define and grade postoperative adverse events
- Based on the type of treatment needed for postoperative complications

Grades	Definition
I	• Any deviation from the normal postoperative course without the need for pharmacological treatment or surgical, endoscopic, and radiological interventions • Allowed therapeutic regimens, including drugs such as antiemetics, antipyretics, analgesics, diuretics, and electrolytes; physiotherapy; and wound infections opened at the bedside
II	• Requiring pharmacological treatment with drugs other than those allowed for Grade I complications • Blood transfusions and total parenteral nutrition also included
IIIa	• Requiring surgical, endoscopic, or radiological intervention without general anesthesia
IIIb	• Requiring surgical, endoscopic, or radiological intervention under general anesthesia
IVa	• Single-organ life-threatening complication (including central nervous system [CNS] complications such as stroke, transient ischemic attack [TIA], brain hemorrhage) requiring intermediate care or intensive care management
IVb	• Multiorgan life-threatening complication (including CNS complications such as stroke, TIA, brain hemorrhage) requiring intermediate care or intensive care management
V	• Death of patient

CHAPTER 38

Medications in Emergency Trauma Management

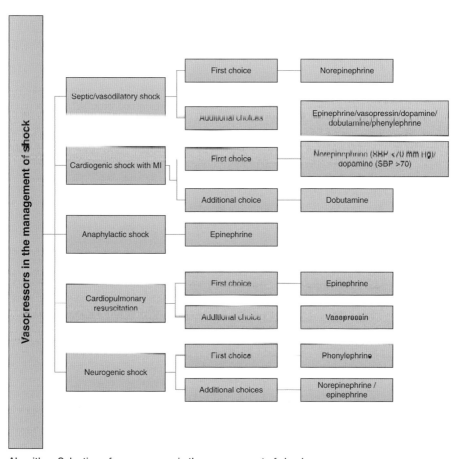

Algorithm: Selection of vasopressors in the management of shock

Must-Know Essentials: Vasopressor Agents

SELECTION OF VASOPRESSORS IN SHOCK

- Septic/vasodilatory shock
  - First choice
    - Norepinephrine

- Additional choices
  - Epinephrine may be added to or replaced the Norepinephrine.
  - Vasopressin
    - Low-dose vasopressin may be added to decrease requirements for other adrenergic agents.
    - It is not recommended as a single agent.
    - Recommended in patients unresponsive to catecholamines or in the presence of acidosis/hypoxia
  - Dopamine
    - May be considered in patients with bradycardia or in patients without risk for or presence of tachyarrhythmias
  - Dobutamine
    - Norepinephrine with Dobutamine can be used in patients with myocardial dysfunction resulting in low cardiac output.
  - Phenylephrine
    - May be considered in patients with serious tachyarrhythmias due to norepinephrine
    - May be considered in patients with persistent hypotension with high cardiac output
- Cardiogenic shock with myocardial infarction (MI)
  - First choice
    - Norepinephrine
      - Patients with severe hypotension (systolic blood pressure [SBP] <70 mm Hg)
    - Dopamine (Intropin)
      - Patients with SBP between 70–100 mm Hg
      - May increase the risk of arrhythmias
  - Additional choice
    - Dobutamine
      - May be given to improve cardiac output, but not recommended for patients with hypotension
      - Agent of choice in low output with increased afterload
- Anaphylactic shock
  - First choice
    - Epinephrine
- Cardiopulmonary resuscitation (CPR)
  - First choice
    - Epinephrine
  - Additional choice
    - Vasopressin for refractory pulseless cardiac arrest
- Neurogenic shock
  - First choice
    - Phenylephrine
      - Commonly used
      - Causes peripheral vasoconstriction due to alpha-1 effect
      - May cause reflex bradycardia due to lack of beta activity and unopposed vagal tone
  - Additional choice
    - Norepinephrine
      - Preferred in patients with hypotension and bradycardia due to its alpha and beta activities
    - Epinephrine
      - May be considered in refractory hypotension

RECEPTORS FOR VASOACTIVE DRUGS

- Alpha-1 adrenergic receptors
  - Peripheral arterial and venous vasoconstriction
  - Constriction of gastrointestinal and urinary sphincters
- Alpha-2 adrenergic receptors
  - Reduce central and peripheral sympathetic outflow
  - Mainly found in the brain
- Beta-1 adrenergic receptors
  - Increase the strength of cardiac contractions (inotropic effect)
  - Increase heart rate (chronotropic effect)
- Beta-2 receptors
  - Mainly located in bronchioles and skeletal muscles
  - Causes vasodilation and bronchodilation
- Dopamine receptors
  - Renal and splanchnic vasodilation
- Vasopressin receptors
  - V-1
    - Causes vascular smooth muscle contraction leading to vasopressor effect
  - V-2
    - Located primarily in the kidney, causing water retention due to its antidiuretic effect
  - V-3:
    - Located in the central nervous system, modulates corticotrophin secretion

CARDIOVASCULAR EFFECTS OF COMMONLY USED VASOPRESSORS

Cardiovascular Effects of Commonly Used Vasopressors

Agents	Alpha-1 effect	Beta-1 effect	Beta-2 effect	Dopamine effect	Heart Rate	Mean Arterial Pressure (MAP)	Cardiac Output	Systemic Vascular Resistance
Epinephrine	| | |	++++	+++	-	++	++	+++	++
Norepinephrine	++++	+++	-	-	+/-	+++	-	+++
Dopamine	++	++++	++	++++	-/+/++	-/+	+/++	-/+
Dobutamine	+	++++	++	-	+	+	+	-
Phenylephrine	++++	-	-	-	-	+	+/-	+
Vasopressin	-	-	-	-	-	+	-	++

EPINEPHRINE

- Alpha, beta-1, and beta -2 effects
- Cardiovascular effects
  - Increase in heart rate (HR)
  - Increase in mean arterial pressure (MAP)
  - Increase in cardiac output (CO)
  - Increase in systemic vascular resistance (SVR)
- Effects are dose dependent.
- Increasing the dose is predominantly associated with the alpha effect.
- Dose

- Shock
  - Starting dose 0.1 µg/kg/min, titrated to achieve the target effect
- Cardiopulmonary resuscitation (CPR):
  - Dose: 1 mg intravenous (IV) or intraosseous (IO), predominantly alpha effects
  - Shockable rhythm: ventricular fibrillation/primary ventricular fibrillation (VF/pVF)
    - First should be given after the second defibrillation
  - Nonshockable rhythm: pulseless electrical activity (PEA; asystole)
    - First dose should be given at the onset of cardiac resuscitation.
  - Continued 1 mg IV/IO every 3–5 min until return of the circulation
- Side effects
  - Increase in myocardial oxygen demand
  - Mesenteric ischemia
    - More common than other vasopressors
  - Increase in lactate regardless of hypoxia/hypoperfusion
    - Increase in adenosine triphosphatase (ATPase)
    - Increase in adenosine triphosphate (ATP) production from glycolysis for the ATPase activity.
    - Glycolysis produces lactic acid.
  - Vasoconstriction of the uteroplacental vasculature leading to placental hypoperfusion and fetal hypoxia; should be avoided in pregnancy

NOREPINEPHRINE

- Alpha and beta-1 effects
- A low dose stimulates both alpha- and beta-adrenergic receptors, causing:
  - an increase in MAP.
  - an increase in HR.
  - an increase in SVR.
- A high dose predominantly stimulates alpha receptors, causing:
  - minimal effect on the HR.
  - bradycardia.
  - an increase in SVR.
  - a reduction in cardiac output due to increase in afterload.
- Dose
  - Starting dose
    - 0.05 µg/kg/min, titrated to achieve the target effect
  - Low dose
    - 2.5–5 mcg/min
  - High dose
    - >5 mcg/min
- Side effects
  - Inadvertent boluses may precipitate profound hypertension that may cause myocardial infarction and cerebral ischemia.
  - Tachycardia is uncommon in adequately resuscitated patients.
  - Reflex bradycardia
  - Renal ischemia resulting in decreased urine output
  - Mesenteric ischemia
  - Increase in blood glucose
  - Extravasation of norepinephrine may cause tissue necrosis.
    - Treated with phentolamine 5–10 mg in 10 mL of normal saline injection into the area of extravasation within 12 hr

■ Vasoconstriction of the uteroplacental vasculature leading to placental hypoperfusion and fetal hypoxia. It should be avoided in pregnancy.

DOPAMINE

- Dopaminergic, alpha-1, and beta-1 effects
- Not the first-line agent for the alpha effect
- Dose
  - Range
    - 2–25 µg/kg/min
  - Beta dose
    - 5–10 mcg/kg/min, titrated to target HR, BP, or cardiac output
  - Alpha dose
    - >10 mcg/kg/min, titrated to target BP
  - Low dose (dopaminergic)
    - Does have renal protection effect
    - Does not improve renal function
    - May have some diuretic effect
- Side effects
  - Tachycardia
  - Arrhythmias
  - Wide QRS
  - Increase in myocardial oxygen consumption
  - Decrease in peripheral perfusion
    - Acute kidney injury (doses >20 hlsug/kg/min)
    - Mesenteric ischemia
  - Increase in blood glucose
  - Fixed, dilated pupils
  - Extravasation of dopamine (Intropin) can cause tissue necrosis.
    - Treated with injection of phentolamine 5–10 mg in 10 mL of normal saline injection into the area of extravasation within 12 hr

DOBUTAMINE

- Synthetic catecholamine, which is similar in structure to dopamine
- Beta-1, beta-2, and ± alpha adrenergic effects
- No dopaminergic effect
- More prominent inotropic effects than chronotropic effects
- Beta-2 vasodilator effect dominates over the alpha-1 constrictor effect in higher doses, causing reduction in SVR
- Increase CO due to:
  - positive inotropic effect.
  - decrease in peripheral resistance from vasodilatory effect.
- Dose
  - Initial infusion: 1–2 mcg/kg/min, titrated to the response
  - Maximum does: 20 mcg/kg/min
- Side effects
  - Significant tachycardia and hypertension
  - Hypotension in inadequately resuscitated patients

- Ectopic heartbeats
- Extravasation causes local blanching, tissue ischemia, or necrosis. It is treated with phentolamine.

PHENYLEPHRINE

- Alpha-adrenergic effect
- May be used in patients with hypotension due to vasodilation and adequate cardiac output
- It causes the following:
  - Increase in MAP
  - Increase in SVR
  - Increase in central venous pressure (CVP)
- Dose
  - Shock
    - 0.1–0.5 mg as slow IV direct injection every 10–15 min (or 1–10 mg intramuscular/subcutaneous every 1–2 hr)
  - Paroxysmal supraventricular tachycardia (PSVT)
    - 0.5–1 mg as rapid intravenous injection every 60–90 sec
- Side effects
  - Bradycardia
  - Arrhythmias
  - Increase in myocardial oxygen consumption
  - Peripheral or mesenteric ischemia

VASOPRESSIN

- V-1 receptors effect
  - Vasoconstriction of the systemic, splanchnic, renal, and coronary vessels via noradrenergic pathway
  - Increase in MAP
  - Increase in SVR
- V-2 receptors effect
  - Antidiuretic effect in the kidney causing water retention
- V-3 receptors effect
  - Modulates corticotropin secretion in the central nervous system
- Dose
  - Shock
    - 0.03 U/min; titrate to response
  - Septic shock:
    - 0.9–1.8 U/hr, run at a fixed rate
  - Refractory pulseless cardiac arrest
    - 40 units IV X 1 dose
- Side effects
  - GI ischemia
  - Cardiac effects
    - Coronary ischemia
    - Bradycardia
    - Arrhythmias

- Decrease in cardiac output
- Fluid retention

MILRINONE

- Phosphodiesterase inhibitor acts by causing an increase in intracellular cyclic adenosine monophosphate (cAMP) and calcium.
- Effects
  - Improves cardiac output due to inotropic effect, and reduces afterload
  - Improves right heart function due to:
    - diastolic relaxation leading to right heart filling.
    - reduction in right atrial pressure and mean pulmonary artery pressure.
    - dilation of coronary arteries.
  - Pulmonary vasodilator
- Uses
  - To improve cardiac output in patients with:
    - adrenergic receptors dysfunction due to downregulation or deacnsitization from chronic heart failure or use of beta blockers.
    - pulmonary hypertension.
    - severe congestive heart failure (CHF) refractory to other medical therapy.
  - Due to risk of worsening outflow obstruction, it is not recommended in patients with:
    - hypertrophic cardiomyopathy.
    - significant aortic valve disorder.
    - significant pulmonary valve disorder.
- Dose
  - Hemodynamic effects are dose related.
  - 50 mcg/Kg bolus over 10 min, followed by an infusion, or an infusion without a bolus
  - Infusion: 0.25–0.75 mcg/kg per min
- Side effects
  - Ventricular arrhythmias
  - Supraventricular arrhythmias
  - Hypotension due to decreased peripheral vascular resistance
  - Hypokalemia
  - Thrombocytopenia

MIDODRINE

- An alpha receptors agonist causing vasoconstriction
- Given orally
- Side effects
  - Bradycardia
  - Fainting
  - Dizziness

Must-Know Essentials: Medications in the Management of Cardiac Arrhythmias

CARDIAC RHYTHM DISORDERS

- Bradycardia
  - Sinus bradycardia
  - First-degree AV block

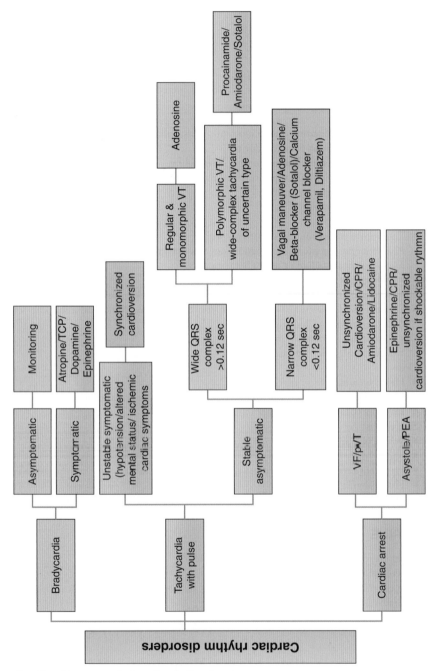

Algorithm: Management of cardiac rhythm disorders

- Second-degree AV block:
    - Mobitz type I (Wenckebach phenomenon)
    - Mobitz type II
- Third-degree atrioventricular (AV) block
- Tachycardia
    - Narrow QRS complex (<0.12 sec) supraventricular tachycardia
        - Regular rhythm
            - Sinus tachycardia
            - Atrial flutter
            - AV nodal reentry
        - Irregular rhythm
            - Atrial fibrillation (AF)
            - Atrial flutter with variable block
            - Atrial tachycardia with variable block
            - Multifocal atrial tachycardia
    - Wide QRS complex (≥0.12 sec) tachycardia
        - Regular rhythm
            - Monomorphic ventricular Tachycardia (VT)
            - Supraventricular tachycardia (SVT) with aberrancy
        - Irregular rhythm
            - AF with aberrancy
            - Preexcited AF (AF + Wolff-Parkinson-White syndrome [WPW])
            - Polymorphic VT
            - Torsades de pointes
            - Ventricular fibrillation (VF)

MANIFESTATIONS OF CARDIAC RHYTHM DISORDERS

- Asymptomatic
- Unstable patients with acute signs/symptoms
    - Ischemic chest discomfort
    - Hypotension
    - Cardiogenic shock
    - Acute heart failure
- Acute cardiac arrest
    - VF
    - Pulseless ventricular tachycardia (pVT)
    - Asystole
    - Pulseless electrical activity (PEA)

MANAGEMENT OF BRADYCARDIA

- Atropine
    - First choice
    - Dose: 1 mg IV bolus, repeated every 3–5 min until maximum dose of 3 mg
    - Mechanism of action
        - Anticholinergic (parasympatholytic) drug
        - Inhibits muscarinic acetylcholine receptors

- Dopamine
  - May be used if atropine does not work
  - May be considered with or without transcutaneous pacemaker
  - Dose: 5–20 mcg/min infusion, titrated to patient response, tapered slowly
  - Mechanism of action
    - Chronotropic effect
- Epinephrine
  - May be used if atropine does not work
  - May be considered with or without transcutaneous pacemaker (TCP)
  - Dose: 2–10 mcg/min infusion, titrated to patient response
  - Mechanism of action
    - Chronotropic effect

MANAGEMENT OF TACHYCARDIA WITH PULSE

- Unstable symptomatic patient
  - Synchronized cardioversion
  - Refractory to synchronized cardioversion
    - Synchronized cardioversion with increased level of energy
    - Antiarrhythmic drugs infusion
      - Procainamide
      - Amiodarone
      - Sotalol
- Stable wide QRS complex with regular monomorphic VT
  - Adenosine
    - First dose: 6 mg rapid IV push followed by 20 mL normal saline IV flush
    - Second dose: if no conversion to sinus rhythm within 1–2 min: 12 mg IV push
    - If necessary: another 12 mg IV
    - Maximum total recommended dose: 30 mg
- Stable wide QRS complex polymorphic VT, uncertain type of VT
  - Procainamide
    - Antiarrhythmic effect
    - Dose
      - Infusion: 20–50 mg/min until arrhythmia is terminated
      - Maximum dose: 17 mg/kg
      - Maintenance dose: 1–4 mg/min
    - Infusion should be stopped for any of the following:
      - Hypotension
      - 50% increase in QRS duration
      - Contraindicated in patients with prolonged QT interval, torsades de pointes, second- or third-degree AV block
  - Amiodarone
    - Antiarrhythmic effect
    - Dose
      - First dose: 150 mg IV bolus over 10 min
      - Repeated every 10–30 min as needed for VT recurrence
      - Maintenance: Infusion of 1 mg/min IV for first 6 hr

- Sotalol
  - Antiarrhythmic effect
  - Dose: 100 mg (1.5 mg/kg) IV over 5 min.
  - Avoid if prolonged QT interval
- Stable narrow QRS complex
  - Regular rhythm
    - Vagal maneuver
    - Adenosine
      - First dose: 6 mg rapid IV push followed by 20 mL normal saline IV flush
      - Second dose: 12 mg IV push if no conversion to sinus rhythm within 1–2 min
      - Another 12 mg IV if necessary
      - Maximum total recommended dose: 30 mg
  - Irregular rhythm
    - Sotalol
      - Long-acting AV nodal beta blocker
      - Dose: 100 mg (1.5 mg/kg) IV over 5 min
    - Verapamil
      - Long-acting AV nodal blocking agent
      - Nondihydropyridine calcium channel blocker
      - Dose
        - Initial dose: 2.5–5 mg IV bolus over 2 min
        - Second dose: 5–10 mg (approximately 0.15 mg/kg) may be given after 15–30 min if no response to initial treatment
        - Maximum total dose: 20–30 mg
    - Diltiazem
      - Long-acting AV nodal blocking agent
      - Nondihydropyridine calcium channel blocker
      - Dose
        - Bolus: 0.25 mg/kg (average adult dose, 20 mg) IV bolus over 2 min
        - Repeat dose: 0.35 mg/kg (average adult dose, 25 mg) IV bolus over 2 min if inadequate response after the first dose
        - IV infusion: 10–15 mg/hr up to 24 hr

MANAGEMENT OF CARDIAC ARREST

- VF/pVT
  - CPR per Advanced Cardiac Life Support (ACLS) protocol
  - Drugs used during CPR
    - Epinephrine (Adrenalin)
      - 1 mg every 3–5 min IV/IO
    - Amiodarone
      - First dose: 300 mg bolus IV/IO
      - Second dose: 150 mg IV/IO
    - Lidocaine
      - Alternative to amiodarone
      - Mechanism of action
        - Suppresses the automaticity of conduction tissue
        - Inhibits depolarization and conduction by blocking sodium permeability of the neuronal membrane

- Dose
  - First dose: 1–1.5 mg/kg IV/IO
  - Second dose: 0.5–0.75 mg/kg IV/IO
- Magnesium sulfate
  - Used for torsades de pointes with prolonged QT interval during CPR
  - Mechanism of action
    - Sodium/potassium pump agonist
    - Suppression of calcium channels
    - Suppression of ventricular tachyarrhythmias after depolarization
- Dose
  - Loading dose: 1–2 g diluted in 10 mL of normal saline/dextrose 5% solution (D5W) IV/IO bolus over 20 min
- Asystole /PEA
  - Epinephrine
    - 1 mg every 3–5 min IV/IO
  - CPR
    - Per ACLS protocol

ADENOSINE

- Mode of action
  - Reduction of conduction time of the AV node by activation of potassium efflux, and inhibition of calcium influx in the nodal cardiac cells
  - Terminates 90% of reentry arrhythmias within 2 min
  - Adenosine does not terminate atrial flutter and AF but slows AV conduction.
- Uses
  - Regular wide QRS complex monomorphic VT
  - Regular narrow QRS complex tachycardia
- Dose
  - First dose: 6 mg rapid IV push followed by 20 mL normal saline IV flush
  - Second dose: if no conversion to sinus rhythm within 1–2 min: 12 mg IV push
  - Another dose: 12 mg IV if necessary
  - Maximum total recommended dose: 30 mg
- Side effects
  - Transient facial flushing
  - Transient dyspnea
  - Bronchoconstriction in patients with asthma
  - Heart block

AMIODARONE

- Mechanism of action
  - Action similar to beta blocker and calcium channel blocker on sinoatrial (SA) and atrioventricular (AV) nodes:
    - Slows heart rate
    - Slows AV nodal conduction
  - Prolongs the refractory periods of the ventricles, bundles of His, and Purkinje fibers via potassium and sodium channel blockade
  - Slows intracardiac conduction via sodium channel blockade
  - Prolongs QT interval

- Uses:
  - Stable VT
  - VF
  - AF
  - PSVT
  - Secondary prevention of life-threatening ventricular arrhythmias
  - Long-term treatment of AF
- Doses
  - Life-threatening arrhythmias
    - Bolus: 150 mg IV over 10 min, if necessary repeated in 10–30 min
    - Maintenance
      - 1 mg per min for 6 hr
      - 0.5 mg per min for 18 hr
    - Reduce IV dosage or convert to oral dosing when possible
  - Secondary prevention of ventricular arrhythmia
    - Dose
      - Initial: 800–1600 mg/day oral in divided doses until a total of 10 g has been given
      - Maintenance: 200–400 mg/day oral
  - Atrial fibrillation
    - Dose
      - Initial: 600–800 mg/day oral in divided doses until a total of 10 g has been given
      - Maintenance: 200 mg/day oral
- Side effects
  - Tremor
  - Nausea
  - Constipation
  - Bradycardia
  - QT prolongation
  - Torsades de pointes
  - Interstitial pneumonitis
  - Pulmonary fibrosis
  - Thyroid dysfunction
    - Hypothyroidism: more common
    - Hyperthyroidism: less common
  - Corneal micro deposits (whorl keratopathy)
    - Optic neuropathy
    - Light-sensitive blue-grey discoloration
    - Peripheral neuropathy
- Contraindications
  - Pregnancy
  - Breast-feeding women
  - Sinus nodal bradycardia
  - Atrioventricular block
  - Polymorphic ventricular tachycardia due to worsening of prolonged QT interval
  - Second- and third-degree heart block
  - Digitalis-induced toxicity

PROCAINAMIDE

- Mechanism of action

- Inhibits recovery after repolarization by binding fast sodium channels
- Reduces impulse conduction and decreases myocardial contractility
- Uses
  - Stable wide QRS complex polymorphic VT
  - Stable wide QRS complex tachycardia of uncertain type
- Dose
  - Infusion: 20–50 mg/min until arrhythmia is terminated
  - Maximum dose: 17 mg/kg
  - Maintenance dose: 1–4 mg/min
  - Infusion should be stopped for any of the following:
    - Hypotension
    - 50% increase in QRS duration
- Side effects
  - Bradycardia
  - Hypotension
  - Drug-induced lupus erythematosus–like syndrome
  - Prolonged QRS complex
  - Prolonged QT interval
  - PR prolongation (time from the onset of the P wave to the start of the QRS complex)
  - Contraindicated in patients with prolonged QT interval, torsades de pointes, second- or third-degree AV block.

VERAPAMIL

- Mechanism of action
  - Nondihydropyridine calcium channel blocker at the AV node and slows AV conduction
- Uses
  - PSVT
  - AF
  - Atrial flutter
  - Preexcited AF (AF + WPW)
- Dose
  - 2.5–5 mg IV bolus over 2 min
  - Second dose: 5–10 mg (approximately 0.15 mg/kg) may be given after 15–30 min if no response to initial treatment
  - Maximum total dose: 20–30 mg
- Side effects
  - First-degree AV block
  - Hypotension
  - Should not be used in patients with severe left ventricular dysfunction or hypertrophic cardiomyopathy due to negative inotropic effects

DILTIAZEM

- Mechanism of action
  - Nondihydropyridine calcium channel blocker
  - Inhibits calcium influx into cardiac and vascular smooth muscle during depolarization
  - Slows AV conduction

- Uses
  - AF
  - Atrial flutter
  - PSVT
  - Preexcited AF (AF + WPW)
- Dose
  - Bolus
    - First dose: 0.25 mg/kg (average adult dose, 20 mg) IV bolus over 2 min
    - Repeat dose if inadequate after the first dose: 0.35 mg/kg (average adult dose, 25 mg) IV bolus over 2 min
    - IV infusion: 10–15 mg/hr up to 24 hr
- Side effects
  - AV block
  - Bradyarrhythmia
  - Hypotension
  - CHF
- Contraindications
  - Congestive heart failure
  - SA node or AV conduction disturbances
  - Peripheral artery occlusive disease
  - Drug-induced lupus
  - Chronic obstructive pulmonary disease (COPD)

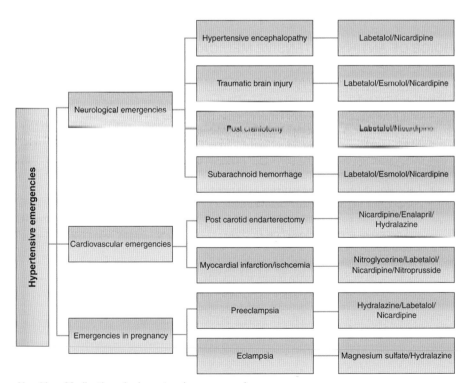

Algorithm: Medications for hypertensive emergencies

Must-Know Essentials: Antihypertensive Medications

DEFINITION OF HYPERTENSIVE EMERGENCIES

- Hypertensive emergency
  - Severe hypertension (BP >180/110 mm Hg) with acute end organ damage (actual or threatened)
- Severe hypertension (BP >180/110 mm Hg) with:
  - neurological emergencies:
    - Hypertensive encephalopathy
    - Traumatic brain injury
    - Post craniotomy
    - Subarachnoid hemorrhage
    - Intracranial hemorrhage
    - Thrombotic stroke
  - cardiovascular emergencies:
    - Left ventricular failure
    - Unstable angina
    - Myocardial infarction
    - Aortic dissection
    - Post cardiac and vascular surgery (threatened suture line)
  - emergency in pregnancy:
    - Preeclampsia
    - Eclampsia

CHOICE OF ANTIHYPERTENSIVE MEDICATIONS IN NEUROLOGICAL EMERGENCIES

- Hypertensive encephalopathy
  - Labetalol or Nicardipine is the drug of choice.
  - Nitroprusside can be used but may increase intracranial pressure (ICP).
  - Phentolamine in patients with pheochromocytoma
  - MAP should not be reduced more than 20%–25% during first 1–2 hr.
  - Aggressive lowering of BP can cause ischemic events.
- Traumatic brain injury
  - Labetalol and Esmolol in patients with tachycardia
  - Nicardipine in patients with bradycardia
  - Nitroprusside not recommended in patients with brain injury because it increases ICP and decreases cerebral blood flow (CBF).
- Post craniotomy
  - Labetalol in patients with tachycardia
  - Nicardipine in patients with bradycardia, CHF, COPD, or asthma
- Subarachnoid hemorrhage (SAH)
  - Labetalol or Esmolol in patients with tachycardia
  - Nicardipine in patients in bradycardia, CHF, COPD, or asthma

CHOICE OF ANTIHYPERTENSIVE MEDICATIONS IN CARDIOVASCULAR EMERGENCIES

- Post carotid endarterectomy
  - Choices
    - Nicardipine
    - Enalapril
    - Hydralazine
- Myocardial ischemia/infarction
  - First choice: Nitroglycerine
  - Alternatives:
    - Labetalol
    - Nicardipine
    - Nitroprusside
  - Hydralazine is not recommended.

CHOICE OF ANTIHYPERTENSIVE MEDICATIONS IN PREGNANCY

- Angiotensin-converting enzyme (ACE) inhibitors are contraindicated in pregnancy
- Preeclampsia
  - Hydralazine
  - Labetalol
  - Nifedipine and Nicardipine are preferred.
- Eclampsia
  - Magnesium sulfate
    - Drug of choice
    - Peripheral and cerebral vasodilator
    - Anticonvulsant effect due to cerebral vasodilation
    - Dose
    - 4–6 g IV bolus over 5 min followed by 1–2 g/hr IV infusion

ENALAPRIL

- Action
  - ACE inhibitor
- Effects
  - Decrease in sympathetic response causing reduction in MAP, SBP, and DBP
  - Reduction in preload
  - Variable effect on cardiac output
  - Reduction in renal efferent arteriolar vasodilation
- Dose
  - Bolus: 0.625–5 mg IV over 5 min, repeated every 6 hr for the desired goal
  - Onset: 15 min
  - Duration: 4–6 hr
  - Maximum dose 5 mg every 6 hr
  - Its effect is not dose dependent.

- Side effects
  - Prolonged hypotension
  - Decreased renal function
  - Sodium retention
  - Hyperkalemia
  - Angioedema
  - Bradykinin release, which may also cause vasodilation
- Contraindications
  - Patients with bilateral renal artery stenosis
  - Pregnant patients
  - Patients with hypovolemia

ESMOLOL

- Action
  - Cardioselective beta receptor antagonist
  - Equivalent efficacy as labetalol
- Effects
  - Reduction of MAP and SBP
  - Reduction of cardiac output and stroke volume
  - Slight increase in preload
  - Slight increase in SVR
  - Significant reduction in left ventricular stroke work leading to reduction of myocardial oxygen demand
- Dose
  - Bolus: 500 mcg/kg over 1 min, followed by continuous infusion 50–100 mcg/kg/min until BP goal is achieved
  - Maximum dose: 300 mcg/kg/min
  - Onset of action: 1–2 min
  - Duration of action: 10–30 min
- Side effects
  - Hypotension
  - Bradycardia
  - Conduction delay
  - Left ventricular dysfunction
  - Bronchospasm
- Caution in patients with:
  - left ventricular dysfunction.
  - CHF.
  - bronchospasm, such as asthma.

LABETALOL

- Action
  - Alpha-1 receptor antagonist that causes vasodilation
  - Beta-1 receptor antagonist that prevents reflex tachycardia
  - Beta-2 receptor antagonist that causes vasodilation and inhibition of neuronal uptake of norepinephrine.

- Effects
  - Reduction of the following:
    - MAP
    - SBP
    - HR
    - CO
  - No significant change in SVR
  - Cerebral, renal, and coronary blood flows maintained
- No effect on ICP and cerebral blood flow
- Agent of choice in suspected myocardial ischemia and neurosurgical patients
- Dose
  - Bolus 10–20 mg IV over 2 min, followed by increasing doses 40–80 mg every 10 min, until the desired blood pressure is achieved
  - Continuous infusion 0.5–2 mg/min titrated to the desired effect
  - Onset of action: 2–5 min
  - Duration of action: 3–6 hr
  - Maximum dose: 300 mg/24 hr
- Side effects
  - Bronchospasm
  - Impaired cardiac conduction
  - Left ventricular dysfunction
- Caution in patients with:
  - left ventricular dysfunction.
  - CHF.
  - bronchospasm such as asthma.

NICARDIPINE

- Action
  - Calcium channel blocker
- Effects
  - Arterial vasodilation due its relatively selective effect on vascular smooth muscles causing:
    - reduction in SVR.
    - reduction in MAP.
  - Small increase in HR
  - Small increase in CO
  - Variable effect on preload
- No effect on ICP and cerebral blood flow
- Agent of choice in neurosurgical emergencies
- Doses
  - Infusion: 5 mg/h, 3 mg/h in patients with renal insufficiency, adjusted by 1–2.5 mg/h every 15 min until desired blood pressure is achieved
  - Onset of action: 1–5 min
  - Duration of action: 30 min
  - Maximum infusion rate: 15 mg/hr
  - More consistent reduction of MAP with minimal dose adjustment
- Side effects
  - Hypotension

- Sinus tachycardia
- Swelling of feet and ankle
- Constipation

HYDRALAZINE

- Action
  - Direct relaxation of arteriolar smooth muscle causing vasodilation
  - No effect on venous smooth muscle
- Effects
  - Reduces systolic, diastolic, and mean arterial blood pressures
  - Causes baroreceptor-mediated increase in sympathetic activity and release of norepinephrine from nerve terminals resulting in:
    - increased heart rate.
    - increased myocardial contractility.
    - increased HR.
  - No effect on coronary arteries.
- Recommended for
  - hypertension in patients after carotid endarterectomy.
  - hypertension in pregnancy.
- Dose
  - 5–10 mg IV over 2 min, repeated every 6 hr, dose and frequency adjusted to achieve required goals
  - Onset of action: 5–20 min
  - Duration of action: 2–12 hr
- Side effects
  - Coronary steal syndrome
    - Not recommended in patients with coronary artery disease, cardiac ischemia, and myocardial infarction
  - Lupus like syndrome
  - Pericarditis
  - Pyridoxine-responsive peripheral neuropathy

SODIUM NITROPRUSSIDE

- Action
  - Direct-acting vascular smooth muscle relaxation causing vasodilation of the arteries and vein resulting in reduction of preload and afterload
  - Converts cysteine to nitrocysteine, which stimulates the formation of cyclic guanosine monophosphate (cGMP), causing muscle relaxation
- Effects
  - Reductions
    - SVR
    - MAP

- Pulmonary vascular resistance
- Left ventricular filling pressure
- CO and stroke volume are usually mainlined or increased.
- Minimal effect on HR
- Dose-dependent reduction in cerebral blood flow
- Acute increase in ICP in patients with elevated ICP
- Dose
  - Initiated at 0.25–5 mcg/kg/min, can be increased by 0.5–1 mcg/kg/min every 5–10 min until desired level is achieved.
  - Rapid onset of action: within 30 sec
  - Short duration: 1–10 min
  - Maximum recommended dose: 10 mcg/kg/min
- Side effects
  - Rebound hypertension due to very short half-life
  - Potent and labile hypotension
  - Myocardial ischemia
  - Coronary steal syndrome
  - Worsening hypoxia due to pulmonary hypoxic vasoconstriction and ventilation perfusion imbalance
  - Ototoxicity
  - Cyanide and thiocyanate toxicity
    - Nausea
    - Weakness
    - Anion gap acidosis
    - Seizures
  - Caution in patients with hypoxia, renal failure, and hepatic insufficiency

NITROGLYCERINE

- Action
  - Predominantly venous vasodilation
    - Increases venous capacitance
    - Reduces preload
    - Lowers cardiac filling pressure
  - Variable effect on arterial pressure
  - Direct coronary vasodilation
- Dose
  - Infusion 20–300 mcg/min
  - Onset of action: 1–2 min
  - Duration of action: 3–10 min
- Side effects
  - Tachyphylaxis
  - Headache
  - Methemoglobinemia

Must-Know Essentials: Sedatives & Analgesics

Commonly used sedatives

Agents	Mechanism of Action	Uses/Doses
Ketamine	N-methyl-D-aspartate (NMDA) receptor antagonist	Induction agent for intubation: 1–2 mg/kg IV Sedation: 0.2–0.5 mg /kg IV followed by continuous infusion of 0.3–1.2 mg/kg/hr Status asthmaticus: 1.0–2.0 mg/kg followed by 0.1–0.5 mg/kg/hr infusion
Propofol	Predominantly Gamma-aminobutyric acid (GABA) receptor agonist	Induction of general anesthesia: 1.0–2.5 mg/kg IV Short-acting general anesthesia: 6–12 mg/kg/hr IV Sedation in head injury/refractory seizures in status epilepticus/status asthmaticus: 1.0–3.0 mg/kg/hr
Lorazepam	GABA receptor agonist	Sedation in alcohol withdrawal–associated agitation: 0.25–1 mg IV every 5–30 min Status epilepticus: 1–4 mg IV
Midazolam	GABA receptor agonist	Sedation for intubation: 0.1–0.3 mg/kg IV Rapid sedation for short duration: 2–5 mg/hr or 0.02–0.1 mg/kg/hr IV infusion or 0.5–1 mg every 5–30 min
Dexmedetomidine	Highly selective alpha-2 adrenergic agonist	Preferred sedative in head injury/alcohol withdrawal–associated agitation Loading dose: 0.1 μg/kg IV over 10 min followed by 0.2–0.7 μg/kg per hr
Haloperidol	Central postsynaptic dopamine (D2) receptor antagonist Blocks acetylcholine, serotonin, histamine, and adrenergic receptors	Sedative for patients with hallucinations, psychosis, and agitation associated with delirium: 1–5 mg IV every hr Infusion: 300 mg every 24 hr
Etomidate	GABA receptor agonist	Sedation during intubation in trauma patients with hypotension, head injury patients with suspected elevation of ICP: 0.3 mg/kg
Pentobarbital	GABA receptor agonist	Refractory intracranial hypertension, Refractory status epilepticus: 10 mg/ kg IV loading dose, followed by infusion of 1–2 mg/kg per hr.

KETAMINE

- Action
  - Phencyclidine derivative
  - Primarily NMDA receptor antagonist
  - Also acts on opioid, monoaminergic, muscarinic, voltage-sensitive calcium and sodium channel receptors
- Effects
  - Neurological effects
    - Potent anesthetic agent
    - Hypnosis
    - Amnesia

- Analgesia
- Dissociative state by stimulating limbic system
- Increase in cerebral blood flow
- Increase in cerebral metabolic rate of oxygen ($CMRO_2$)
- Increases ICP
- Decrease in cerebral perfusion pressure (CPP)
- Cardiovascular effects due to sympathetic stimulation
  - Increases MAP
  - Increases SVR
  - Increases HR
  - No change in CO
- Pulmonary effects
  - Does not affect spontaneous ventilation
  - Bronchodilation
- Rapid action
  - Within seconds when given IV
- Duration of action
  - 15–30 min
- Eliminated from the system in 2–3 hr
- Clinical uses
  - Induction agent for intubation
    - Dose: 1–2 mg/kg IV or 5–10 mg/kg IM
  - Anesthesia/sedation
    - Dose: 0.2–0.5 mg/kg IV followed by continuous infusion of 0.3–1.2 mg/kg/hr as required
  - Bronchodilator agent in patients with bronchospasm such as status asthmaticus
    - Dose: 1.0–2.0 mg/kg induction followed by 0.1–0.5 mg/kg/hr infusion
  - Ideal agent for sedation in patients with hypotension in hemorrhagic, hypovolemic, or septic shock due to its sympathetic stimulation effect
- Side effects
  - Hypertension
  - Tachycardia
  - Delirium
  - Seizures
  - Increase in ICP
  - Excessive salivation
  - Excessive lacrimation
  - Emergent phenomena
    - Postanesthesia visual, auditory, and proprioceptive hallucinations
    - Can be blunted with concomitant use of a benzodiazepine
    - Rare in children
    - 30% incidence in adults
- Contraindications
  - Uncontrolled hypertension
  - Where hypertension should be avoided
    - Aortic dissection
    - Aortic aneurysm
    - Myocardial infarction
    - Ischemic heart disease

- Head injury due to risk of ICP elevation
- Seizure disorders

PROPOFOL

- Action
  - Predominantly GABA receptors agonist
  - Other actions
    - NMDA receptors antagonist
    - Some effects on cannabinoid and glutamate receptors
- Effects
  - Neurological effects
    - Dose-dependent sedation
    - No analgesic property
    - Antegrade amnesia
    - Due to decrease in MAP
      - Decrease in ICP
      - Decrease in $CMRO_2$
      - Decrease in CPP
      - Decrease in CBF
  - Cardiovascular effects
    - Decreases MAP, SVR, CVP, CO, and HR
    - Hypotension due to reduced SVR and venodilation
  - Pulmonary effects
    - Respiratory depression
    - Bronchodilator
  - Onset of action: 1–2 min
  - Short duration of action: 10–15 min
- Clinical uses
  - Induction of general anesthesia
    - Dose: 1.0–2.5 mg/kg IV
  - Short-acting general anesthesia
    - Dose: 6–12 mg/kg/hr IV
  - Sedation in ICU
    - Dose: 1.0–3.0 mg/kg/hr
    - If patient is not hypotensive: May be given as boluses of 10–20 mg to rapid sedation
    - Sedative of choice in neuro ICU patients on ventilation due to its short duration of action and rapid awakening
    - Preferred sedative in patients with elevated ICP
  - Refractory seizures in status epilepticus
  - May be used in status asthmaticus due to its bronchodilator property
- Contraindications
  - Patients allergic to soybean oil or egg lecithin
  - Continuous infusion not recommended in children <18 years of age
- Side effects
  - Respiratory depression
  - Hypotension, especially in hypovolemic patients
  - Bradycardia
  - Causes (rarely) green discoloration of urine, hair, and nail beds
  - Tonic–clonic seizures when abruptly stopped after days of infusion

- Hypertriglyceridemia after >72 hr of infusion
- Pancreatitis
- Propofol infusion syndrome (PRIS)
  - Mechanism
    - Blockade of mitochondrial fatty oxidation and accumulation of free fatty acid
  - Risk factors
    - Associated with high dose and long term (>5 mg/kg/hr for more than 48 hr)
    - Common in children
    - Low body mass index (BMI)
    - Concomitant use of vasopressors
  - Manifestation
    - Cardiac arrhythmia, bradycardia, asystole, and cardiac failure
    - Metabolic acidosis
    - Rhabdomyolysis: Elevated creatine phosphokinase (CPK)
    - Renal failure
    - Hyperkalemia
    - Hyperlipidemia
  - Associated with high mortality

BENZODIAZEPINES

- Action
  - GABA receptors agonist
- Effects
  - Sedative and anxiolytic
  - No analgesic effect
  - Potentiate effects of narcotics when given together
  - Produces anterograde amnesia
    - Anticonvulsant
    - Decrease in CBF
    - Decrease in $CMRO_2$
    - No change in ICP
    - Central muscle relaxation
- Onset of action: 5 min
- Elimination half-life: 60 min
- Duration of action: 0.5–3.5 hr
- Side effects
  - Respiratory depression
  - Hypotension or hypertension
  - Withdrawal in benzodiazepine-dependent patients
  - May precipitate seizures or status epilepticus after acute cessation
  - Tachyphylaxis with prolonged use
  - Reversible encephalopathy
  - Paradoxical reactions causing increased agitation and delirium in patients with preexisting central nervous system (CNS) pathology can occur due to altered sensory perception.
- Reversal of benzodiazepines
  - Flumazenil

- Acts by binding GABA receptors
- Dose: 0.2–1.0 mg IV
- Maximum dose: 3 mg IV
- Synergistic sedative effect with benzodiazepines
  - Combination of haloperidol and BZ
    - Lowers the doses of BZ and haloperidol
    - Lowers the risk of respiratory depression
    - Lowers the risk of extrapyramidal manifestations of haloperidol
  - Combination of propofol and BZ
    - Results in better hemodynamic stability due to reduced dose of propofol

COMMONLY USED BENZODIAZEPINES

- Lorazepam
  - Most potent benzodiazepine
  - Six times more potent than diazepam
  - Slower onset of action (5–10 min) due to lower lipid solubility
  - Elimination half-life: 10–20 hr
  - Clinical uses
    - Sedation such as in alcohol withdrawal
      - Dose: 0.25 mg–1 mg IV every 5–30 min
    - Status epilepticus
      - Dose: 1–4 mg IV
  - Side effects
    - High-dose infusion for more than 2 days may lead to propylene glycol toxicity, with features including the following:
      - Lactic acidosis
      - Delirium
      - Hallucinations
      - Hypotension
      - Bradycardia
- Diazepam
  - Rapid onset of action: 2–5 min
  - Long half-life: 60–120 min due to its potent active metabolites (desmethyldiazepam and oxazepam)
  - Uses
    - Sedation in the ICU
      - Dose: 5–10 mg IV bolus followed by a maintenance dose of 0.05–0.10 mg/kg every 2–4 hr
    - Status epilepticus
      - Dose: 0.15–0.20 mg/kg IV per dose as needed
  - Resedation occurs after reversal with flumazenil because of its long duration of action.
- Midazolam
  - Commonly used benzodiazepines BZ in the ICU
  - Is 3–4 times more potent than diazepam
  - Rapid onset of action: 2–3 min
  - Short duration of action due to rapid metabolism by the liver to an inactive metabolite
  - Elimination half-life: 2–2.5 hr

- Mild decreases in CPP
- Minimal cardiovascular and respiratory effects
- Clinical use
  - Intubation
    - Dose: 0.1–0.3 mg/kg IV
    - Usually not recommended for intubation because of its delayed induction time, hypotension at induction doses, and prolonged duration of action
  - Rapid sedation in ICU
    - Dose: 2–5 mg/hr or 0.02–0.1 mg/kg/hr IV infusion or 0.5–1 mg every 5–30 min
- Special precautions
  - Increased effect in patients with:
    - liver disease.
    - renal failure.
  - Prolonged sedation after repeated doses or continuous IV due to sequestration fat stores with slow release

DEXMEDETOMIDINE

- Action
  - Highly selective alpha-2 adrenergic agonist
  - Decreases sympathetic activity
  - Elimination half-life: 2 hr
  - Duration of action: 2–6 hr
- Effects
  - Sedative and analgesic
  - No amnestic effect
  - Decreases seizures threshold
  - May decrease ICP and CBF due to alpha-2 receptor-induced cerebral arteriolar vasoconstriction
  - No respiratory depression
- Clinical use
  - Preferred agent in neuro ICU as it facilitates neurologic exams
  - May reduce BZ requirement in patients with:
    - alcohol withdrawal–associated agitation.
    - Autonomic hyperreactivity.
  - Recommended for short-term sedation <24 hr
- Dose
  - Loading dose: 0.1 µg/kg IV for 10 min, then 0.2–0.7 µg/kg per hr
  - Bolus dose can cause hypotension.
- Side effects
  - Hypotension
  - Bradycardia

HALOPERIDOL

- Action
  - Central postsynaptic dopamine (D2) receptors antagonist
  - Also blocks acetylcholine, serotonin, histamine, and adrenergic receptors

- Effects
  - Sedation
  - No analgesia
  - No amnesia
  - No respiratory depression
- Clinical uses
  - Sedative for patients with hallucinations, psychosis, and agitation associated with delirium
  - Antipsychotic for symptomatic schizophrenia
- Dose
  - Delirium
    - 1–5 mg IV every hr
    - Infusion: 300 mg/24 hr
- Contraindications
  - Parkinson disease
  - Pregnancy
  - Seizures
  - Caution in patients with head injury because of potential to increase seizure threshold
- Side effects
  - Extrapyramidal acute dystonic symptoms; treated with diphenhydramine
  - Hypotension due to alpha-blocking property
  - Prolongation of QT interval: torsades de pointes
  - Neuroleptic malignant syndrome (NMS)
    - Manifestations
      - Hyperthermia
      - Muscle rigidity
      - Autonomic instability
      - Elevated CPK
      - Hyperglycemia
    - Treatment
      - Discontinuation of medication
      - Dantrolene for muscle rigidity
      - Bromocriptine or amantadine for dopamine production

ETOMIDATE

- Action
  - Agonist of GABA receptors
- Effects
  - Neurological effects
    - Sedation
    - Decreases CBF
    - Decreases $CMRO_2$
    - Decreases ICP
    - Increases CPP
    - Lowers threshold for seizures
  - No change in CO and HR
  - Rapid onset: 5–15 sec
  - Short duration: 5–15 min

- Clinical use
  - Sedation during intubation:
    - trauma patients with hypotension.
    - patients with head injury with suspected elevation of ICP.
  - Dose: 0.3 mg/kg
- Contraindications
  - Acute intermittent porphyria
  - Seizures
- Side effects
  - Generalized seizures
  - Myoclonus
  - Laryngeal spasm
  - Adrenal suppression
    - Reduced cortisol level due to blockage of the conversion of 11-deoxycortisol into cortisol from direct inhibition of 11-beta-hydroxylase
    - Decreased response to cosyntropin stimulation on adrenal gland
    - Transient and dose-dependent effects
    - May last 5–15 hr
    - Clinically insignificant effect when used as an induction agent
  - Increased intraocular pressure (IOP)

BARBITURATES

- Action
  - Enhances GABA receptors and opens the chloride channels
- Effects
  - Neurological effects
    - Sedation
    - Decrease in CBF, $CMRO_2$, ICP, and CPP
  - Cardiovascular effects
    - Decrease in MAP
    - Decreases in SVR
    - Increase in HR
    - Hypotension
  - Metabolism effects
    - Hepatic; enzyme inducer with effects on the metabolism of other drugs
- Clinical uses
  - Sedation in ICU patients
  - Head injury with severe intracranial hypertension
  - Refractory status epilepticus
- Commonly used barbiturates
  - Phenobarbital
    - Used for short-term sedation
    - Duration of action: 10–24 hr
    - Dose for sedation: 1–3 mg/kg IV, up to 200 mg in 24 hr
  - Pentobarbital
    - Used to induce coma in:

     refractory intracranial hypertension.
     refractory status epilepticus.
  - Dose: 10 mg/ kg IV loading dose, followed by infusion of 1–2 mg/kg per hr
- Side effects
  - Hypoventilation
  - Bronchospasm
  - Laryngeal spasm
  - Hypersalivation
  - Vasoconstriction of renal artery leading to decrease in urine output

OPIOIDS

- Action
  - Mu receptors agonist
  - Metabolized in the liver
  - Excreted in the kidneys
- Effects
  - Neurological effects
    - Primarily analgesic
    - Low sedative
    - No amnesia
    - Decrease in CBF, $CMRO_2$, ICP
  - Cardiovascular effects
    - Decrease in MAP due to:
      venodilation.
      decrease in sympathetic tone.
      histamine release with morphine
    - Dose-dependent vagal-mediated bradycardia
  - Respiratory effects
    - Respiratory depression
  - Gastrointestinal effects
    - Delay in gastric emptying
    - Ileus
    - Spasm of the sphincter of Oddi
- Opioid reversal
  - Naloxone
    - Opioid antagonist
    - Acts by blocking the Mu receptors
    - Onset of action: 1–2 min
    - Can be administered by intranasal spray, and intramuscular, subcutaneous, and intravenous injections
    - Dose
      Initial dose: 0.4–2 mg IV
      May be repeated every 2–3 min as required
    - Side effects
      Hypertension
      Dysrhythmias
      Pulmonary edema
      Cardiac arrest

- Commonly uses opioids
  - Fentanyl
    - Synthetic opioid 75–100 times more potent than morphine
    - Rapid onset and shorter duration of action
    - May accumulate in fat stores, resulting in prolonged effect in patients with infusion
    - No histamine release
    - Less hemodynamic instability
    - Preferred analgesic in patients with hypotension
    - Metabolized to norfentanyl in the liver, which has its own analgesic properties
    - Dose
      Should be individualized based on age, body weight, physical status, and the pathology condition
      Low dose: 2 mcg/kg IV
      Moderate dose: 2–20 mcg/kg IV
      High dose: 20–30 mcg/kg IV
      Patient-controlled analgesia (PCA)
          Demand: 10–50 mcg, lockout interval: 5–10 min
          Basal rate: 50 mcg/hr
  - Morphine
    - Apart from mu receptor, also acts as delta and kappa receptors agonist
    - Slow CNS entry due to lowest lipid solubility
    - Metabolized by conjugation with glucuronic acid in hepatic and extrahepatic sites, especially kidneys
    - Releases histamine causing:
      hypotension.
      flushing.
      bradycardia.
      pruritis.
      urticaria.
      edema.
      other skin rashes.
    - Dose:
      Analgesic: 2–10 mg IV every 4 hr as required
      PCA
          Demand dose: 1–2 mg, lockout interval 5–10 min
          Basal rate: 0.5 mg/hr
  - Hydromorphone
    - Morphine derivative
    - 6–8 times more potent than morphine
    - Metabolized as an inactive glucuronide
    - Preferred in patients with renal dysfunction
    - Dose
      PCA
          Demand dose: 0.20–0.5 mg, lockout interval: 5–10 min
          Basal infusion rate: 0.4 mg/hr

Must-Know Essentials: Paralytic Agents

SUCCINYLCHOLINE

- Depolarizing paralytic agent
- Acetylcholine (ACh) agonist, stimulates all nicotinic and muscarinic cholinergic receptors
- Paralytic effect due to depolarization at postsynaptic nicotinic acetylcholine receptor at the neuromuscular junction
- Causes transient fasciculation due to stimulation of nicotinic ACh receptors
- Metabolism: Hydrolysis by pseudocholinesterase enzyme
- Rapid onset of action: 10–15 sec
- Duration of action: 10–15 sec
- Dose
  - 1.5 mg/kg in adults
  - 2 mg/kg in children younger than 5 years
- Side effects
  - Insignificant increase in ICP
  - Insignificant increase in intraocular pressure
  - Hyperkalemia in patients with:
    - crush injury.
    - major burns.
    - electric injury.
    - chronic renal failure.
    - chronic paralysis.
    - chronic neuromuscular diseases.
  - Bradycardia
    - Common in children
    - Risk increases with second dose
    - In children <7 years, atropine recommended to prevent bradycardia
      - Dose of atropine: 0.01 mg/kg in infants, and 0.02 mg/kg in older children
  - Masseter muscle spasm
    - Seen in 0.3%–1% children
    - Risk of development of malignant hyperthermia
  - Malignant hyperthermia
    - Etiology
      - Autosomal dominant
      - Genetic defect (RYR1) on the long arm of chromosome 19 involving ryanodine receptors
      - More common in men
      - May be triggered by:
        - volatile anesthetic agents such as halothane, isoflurane, and enflurane
        - physical exercise.
        - heat exposure.
    - Manifestation is caused by release of calcium from the muscle cells resulting in contraction of muscle fibers.

- Clinical features
  - Tachycardia
  - High fever
  - Muscle rigidity
  - Rhabdomyolysis
  - Hyperkalemia
- Susceptible individuals should be tested with muscle biopsy for:
  - caffeine-halothane contracture test.
  - genetic testing for RYR1 mutation.
- Treatment
  - Dantrolene
    - Acts on ryanodine receptors to prevent the release of calcium
    - 2.5 mg/kg IV bolus, followed by 1 mg/kg IV every 4–6 hr for 36 hr
- Contraindication
  - Personal or family history of malignant hyperthermia

NONDEPOLARIZING AGENTS

- Competitive antagonist of ACh
- Blocks the binding of ACh at the postsynaptic receptors and prevents depolarization
- Slower onset: 1–4 min
- Longer duration of action: 20–60 min
- Rocuronium
  - Fastest action compared to other nondepolarizing agents
  - Effective and safe alternative to succinylcholine
  - Low incidence of histamine release
  - Accumulates in hepatic dysfunction
  - Some vagolytic properties
  - Dose: 1–1.2 mg/kg IV
- Pancuronium
  - Slow onset of action compared to other nondepolarizing agents
  - Onset of action: 3 min
  - Duration of action: 60 min
  - Causes histamine release
  - Accumulates in hepatic and renal dysfunction
  - Vagolytic properties
  - Most common side effect: Tachycardia
  - Useful in postintubation paralysis
  - Dose: 0.06–0.1 mg/kg
  - Cumulative effect with increasing doses
- Atracurium or cisatracurium
  - Organ-independent elimination; degradation by plasma esterase hydrolysis (Hofmann elimination)
  - Agent of choice in patients with renal or hepatic dysfunction
  - Development of tolerance
  - Histamine release with atracurium but not with cisatricurium
  - Predisposes to seizures due to accumulation of laudanosine metabolites of atracurium and cisatracurium

Must-Know Essentials: Medications for Seizure Prophylaxis

FOSPHENYTOIN

- Prolongs recovery of activated voltage-gated Na+ channels in neuron to stabilize against repetitive neuronal firing
- Is a water-soluble phenytoin for IV use
- Potentially safer than IV phenytoin
- Fosphenytoin is dosed as phenytoin equivalents (PE): 1 PE fosphenytoin = 1 mg phenytoin sodium = 1.5 mg fosphenytoin sodium
- Dose
  - Loading dose: 10–20 mg PE/kg IV; should not exceed 150 mg PE/min
  - Maintenance dose: 4–6 mg PE/kg/day IV in divided doses; should not exceed 150 mg PE/min
  - Serum concentrations should be monitored for therapeutic concentration.
- Side effects
  - Arrhythmias
  - Hypotension (especially rapid IV administration)
  - Injection site pain, phlebitis, tissue necrosis
  - Fosphenytoin converts to phenytoin in 15 min.

LEVETIRACETAM

- An alternative to phenytoin
- No clear mechanism of action, possible presynaptic calcium channel modulator and regulation of neurotransmitter release
- Potential advantages of Levetiracetam
  - No drug–drug interactions
  - No need for serum monitoring
  - No significant advantage of seizure prevention rate compared to phenytoin in patients with severe traumatic brain injury (TBI)
  - Dose
    - 500–1000 mg twice daily with or without a 20 mg/kg–1 g loading dose; can be given oral or IV
    - 250 mg BID in patients with renal failure on hemodialysis
  - Side effects
    - Behavioral abnormalities
      - Agitation
      - Irritability
      - Depression
      - Somnolence
      - Asthenia
      - Dizziness
    - Caution in patients with psychiatric disorders

SELECTED RESOURCES

1. ATLS (Advanced Trauma Life Support) Student Course Manual (10th Edition, 2018); American College of Surgeons.
2. Trauma (9th Edition, 2021); Editors: David V. Feliciano, MD, Kenneth L. Mattox, MD, Ernest E. Moore, MD.
3. Atlas of Surgical Techniques in Trauma (2015); Editors: Demetrios Demetriades, MD, Kenji Inaba, MD, George Velmahos, MD.
4. Grant's Atlas of Anatomy (12th Edition, 2009); Editors: Anne M. R Agur, Arthur F. Dalley.
5. Top Knife: Art and Craft in Trauma Surgery (2005); Asher Hirshberg MD, Kenneth L. Mattox MD.
6. American College of Surgeons Committee on Trauma Guidelines.
7. Current Therapy of Trauma and Surgical Critical Care (2nd Edition, 2015); Juan A. Asensio, MD, Donald D. Trunkey, MD.
8. Western Trauma Association Algorithms.
9. The Eastern Association for the Surgery of Trauma (EAST) Guidelines.
10. The American Association for the Surgery of Trauma.

Fractures
  evaluation of, 147
  pattern, based on mechanism, 148–149
  pelvic
    classification of, 373–376
    complications of, management of, 384–385
    evaluation of, 377–378
  thoracolumbar spine, 151–153
    burst fractures, 151–152
    Chance fracture, 149, 151
    Denis three-column concept of, 149–150
    and dislocations, 152–153
    McAfee classification of, 150
    unstable, 151
    wedge fracture, 152
Frailty score, 451–452, 452t
Frank-Starling curve, 76
Frontal fracture, 123–124
  complications of, 123–124
  treatment for, 124
  types of, 123
Frontal sinus fractures, 129
Frontotemporoparietal craniectomy. See Unilateral
    craniectomy
Full Outline of Unresponsiveness (FOUR) score,
    84–85, 448, 448t
Fundus, of stomach, 291
FVCA. See Four-vessel cerebral angiography

G

G measurement, 61
Gallbladder injury, treatment for, 276
Gastrosplenic ligament, 287
GCS. See Glasgow Coma Scale
Gestational age
  estimation of, 433
  fetal injury with, risk of, 432–433
Glasgow Coma Scale (GCS), 83–84
  adult, 447, 447t
  grading of traumatic brain injury (TBI) based
    on, 84
  pediatric, 421t, 447–448, 447t
  for severe brain injury, 96
Glossopharyngeal nerve, 184f, 186
Gluteus maximus compartment, 395
Gluteus medius/minimus compartment, 395
Gustilo-Anderson classification, of open fractures,
    405–406, 450–451, 450t

H

Haldol. See Haloperidol
Haloperidol (Haldol), 474t, 479–480
Hand, compartments of, 393–395
Hangman's fracture, 140–141

Head injury
  evaluation of, 81, 83f
    acute epidural hematoma, 88
    acute subdural hematoma, 88–89
    brain injury
      management of, 87–88
      types of, 85
    concussion, 86
    extracerebral hematomas, 85–86
    Full Outline of Unresponsiveness (FOUR)
      score, 84–85
    Glasgow Coma Scale, 83–84
    management guidelines for, 87
    pneumocephalus, 89
    posttraumatic intracerebral hematoma, 85
    second-impact syndrome, 86–87
    traumatic intracerebral hemorrhage, 89
    traumatic subarachnoid hemorrhage, 89
  pediatric, 422–423
  scoring system for, 447–448
Heart
  anatomy of, 197f, 200
  decreased filling pressure in, due to volume loss, 39
  exposure of, 227
Heart rate, 79
Heart tone, fetal, 433–434
HELLP syndrome, in pregnancy, 439
HemCon (Hemorrhage Control Technologies,
    Portland OR, USA), 57
Hemiazygos vein, 200, 338
Hemicraniectomy. See Unilateral craniectomy
Hemodynamic instability
  abdominal trauma with, 58
  pelvic fractures with, 58
Hemodynamically stable abdominal penetrating/
    blunt trauma, 244
  abdomen anatomy in, 245–246
  common organs involved, 246–248, 247f
  evaluation of, 248–250
    algorithm, 244f
    CT abdomen, 250
    diagnostic peritoneal lavage, 249–250
    focused assessment with sonography for
      trauma, 248–249
    physical examination, 248
  management of, 250–252
  mechanism of injury, 246–248
Hemodynamically unstable penetrating abdominal
    trauma, 230
  abdominal compartment syndrome in, 241–243
  damage-control laparotomy for, 236–237
  initial evaluation & management of, 231f,
    232–233
  pelvic packing for, 239

Mandibular fractures, 129–131
complications of, 131
features of, 129
management of, 130–131
types of, 129–130
Mangled extremities, 390
management of, 390–391
Mangled Extremity Severity Score (MESS), 390, 449–450, 450*t*
Mannitol (Osmitrol), 426
for intracranial hypertension, 105–106
Manubrial notch, in penetrating neck injuries, 183*f*
Manubrium, 184*f*, 197*f*
MAP. *See* Mean arterial pressure
Marginal artery of Drummond (MAD), 304–305
Mass reflex. *See* Autonomic hyperreflexia
Masseter muscle spasm, succinylcholine and, 20, 484
Massive transfusion
adjuncts to, 55–56
protocol (MTP), 13, 54–55
Mastoid bone, 184*f*
Mattox maneuver, 258–260, 260*f*
Maxillary sinus fractures, 129
Maxillofacial trauma
airway and C-spine protection in, 115–116
circulation in, 116–117
complex, breathing and ventilation for, 31
definitive airway for, 15
evaluation of, 115–117
Maximum amplitude value, 61
McAfee classification, of thoracolumbar spine fracture, 150
MCT. *See* Medial canthal tendon
Mean arterial pressure (MAP), 79, 91
Medial canthal tendon (MCT), 124
Median nerve, 357, 370–371, 404
Median sacral artery, 337
Median sternotomy, 205
closure of, 207
Mediastinal vascular injuries, treatment of, 227–229
Mediastinal vessels, exposure of, 227
Medications, in emergency trauma management, 453
antihypertensives, 467*f*, 468–474
for cardiac arrhythmias, 459–467, 460*f*
paralytic agents, 484–486
in pediatrics, dosages of, 425–426
sedatives & analgesics, 474–484, 474*t*
for seizure prophylaxis, 486
vasopressor agents, 453–459, 453*f*
MELD. *See* Model for End-Stage Liver Disease
Membranous urethra, 330
Mephentermine (Wyamine), in pregnancy, 430
Mesenteric vascular injuries, 256
Mesentery, of small bowel, 301

MESS. *See* Mangled Extremity Severity Score
Metabolic acidosis
hemorrhagic shock and, 41
progressive, 42
Metabolic parameters, monitoring of, 78–79
Midazolam (Versed), 425, 474*t*, 478–479
for endotracheal intubation, 19
for intracranial hypertension, 105
Middle rectal artery, 308
Middle rectal veins, 308
Middle scalene, 184*f*
Middle suprarenal arteries, 337
Middle thyroid vein, 184*f*
Midface Le Fort fractures, 121–123
classification of, 121, 122*f*
complications of, 121–122
treatment for, 122–123
Midodrine (Orvaten), 459
Milrinone (Primacor), 455*t*, 459
Miscarriage, 436
Mixed venous oxygen saturation (SmvO2), decreased, 42–43
Mobile wad compartment, 393
Model for End-Stage Liver Disease (MELD) score, 446, 446*t*
Monro-Kellie hypothesis, 91
Morphine (Avinza, MS-Contin), 426, 483
Motor vehicle collision (MVC)
mechanism and injuries in, 167
during pregnancy, 427
MRA. *See* Magnetic resonance angiography
MRCP. *See* Magnetic resonance cholangiopancreatography
MRI. *See* Magnetic resonance imaging
MS-Contin. *See* Morphine
Musculoskeletal dysfunction, abdominal compartment syndrome and, 242
Musculoskeletal injuries, scoring & grading for, 449–451
MVC. *See* Motor vehicle collision
Mylohyoid, 184*f*
Myocardial contusion, 223
EAST guidelines for, 226
Myocardial infarction
antihypertensive medications for, 469
cardiogenic shock and, 44
vasopressors for, 454
Myocardial ischemia, antihypertensive medications for, 469
Myotomes, of spinal cord, 157–158

N

Naloxone (Narcan), 482–483
Narcan. *See* Naloxone

Retroperitoneal vascular injuries (*Continued*)
  initial, 340
  must-know essentials in, 339–341
  techniques of exposure of, during exploratory
      laparotomy, 343–345
  zone 1, 341
    exposure of, 344*t*–345*t*
    illustration, 342*f*
    indications for exploration in, during emergent
        exploratory laparotomy, 342–343
    treatment of, 341–350
  zone 2, 341
    illustration, 342*f*
    indications for exploration of, 350
    treatment of, 350–351
  zone 3, 341
    illustration, 342*f*
    sources of bleeding of, 351
    stable patients, 351–352
    treatment of, 351 354
    unstable patients, 351
    vessels, exposure of, 352
Retroperitoneal vessels, anatomy of, 336–339
Revascularization
  for extremity vascular injuries, 388
  for vascular injuries, 366
Rhabdomyolysis, 368, 388–389
  diagnosis of, 388
  etiology of, 388
  management of, 388–389
  pathophysiology of, 388
Rib fractures, 211–213
  complications of, 212
  fixation of, 213
  nonoperative treatment of, 212
  operative treatment of, 212–213
Right brachiocephalic vein, 184*f*, 197*f*, 199
Right bronchial vessels, 197*f*
Right bronchus, 197*f*, 199
Right common carotid artery, 197*f*
Right inferior pulmonary veins, 197*f*
Right phrenic nerve, 197*f*
Right pulmonary artery, 197*f*
Right pulmonary hilum, 197*f*, 200
Right superior pulmonary veins, 197*f*
Right vagus nerve, 197*f*, 200–201
Right ventricular end diastolic volume index
      (RVEDVI), 77
Rocuronium (Zemuron), 426, 485
  endotracheal intubation medication, 20–21
Rouviere's sulcus, 267
R-time, 60
RVEDVI. *See* Right ventricular end diastolic
      volume index

S
Sacral sparing, spinal cord injury and, 159
Sacrococcygeal fractures, 376
SAH. *See* Subarachnoid hemorrhage
Scalene anterior muscle, 197*f*
Scalp
  anatomy of, 117
  laceration, 115, 117
    algorithm for, 115*f*
    repair of, 117
SCI. *See* Spinal cord injury
Sciatic nerve, 403
SCIWORA. *See* Spinal cord injury without
      radiographic abnormality
$S_{cv}O_2$. *See* Central venous oxygen saturation
Seatbelt fractures. *See* Chance fracture
Secondary brain injury, 85
Second-impact syndrome (SIS), 86–87
Sedatives, 474–484, 474*t*
  for intracranial hypertension, 105
Seizure prophylaxis, medications for, 486
Selective urethroscopy, 331
Sepsis, 46
  new definition of, 47, 47*t*
Septic shock, 46
  assessment of, 46*f*
  definitions for, 47, 47*t*
  distributive shock and, 45
  SOFA score in, 445–446, 445*t*–446*t*
Sequential (sepsis related) Organ Failure
      Assessment (SOFA) score, 47*t*, 445–446,
      445*t*–446*t*
Severe sepsis, 46
Shock, 38–39
  assessment of, 37
  cardiogenic, 38, 44–45
    differential diagnosis of, 43*t*
    manifestations in, 44–45
    persistent shock and, 38
  classification of, 38
  distributive, 38, 45
    differential diagnosis of, 43*t*
    manifestations of, 45
  evaluation of, scoring for, 444–446
  hemorrhagic, 38
    classification of, 38–39, 43*t*
    management of, 49–53
      access for fluid resuscitation, 49–51
      adjuncts to massive transfusion, 55–56
      albumin for resuscitation, 53
      algorithm of, 48*f*
      balanced resuscitation, 51–52
      blood and blood products in trauma
        resuscitation, 53–55